PRACTICAL ADVANCED PERIODONTAL SURGERY

PRACTICAL ADVANCED PERIODONTAL SURGERY

Second Edition

Edited by
Serge Dibart, DMD
Professor and Chair
Department of Periodontology
Director Advanced Specialty Program in Periodontics
Boston University Henry M. Goldman School of Dental Medicine
Boston, MA, USA

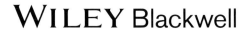

Registered Office(s)
John Wiley & Sons, Inc., 111 River Street, Hoboken, NJ 07030, USA
John Wiley & Sons Ltd, The Atrium, Southern Gate, Chichester, West Sussex, PO19 8SQ, UK
Wiley-VCH Verlag GmbH & Co. KGaA, Boschstr. 12, 69469 Weinheim, Germany
John Wiley & Sons Singapore Pte. Ltd, 1 Fusionopolis Walk, #07-01 Solaris South Tower, Singapore 138628

Editorial Office
111 River Street, Hoboken, NJ 07030, USA

For details of our global editorial offices, customer services, and more information about Wiley products visit us at www.wiley.com.

Wiley also publishes its books in a variety of electronic formats and by print-on-demand. Some content that appears in standard print versions of this book may not be available in other formats.

Library of Congress Cataloging-in-Publication Data

Names: Dibart, Serge, editor.
Title: Practical advanced periodontal surgery / edited by Serge Dibart.
Description: 2 edition. | Hoboken, NJ : Wiley-Blackwell, 2020. | Includes
    bibliographical references and index.
Identifiers: LCCN 2019046551 (print) | LCCN 2019046552 (ebook) | ISBN
    9781119196310 (hardback) | ISBN 9781119196334 (adobe PDF) | ISBN
    9781119196341 (epub)
Subjects: MESH: Periodontium–surgery | Oral Surgical Procedures,
    Preprosthetic–methods | Periodontics–methods | Atlas
    Classification: LCC RK361 (print) | LCC RK361 (ebook) | NLM WU 317 | DDC
    617.6/32–dc23
LC record available at https://lccn.loc.gov/2019046551
LC ebook record available at https://lccn.loc.gov/2019046552

Cover Design: Wiley
Cover Image: Courtesy of Serge Dibart

Set in 9.5/12pt Helvetica Light by SPi Global, Pondicherry, India
Printed and bound in Singapore by Markono Print Media Pte Ltd

10 9 8 7 6 5 4 3 2 1

Ziedonis (Zie) Skobe, PhD

29 April 1941–5 August 2018

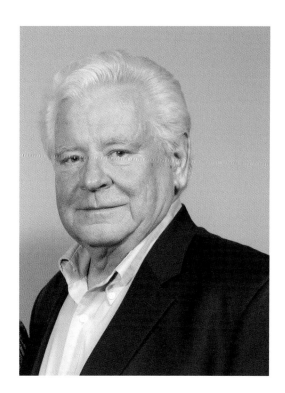

Known as a "gentle giant" who had "a remarkable life and career," Zie guided and supported hundreds of projects and grants, and countless young scientists, during his 40 plus years career at the former Forsyth Dental Institute.

Always proud of his immigrant background, he arrived in the USA from Latvia as a refugee during World War II, overcoming language barriers while learning English then working in the construction industry as a laborer while studying for his PhD

Throughout his long career, he always had a welcoming smile and encouraging words for the young scientists whom he mentored. His early experience with learning English prepared him to enthusiastically help those for whom English was not a first language. He is remembered by all those whose lives he touched for being a great friend, scientist, and mentor with a kind and generous heart. You will not be forgotten, Zie. Rest In Peace.

Contents

List of Contributors

Nawaf J. Al-Dousari, DDS, MSD
Practice Limited to Prosthodontics
Armed Forces Hospital
Ministry of Defense
Shamiya, Kuwait City, Kuwait

Haneen N. Bokhadoor, DDS, MSD
Practice Limited to Periodontics and Dental Implants
Bneid Al Gar Specialty Dental Center
Ministry of Health
Shamiya, Kuwait City, Kuwait

Rokas Borusevičius, DDS
Division of Periodontology, Institute of Odontology
Faculty of Medicine
Vilnius University, Vilnius, Lithuania

Jean-Pierre Dibart, MD
Rheumatology and Sport Medicine
Marseilles, France

Serge Dibart, DMD
Professor and Chair
Department of Periodontology
Director Advanced Specialty Program in Periodontics
Boston University Henry M. Goldman School of
Dental Medicine
Boston, MA, USA

Thomas Van Dyke, DDS, PhD
Vice President and Senior Member of Staff
Forsyth Institute
Professor of Oral Medicine, Infection and Immunity
Faculty of Medicine, Harvard University
Boston, MA, USA

Agnė Gečiauskaitė, DDS
Division of Prosthodontics, Institute of Odontology,
Faculty of Medicine
Vilnius University, Vilnius, Lithuania

Sadru Kabani, DMD, MS
Co-Director of Oral Pathology
STRATADX
Lexington, MA, USA

Elif Keser, DDS, PhD
Private Practice, London, UK
Adjunct Assistant Professor, Department of
Orthodontics & Dentofacial Orthopedics
Boston University Henry M. Goldman School of
Dental Medicine
Boston, MA, USA

Jess Liu, DDS, MSD
Clinical Assistant Professor
Department of Periodontology
Boston University School of Dental Medicine
Boston, MA, USA

Lorenzo Montesani, DDS
Practice Limited to Prosthodontics and
Implant Dentistry
Rome, Italy

Luigi Montesani, MD, DDS
Practice Limited to Periodontology, Prosthodontics,
and Implant Dentistry
Rome, Italy

Steven Morgano, DMD
Professor and Chair
Department of Restorative Dentistry
Rutgers University School of Dental Medicine
Newark, NJ, USA

Mani Moulazadeh, DMD
Assistant Clinical Professor
Department of Endodontics
Boston University School of Dental Medicine
Boston, MA, USA

Donald Nelson, DMD
Assistant Clinical Professor
Department of Orthodontics
Harvard School of Dental Medicine
Boston, MA, USA

Vikki Noonan, DMD, DMSc
Director and Associate Professor, Division of Oral
Pathology
Boston University Henry M. Goldman School
of Dental Medicine
Boston, MA, USA

Justinas Pletkus, DDS
Division of Prosthodontics, Institute of Odontology
Faculty of Medicine
Vilnius University, Vilnius, Lithuania

Albert Price, DMD, MS
Clinical Professor
Department of Periodontology and Oral Biology
Boston University School of Dental Medicine
Boston, MA, USA

Vygandas Rutkūnas, DDS, PhD
Associate Professor
Division of Prosthodontics, Institute of Odontology
Faculty of Medicine
Vilnius University, Vilnius, Lithuania
ProDentum Clinic, Vilnius, Lithuania

Sherif Said, DDS, MSD
Clinical Assistant Professor
Department of Periodontology
Boston University School of Dental Medicine
Boston, MA, USA

Ulrike Schulze-Späte, DMD, PhD
Diplomate, American Board of Periodontology
Director, Section of Geriodontics
Department of Conservative Dentistry
and Periodontology
Center of Dental Medicine
University Hospital Jena
Jena, Germany

Peyman Shahidi, DDS, MScD
Practice Limited to Periodontology and
Implant Dentistry
Toronto, Ontario, Canada

Ming Fang Su, DMD, MS
Clinical Professor
Department of Periodontology and Oral Biology
Boston University School of Dental Medicine
Boston, MA, USA

Yun Po Zhang, PhD, DDS(hon)
Director
Clinical Dental Research
Colgate-Palmolive Company
Piscataway, NJ, USA

Acknowledgments

I would like to thank my colleagues and students of Boston University Henry M. School of Dental Medicine for their invaluable help. I would also like to thank Ms. Leila Joy Rosenthal for drawing Figures 7.32 and 7.33, Dr. Alessia De Vit Dr. Trevor Fujinaka for the video on Piezocision and Dr. Galip Gurel.

I would also like to thank Ms. Samantha Rose Burke for her invaluable help in formatting this manuscript, Mary Malin for copyediting and to the team at Wiley for bringing the book to Production.

About the Companion Website

This book is accompanied by a companion website:

www.wiley.com/go/dibart/advanced

The website includes 2 videos from Chapter 4.

Introduction

Thomas Van Dyke

As reflected in this Second Edition, the surgical techniques that span the scope of dentistry have continued to evolve. Predictable implant placement and bone augmentation techniques have become a common part of the repertoire of the periodontist. Importantly, these technical developments and the research on which they are based have impacted other specialties, including orthodontics, endodontics, oral and maxillofacial surgery, and prosthodontics.

In *Practical Advanced Periodontal Surgery, Second Edition,* Dr. Serge Dibart has updated, expanded, and improved on the landmark First Edition with a team of experts who have played a major role in the development of these concepts, in some cases, and their implementation, in all cases. It is arranged into 13 chapters that range from a review of the science leading up to new technologies to their implementation and the evidence backing their veracity. The contribution of periodontal concepts to orthodontics and endodontics is just an example of how modern periodontology adds to the armamentarium of all aspects of the dental profession.

The focus of this book is bone – the biology of bone and how an understanding of the basic principles of biology can be used to enhance treatment. The book begins with a review of bone biology and current understanding of wound healing. The discovery that surgically injured bone becomes rapidly osteopenic followed by increased turnover has been updated to include new clinical techniques for rapid tooth movement through *Piezocision*.

Notably, there are three new chapters in the Second Edition. The topics are vital to modern practice, including IV sedation by Dr. Jess Liu, Digital Technologies in Clinical Restorative Dentistry by Dr. Vygandas Rutkūnas and colleagues, and Extraction Site Management in the Esthetic Zone: Hard and Soft Tissue Reconstruction by Dr. Sherif Said. The final five chapters of the book are devoted to exploring the specialized needs of complex cases. The problems of inadequate vertical bone height and soft tissue defects can now be predictably addressed in most cases. In particular, the esthetic issues of lack of papillary redevelopment between adjacent implants are addressed by established investigators in the field. Distraction osteogenesis and papilla regeneration techniques now provide a means to enhance the esthetics of the most complicated cases.

Periodontal medicine has its roots in oral pathology/oral medicine. The forefathers of periodontics, physicians such as Gottlieb, Orban, and Goldman, were oral pathologists first. No book of advanced periodontal techniques would be complete without a review of the most common oral lesions that face the periodontist and their treatment, along with proper biopsy techniques.

The look to the future has also changed between the First and Second Editions. The future of periodontology is bright; we are provided an exciting glimpse of what is next.

Dr. Dibart has again brought together the subject, the team, and the expertise to produce a most valuable compilation of advanced techniques of modern periodontics. The content is based in science and is well-balanced, providing a reference work and guide for the practitioner of advanced dentistry.

Practical Advanced Periodontal Surgery, Second Edition. Edited by Serge Dibart.
© 2020 John Wiley & Sons, Inc. Published 2020 by John Wiley & Sons, Inc.
Companion website: www.wiley.com/go/dibart/advanced

Chapter 1 Conscious IV Sedation Utilizing Midazolam

Jess Liu

INTRODUCTION

Dental fear and anxiety are the common reasons why patients avoid seeking proper dental care. A survey conducted in the US has reported up to 30.5% of both US adults and adolescents experience a moderate to high dental fear (Gatchel 1989). Therefore, it is important for dentists to understand the management of dental fear and anxiety as an integral component of the overall treatment.

As defined by the American Society of Anesthesiologists (see Table 1.1), the continuums of depth of sedation are:

- Minimal Sedation: Normal response to verbal stimulation.

- Moderate Sedation: Purposeful response to verbal or tactile stimulation.

- Deep Sedation: Purposeful response following repeated or painful stimulation.

- General Anesthesia: Unarousable even with painful stimulus.

According to the American Society of Anesthesiologists moderate sedation is also known as "Conscious Sedation," and by definition, conscious sedation is "a drug-induced depression of consciousness during which patients respond purposefully to verbal commands, either alone or accompanied by light tactile stimulation. No interventions are required to maintain a patent airway, and spontaneous ventilation is adequate. Cardiovascular function is usually maintained."

Conscious sedation can be achieved by different routes of administration such as enteral or parenteral administration. For the purpose of this chapter, parenteral administration of conscious sedation limited to intravenous administration of Midazolam (Versed) will be reviewed.

Training in Intravenous Conscious Sedation

While IV conscious sedation is relatively safe to practice, only a qualified and well-trained healthcare provider who is able to manage emergency complications should perform the practice. Dentists who practice IV conscious sedation are mandated by all states to be certified by an approved continuing education program. Furthermore, each state is governed by its own rules and regulations for the administration of conscious sedation, therefore it is important to verify with the individual state dental board for the proper requirements to obtain a permit to practice IV conscious sedation.

MIDAZOLAM (VERSED)

Midazolam is a water soluble, short acting benzodiazepine central nervous system (CNS) depressant. Pharmacologically, it produces anxiolytic, hypnotic, anterograde amnestic, muscle relaxation, and anticonvulsant effects (Reves et al. 1985). Metabolized in the liver by cytochrome P450 enzymes, its mechanism of action is through binding of the $GABA_A$ receptors, (causing an influx of chloride ion which causes hyperpolarization of the neuron's membrane potential) creating a neural inhibition effect.

The onset of intravenous administration of midazolam is relatively fast with a short acting duration. Intravenous administration of 5 mg of midazolam in healthy adults has shown to take effect one to two minutes after administration and has a half-life of approximately one to three hours (Smith et al. 1981).

It is important to understand that the use of midazolam is to produce conscious sedative effects and does not replace the need for proper local anesthesia. Therefore proper anesthetic should be administered prior to the starting of the dental procedure.

Practical Advanced Periodontal Surgery, Second Edition. Edited by Serge Dibart.
© 2020 John Wiley & Sons, Inc. Published 2020 by John Wiley & Sons, Inc.
Companion website: www.wiley.com/go/dibart/advanced

Table 1.1 Continuum of sedation: definition and levels (2004).

Continuum of depth of sedation: definition of general anesthesia and levels of sedation/analgesia

	Minimal sedation (Anxiolysis)	Moderate sedation/analgesia (Conscious sedation)	Deep sedation/Analgesia	General anesthesia
Responsiveness	Normal response to verbal stimulation	Purposeful[a] response to verbal stimulation	Purposeful[a] response following repeated or painful stimulation	Unarousable even with painful stimulus
Airway	Unaffected	No intervention required	Intervention may be required	Intervention often required
Spontaneous Ventilation	Unaffected	Adequate	May be inadequate	Frequently inadequate
Cardiovascular Function	Unaffected	Usually maintained	Usually maintained	May be impaired

[a] Reflex withdrawal from a painful stimulus is NOT considered a purposeful response.

ARMAMENTARIUM

Monitoring equipment for:

- Non-invasive Blood Pressure (NIBP)
- Electrocardiogram (EKG)
- Pulse Oximetry
- Capnography

IV Supplies:

- 0.9% Sodium Chloride Injection 250 ml bag
- Primary IV set (100″)
- 22 Gauge × 1″ Introcan Safety® IV Catheter
- 24 Gauge × ¾″ Introcan Safety IV Catheter

Basic Supplies:

- 1 ml Insulin Syringe
- Blunt Plastic Cannula
- Nasal Cannula
- Supplemental Oxygen
- 1″ Latex free Tourniquet
- 3M Tegaderm Film Transparent Film Dressing
- 3M Transpore Tape
- Gauze
- Band-Aids
- Alcohol Wipes

Basic Medications:

- Midazolam 5 mg/1 cc
- Flumazenil 5 cc
- ACLS Emergency Medical Kit (HealthFirst)

Please see Figure 1.1.

STEPS IN IV SEDATION

Patient pre-op evaluation: As with all dental procedures, a thorough review of the patient's medical history is essential to ensure safe and successful treatment. Review of the patient's medical history with complete review of the system, current medications, as well as drug allergies will provide you the necessary information to assess the patient utilizing the ASA Physical Status Classification System (see Table 1.2). The authors recommend limiting the administration of conscious sedation with patients with ASA Physical status of 2 or less to reduce the chance of medical emergencies.

Contraindication:

- Hypersensitivity
- Acute narrow-angle glaucoma
- Hypotension
- Pregnancy
- Renal disease
- Critically ill patients

Pre-op instructions

- No food or drinks eight hours prior to procedure.
- Please wear comfortable loose-fitting clothing with short sleeves to allow for monitoring of your blood pressure.
- Must be accompanied by a person of legal age to escort you home.
- No sedatives for 24 hours before appointment.

Day of Procedure:

- Seat the patient
- Review medical history. *If patient has medical history of asthma instruct patient to take two puffs of asthma inhaler prior to starting of procedure.*

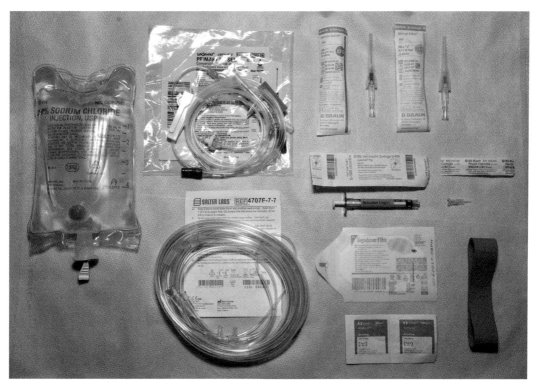

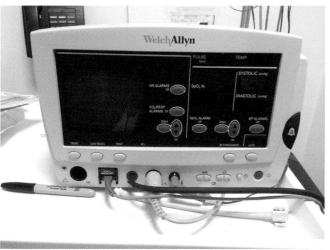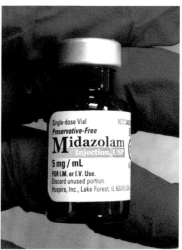

Figure 1.1 Armamentarium needed to provide sedation: monitor, drug, IV sedation set.

Table 1.2 ASA physical status classification (American Society of Anesthesiologists 2015).

ASA physical status classification system

ASA Physical Status 1	A normal healthy patient
ASA Physical Status 2	A patient with mild systemic disease
ASA Physical Status 3	A patient with severe systemic disease
ASA Physical Status 4	A patient with severe systemic disease that is a constant threat to life
ASA Physical Status 5	A moribund patient who is not expected to survive without the operation
ASA Physical Status 6	A declared brain-dead patient whose organs are being removed for donor purposes

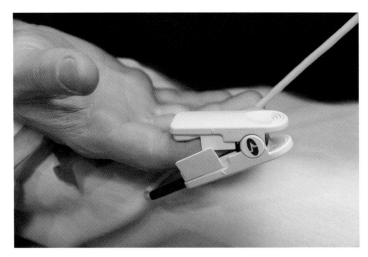

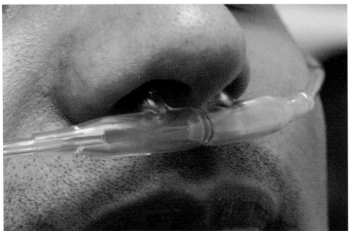

Figure 1.2 Pulse oximetry, oxygen cannula, blood pressure cuff.

- Attach patient monitors (See Figure 1.2) for:

  ○ Blood pressure

  ○ Electrocardiography (EKG)

  ○ Pulse oximetry (Oxygen saturation)

  ○ Capnography (CO2 partial pressure) Give earliest warning of respiratory distress

- Record pre-operatory vital signs: Blood pressure, pulse, respiratory rate, oxygen saturation, end tidal CO_2 level. If vital signs not within normal range re-evaluate patient for the procedure.

Pre-operative vital signs chart

Diagnosis	Systolic (mm Hg)	Diastolic (mm Hg)
Normal	Less than 120 and	Less than 80
Prehypertension	120–139 or	80–89
Hypertension Stage 1	140–159 or	90–99
Hypertension Stage 2	160 or higher or	100 or higher

	Average range
Pulse Rate	Adult 60–80 beats/min
Respiratory Rate	12–20 breaths/min
Oxygen Saturation	95–100%
End tidal CO_2	35–45 mm Hg

- Starting of IV:

  ○ Complete assemble of Primary IV infusion set with 0.9% Sodium Chloride Injection bag See Figure 1.3.

  ○ Exam and select visible superficial vein for venepuncture: Location: Dorsum of hand/wrist, Ventral Forearm, or Antecubital Fossa.

    ▪ Contraindication for venepuncture site are:

      • Mastectomy

      • Cannulas

      • Scarring

      • Vein with valves or bifurcations

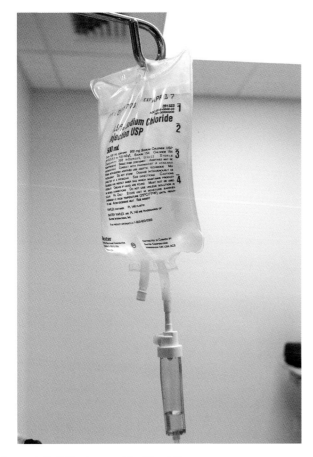

Figure 1.3 Saline bag used for IV sedation.

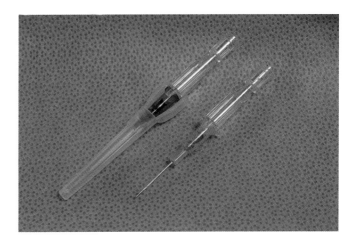

Figure 1.4 IV catheters of various size.

- Methods of venous distension to facilitate venepuncture.
  - Application of tourniquet 3–4 in. above collection area with appropriate compression
  - Opening and closing of hand
  - Hanging of the arm below heart
  - Light slapping or rubbing of the area with alcohol wipe
- Select appropriate Introcan Safety I.V. Catheter *(22/24 gauge is recommended)*. See Figures 1.4 and 1.5.
- Disinfect selected area of venepuncture with 70% isopropyl alcohol wipe
- Insertion of needle and observe for blood return in the flashback chamber
  - *Caution: At no time should venepuncture be performed on an artery*
- Remove tourniquet
- Attach infusion set to catheter adaptor
- Start IV drip, constant drip should be observed. See Figure 1.6.

- *Caution: Initially exam the area of venepuncture after starting IV drip for swelling to ensure proper venepuncture has been performed*
- Stabilize the catheter with 3M Tegaderm Film Transparent Film Dressing and 3M Transpore Tape. See Figure 1.7.

- **Dosage and Administration**
  - Use the 1 ml Insulin Syringe U-100 to draw up 1 ml of 5 mg/ml midazolam. See Figure 1.8.
  - Dosage and administration indicated for the intravenous administration of midazolam as provided by pharmaceutical company Hospira Inc. is as follows:
    - **Healthy Adults Below the Age of 60:** Titrate slowly to the desired effect (e.g. the initiation of slurred speech). Some patients may respond to as little as 1 mg. No more than 2.5 mg should be given over a period of at least two minutes. Wait an additional two or more minutes to fully evaluate the sedative effect. If further titration is necessary, continue to titrate, using small increments, to the appropriate level of sedation. Wait an additional two or more minutes after each increment to fully evaluate the sedative effect. A total dose greater than 5 mg is not usually necessary to reach the desired endpoint.
    - **Patients Age 60 or Older, and Debilitated or Chronically Ill Patients:** Because the danger of hypoventilation, airway obstruction, or apnea is greater in elderly patients and those with chronic disease states or decreased pulmonary reserve, and because the peak effect may take longer in these patients, increments should be smaller and the rate of injection slower. Titrate slowly to the desired effect (e.g. the initiation of slurred speech). Some patients may respond to as little as 1 mg. No more than 1.5 mg should be given over a period of no less than two minutes. Wait an additional two or

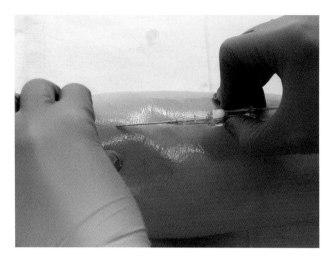

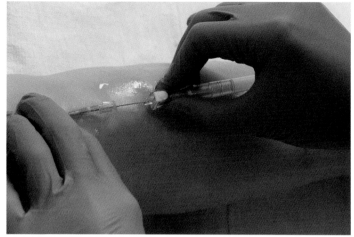

Figure 1.5 Catheter insertion in the vein.

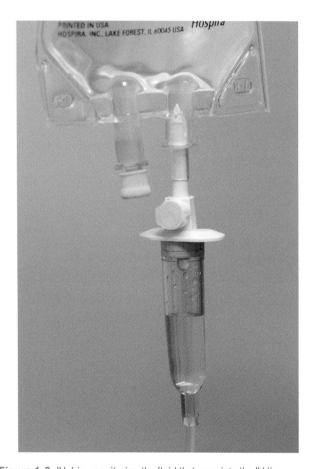

Figure 1.6 IV drip, monitoring the fluid that goes into the IV line.

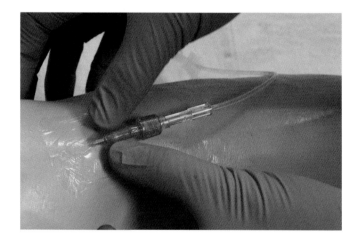

Figure 1.7 IV portal secured with transparent film dressing.

more minutes to fully evaluate the sedative effect. If additional titration is necessary, it should be given at a rate of no more than 1 mg over a period of two minutes, waiting an additional two or more minutes each time to fully evaluate the sedative effect. Total doses greater than 3.5 mg are not usually necessary. If concomitant CNS depressant premedications are used in these patients, they will require at least 50% less midazolam than healthy young unpremedicated patients.

- Starting of procedure is initiated with administering of appropriate local anesthesia after desired sedative effect is achieved.

  o **Maintenance Dose:** Additional doses to maintain the desired level of sedation may be given in increments of 25% of the dose used to first reach the sedative endpoint, but again only by slow titration, especially in the elderly and chronically ill or debilitated patient. These additional doses should be given only after a thorough clinical evaluation clearly indicates the need for additional sedation. For conscious sedation in diagnostic or surgical interventions carried out under local anesthesia (Hospira, Inc., Midazolam Injection 2010).

- Upon completion of the procedure, stop the flow of the IV infusion followed by the removal of the IV catheter.

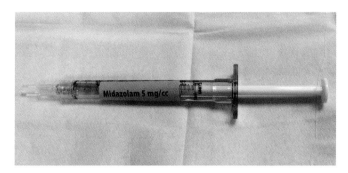

Figure 1.8 Use the 1 ml Insulin Syringe to draw up 1 ml of 5 mg/ml midazolam.

Place sterile gauze over site of venepuncture and apply firm pressure for three to five minutes to prevent hematoma.

- Escort patient to recovery room and continue to monitor patient's vital signs, once recovered release patient to escort.

Post-operative instructions:

a. No sedatives 12 hours after procedure.

b. No consumption of alcoholic beverages after procedure.

c. No stairs without assistance or heavy lifting until completely recovered.

d. Do not drive, operate heavy machinery, or do any dangerous activities for the rest of the day.

e. Do not make important decisions for 24 hours after your appointment.

f. Drink lots of water for at least 12 hours after your appointment.

Reversal agent for midazolam:

In a situation when a patient is oversedated and does not respond purposefully to verbal commands. The reversal agent for benzodiazepine, flumazenil (Romazicon) can be administered. It reverses the effects of benzodiazepines by competitive inhibition at the benzodiazepine binding site on the GABA$_A$ receptor. The initial dose of 0.2 mg of flumazenil can be administered and takes about 2–2.5 minutes to take effect.

Initial dose: 0.2 mg IV one time over 30 seconds.

Repeated doses: 0.5 mg may be given every minute.

Maximum total dose 3 mg. Patients responding partially at 3 mg may receive additional doses up to 5 mg.

Most patients respond to 1–3 mg.

Resedation doses: 0.5 mg every 20 minutes to a total of 1 mg/dose and 3 mg/hour.

Medical Emergencies: As with all medical procedures where drugs are being introduced in the bloodstream while performing dental/surgical therapy, there is a risk of unexpected outcomes. The list below is not exhaustive and the discussion regarding these eventualities and how to deal with them is outside the scope of this chapter.

- Laryngospasm
- Bronchospasm
- Airway Obstruction
- Aspiration
- Angina Pectoris
- Myocardial Infarction
- Hypotension
- Hypertension
- Phlebitis
- Intra-Arterial Injection
- Syncope
- Hyperventilation
- Seizures
- Severe Allergic Reaction
- Bradycardia
- Ventricular Tachycardia
- Ventricular Fibrillation
- Asystole
- Malignant Hyperthermia

REFERENCES

American Society of Anesthesiologists (2015). *ASA Physical Status Classification System*. N.p., n.d. Web. 06 Jan. 2015.

Continuum of Depth of Sedation: Definition of general anesthesia and levels of sedation/analgesia (2009). (pdf). American Society of Anesthesiologists. Approved October 27, 2004, amended October 21, 2009. Retrieved 2010-11-29.

Gatchel, R.J. (1989). The prevalence of dental fear and avoidance: expanded adult and recent adolescent surveys. *J. Am. Dent. Assoc.* 118 (5): 591–593.

Hospira, Inc., Midazolam Injection (1985). USP Revised January 2010.

Reves, J.G., Fragen, R.J., Vinik, H.R. et al. (1985). Midazolam: pharmacology and uses. *Anesthesiology* 62: 310–324.

Smith, M.T., Eadie, M.J., and Brophy, T.O. (1981). The pharmacokinetics of midazolam in man. *Eur. J. Clin. Pharmacol.* 19 (4): 271–278.

Chapter 2 Bone Physiology and Metabolism

Jean-Pierre Dibart

BONE COMPOSITION

Bone consists of three types of cells and a matrix.

Cells: Osteoblasts, Osteoclasts, and Osteocytes

Osteoblasts and osteocytes (mature osteoblasts) are involved in the deposition of bone matrix. Osteoblasts are responsible for the formation of new bone; they secrete osteoid and modulate the crystallization of hydroxyapatite. Osteocytes are mature bone cells; they communicate with each other via gap junctions or canaliculi. Osteoclasts are involved in the resorption of bone tissue; they are responsible for the resorption of bone, which is necessary for its repair in case of fracture or remodeling.

Matrix: Organic and Inorganic

The organic matrix is composed of collagen fibers and a ground substance. The collagen fibers are proteins that give bone its flexibility. The ground substance is made of proteoglycans and glycosaminoglycans: keratin sulfate, chondroitin sulfate, and hyaluronic acid. These components bind cells together and are necessary for the exchange of materials.

The inorganic matrix is composed of hydroxyapatite, calcium carbonate, and calcium citrate. Hydroxyapatite gives bone its strength. Hydroxyapatite is a very hard substance; it is the main mineral component of bone and the enamel of teeth, and it contains calcium, phosphorus, oxygen, and hydrogen.

Bone is the body's major reservoir of calcium (the skeleton contains 99% of the body's calcium, as hydroxyapatite). Mature adults have about 1200 g of calcium.

BONE TYPES

There are two different types of bone:

- Cortical bone, also known as compact bone
- Trabecular bone, also known as cancellous bone

Cortical Bone

Denser and more calcified than trabecular bone, cortical bone is found in the diaphysis of long bones and in the exterior of short bones. It is also called compact bone, and it has a high resistance to bending and torsion. Osteons (Haversian system) are the predominant structures found in compact bone. Each osteon is composed of a central vascular channel, the Haversian canal, surrounded by concentric layers of matrix called lamellae. Osteocytes are found between concentric lamellae. They are connected to each other and the central canal by cytoplasmic processes through the canaliculi. Osteons are separated from each other by cement lines. The space between separate osteons is occupied by interstitial lamellae. Osteons are connected to each other and the periosteum by oblique channels called Volkmann's canals (Marieb 1998).

Trabecular Bone

Trabecular bone is more spongy than cortical bone, it has a lower calcium content and a higher turnover rate, and it is more vulnerable to bone loss. It is found at the metaphysis and diaphysis of long bones and in the interior of the short bones (spine). It is composed of bundles of short and parallel strands of bone fused together. The external layer of trabecular bone contains red bone marrow, where the production of blood cellular components takes place and where most of the arteries and veins of bone organs are located (Tortora 1989).

BONE FORMATION

Intramembranous and Endochondral Ossifications

- Intramembranous ossification: Direct replacement of connective tissue with bone (i.e. mandible and flat bones of the skull).

- Endochondral ossification: Cartilage is replaced by mineralized bone, and the bones become longer, explaining growth during childhood (i.e. femur and humerus).

Bone Remodeling

Remodeling is a sequence of activation, resorption, and formation. The bone is continuously remodeling; osteoclasts become activated and resorb the old bone, and then osteoblasts begin formation of the new bone, giving rise to the Haversian system. The mature osteoclasts resorb bone by forming a space on the matrix surface; then, the osteoids begin to mineralize, regulated by the osteoblasts.

Months later, the crystals are packed closely, and the density of the bone increases.

Remodeling is necessary to maintain bone structure after a fracture or after age-related modifications; osteoclasts resorb aging bone in order to repair damage and maintain the quality of bone and to retain calcium homeostasis.

Bone can also remodel according to stresses, such as orthodontic tooth movement, in which there is resorption on the pressure side and apposition on the traction side.

Complete rest results in accelerated bone loss, whereas weight-bearing activities are associated with bone formation. Peak bone mass is the maximum bone mass achieved by midlife. Exercise programs increase bone mass at all ages; adolescence is a particularly critical period because the velocity of bone growth doubles. When women reach menopause, bone resorption exceeds bone formation, osteoblastic activity cannot keep up with osteoclastic activity, and women begin to lose bone. This puts them at high risk for osteoporosis and fractures.

There are five stages in bone remodeling:

1. Quiescence: Resting state of the bone surface

2. Activation: Recruitment of osteoclasts to a bone surface; osteoblasts secrete collagenase

3. Resorption: Removal of bone by osteoclasts; Howship's lacunae are excavated

4. Reversal: Short phase; cement line is formed; osteoclasts stop removing bone; osteoblasts fill the defect

5. Formation: Laying down of bone; osteoblasts produce osteoid; mineralization begins; then bone is again converted to a resting surface

Bone is remodeled through the following actions:

- Osteoblasts
- Osteoclasts
- Parathyroid hormone (PTH)
- Vitamin D
- Calcitonin (CT)
- Estrogens
- Corticoids
- Growth hormone (GH)
- Thyroid hormone

Bone Remodeling and Periodontitis

After damage to the bone has occurred, the osteocytes send messages to the surface to produce preosteoblasts. They express RANK-L (receptor activator of nuclear factor [NF]-κB ligand). Preosteoclasts have receptors called RANK (receptor activator of NF-κB). RANK-L activates these receptors, which produce mature osteoclasts. RANK, RANK-L, and osteoprotegerin (OPG) (RANK-L inhibitor) are the key factors regulating osteoclast formation in normal bone physiology. The molecular interactions of these molecules regulate osteoclast formation and bone loss in various diseases such as rheumatologic inflammatory diseases, periodontitis, or peri-implantitis (Haynes 2004). The change in the levels of these regulators plays a role in the bone loss seen in periodontitis. Significantly higher levels of RANK-L protein were found to be expressed in the periodontally affected tissues, whereas OPG protein levels are lower. RANK-L protein is associated with lymphocytes and macrophages; many leukocytes expressing messenger RNA (mRNA) are observed in periodontitis tissues (Crotti et al. 2003). RANK-L is a TNF (tumor necrosis factor) receptor–related protein and a major factor for osteoclast differentiation and activation. The levels of RANK-L mRNA are higher in advanced periodontitis; although the levels of OPG mRNA are lower in advanced and moderate periodontitis, the ratio of RANK-L to OPG mRNA is increased in periodontitis. RANK-L mRNA is expressed in proliferating epithelium and in inflammatory cells, mainly lymphocytes and macrophages. Upregulation of RANK-L mRNA is associated with the activation of osteoclastic bone destruction in periodontitis (Liu et al. 2003).

Markers of Bone Formation

Markers of bone formation measure osteoblastic activity: osteocalcin, P1NP (N-terminal propeptide of type 1 procollagen), and bone-specific alkaline phosphatase (BALP).

Markers of Bone Resorption

These markers measure osteoclastic activity: deoxypyridinoline (DPD), pyridinoline, and associated peptides, NTX (cross-linked N-terminal telopeptide of type I collagen), and CTX I (cross-linked C-terminal telopeptide of type I collagen) generated from bone by osteoclasts as a degradation product of type I collagen and released into circulation.

Vitamin C

This vitamin is necessary for the osteocytes to form collagen; in the case of vitamin C deficiency, collagen formation is decreased, and so is the thickness of the bone cortex.

Vitamin D

Vitamin D has an important role in calcium absorption. The two major forms involved in humans are vitamin D_2 (ergocalciferol) and vitamin D_3 (cholecalciferol). 1,25-Dihydroxyvitamin D_3 [1,25-(OH)2 vitamin D_3] is produced by metabolism in the liver and the kidneys. It is the most active form of vitamin D, and it increases calcium absorption from the intestines. Conversion into the active metabolite 1,25-(OH)2 vitamin D_3 from its precursor is affected by cytochrome P450 enzymes in the liver and the kidneys. This is tightly regulated by the plasma levels of calcium, phosphate, PTH, and 1,25-(OH)2 vitamin D_3 itself (Tissandie et al. 2006). It affects the kidneys and the intestines and stimulates the mineralization of bone. Ultraviolet irradiation from the sunlight to the skin will also affect the production of vitamins D_2 and D_3.

Genetic polymorphisms in the vitamin D receptor (VDR) gene are associated with parameters of bone homeostasis and with osteoporosis and rapid bone resorption. Interestingly, some authors have found VDR polymorphism to be associated with localized aggressive periodontal disease (Hennig et al. 1999).

Childhood vitamin D deficiency syndrome is called rickets: unmineralized osteoid accumulates, and the bone formed is weak and can lead to permanent deformities of the skeleton. In adulthood, the absence of adequate amounts of vitamin D leads to osteomalacia: decalcification of bone occurs by defective mineralization of newly formed bone matrix.

What are the sources of vitamin D? Only a few foods contain appreciable amounts of vitamin D – fish liver, fish (i.e. salmon, mackerel, tuna, sardines), eggs, liver, butter, and Shiitake mushrooms.

Vitamin K

This vitamin is required for the production of osteocalcin (a protein produced by the osteoblasts); a good vitamin K status is necessary to prevent osteoporosis. Vitamin K is found in green leafy vegetables.

Calcitonin

This is a hormone secreted by the thyroid gland. Its effects are opposite those of the PTH (lowering of blood calcium). Calcitonin inhibits matrix resorption by inhibiting osteoclast activity; it reverses hypercalcemia.

Parathyroid Hormone

PTH is a hormone produced by the parathyroid glands. It increases ionized blood calcium levels. The fall in ionized blood calcium causes the release of PTH and vitamin D. PTH stimulates osteoclast activity, and calcium is released from the bone. PTH causes resorption of bone, calcium absorption from the kidneys, and synthesis of active vitamin D. Bone calcium mobilization is due to the transfer of calcium ions from hydroxyapatite to blood, to ensure calcium homeostasis.

PTH activates and increases the number of osteoclasts, causing resorption of the bone matrix. PTH also acts on the kidneys to decrease urinary calcium.

Hyperparathyroidism causes increased bone resorption.

Osteoprotegerin

OPG is an inhibitor of bone resorption and is involved in bone density regulation. High levels cause the development of dense bone. OPG blocks the differentiation of osteoclasts and impairs bone resorption.

Low-Density Lipoprotein Receptor–Related Proteins

Recent analyses revealed a new signaling pathway involved in the regulation of osteoblastic cells and the acquisition of peak bone mass. Wnts are soluble glycoproteins that engage receptor complexes composed of low-density lipoprotein receptor–related proteins Lrp 5 and 6 and Frizzled proteins. The loss of function of Lrp 5 causes a decrease in bone formation, and Lrp 5 mutations are associated with high bone mass diseases. These mutations influence the Wnt-beta-catenin canonical pathway that increases bone mass through a large number of mechanisms.

Osteoporosis

Osteoporosis means "porous bone." Calcium deficiency leads to decalcification of bones and aggravated fracture risks (especially vertebrae, hip, and forearm). Hyperparathyroidism can also cause decalcification. Androgens and estrogens (especially before menopause), on the other hand, stimulate bone formation.

Osteoporosis is characterized by low bone mass and micro-architectural deterioration due to decreased bone formation and increased bone resorption; this phenomenon leads to increased bone fragility and fracture. As we age, bone resorption exceeds bone formation and the severe loss of bone mass results in gaps in the bone structure, leading to fractures (hip, spine, and wrist being the most common).

Bone strength is also determined by another important element, which is the trabecular microstructure. In estrogen deficiency, resorption cavities are too deep, and the trabeculae are not well connected, resulting in increased bone fragility.

In women after age 30, bone resorption exceeds bone formation and bone mass decreases slowly. After menopause, because of a decrease in estrogen levels, bone loss is accelerated. Peak bone density is lower in females than in males, and bone mineral status depends on peak bone mass achieved before the age of 30. Optimizing peak bone mass, especially in children and adolescents, between the ages of 10–18, is important in reducing the future risk of osteoporosis.

Although most of the variance in peak bone mass is considered to be genetic, bone mineral density (BMD) is higher with sufficient consumption of calcium, fruits, and vegetables. Calcium-rich foods include dairy products, cereals, nuts, seeds, dried fruits, mineral water, and green-leafed vegetables.

Risk factors include the following:

- Female patients after menopause or age over 60
- First-degree female relative with osteoporosis or fracture
- Personal history of nontraumatic fracture
- Low body mass index (BMI) ($<19\,kg/m^2$)
- Anorexia–amenorrhea episodes
- Excessive sports participation
- Prolonged use of cortisone
- Early menopause before age 40, natural or surgically induced
- Smoking
- Excessive alcohol intake
- Sedentary lifestyle
- Excessive caffeine or salt intake
- Low calcium intake
- Thyroid hormone or PTH abnormalities
- Hypercortisolism
- Prevalent radiographic vertebral fracture

BONE DENSITY MEASURING TECHNIQUES

DEXA: Dual Energy X-Ray Absorptiometry (Bone Densitometry)

In DEXA, an x-ray with two energy peaks is sent through the bones. One is absorbed by the soft tissues, and the other is absorbed by the bones; through subtraction, BMD is measured. This is the most widely used method to measure bone density and provides whole-body scans and detailed measurements of the spine (lumbar spine), the hip (femoral neck), and the forearm (wrist).

The World Health Organization (WHO) definition of *osteoporosis* is based on BMD expressed as T scores and Z scores:

- T score is the comparison with the bone density of young people.
- Z score is the comparison with the bone density of age peers.
- A T score superior to −2.5 standard deviation is the definition of *osteoporosis*. The WHO based the diagnosis of postmenopausal osteoporosis on the presence of a BMD T score that is 2.5 standard deviations or more below the mean for young women.
- A T score between −1 and −2.5 standard deviations is the definition of *osteopenia*.

Quantitative Ultrasound

Quantitative ultrasound (QUS) is a radiation-free reliable technique to evaluate skeletal status. Three parameters are measured: broadband ultrasound attenuation (BUA), speed of sound (SOS), and stiffness index (SI).

This is a technique performed with use of the calcaneous or radial bone; it measures the bone mass on the basis of the bone SOS.

Quantitative Computed Tomography

Quantitative computed tomography (QCT) provides three-dimensional BMD of trabecular and cortical components. It is also used to analyze trabecular microstructure.

This technique measures an imaged slice of the forearm or the leg; it can be used to measure bone size and the width of cortical and trabecular bone. It provides a volumetric density of bone. It can also measure the volume and content of calcium hydroxyapatite.

Cone Beam Computed Tomography

This technique offers a significant advantage because of its three-dimensional capability for osseous defects detection (Misch et al. 2006).

Fractal Analysis of Bone Texture

The analysis of bone texture based on fractal mathematics when applied to bone images on plain radiographs can be considered as a reflection of trabecular bone microarchitecture.

IMPLICATIONS FOR DENTAL TREATMENTS

Osteonecrosis of the Jaws

Bisphosphonates are used in treatment of cancers and osteoporosis; as a side effect, they may cause jaw necrosis. These necroses mostly appear after administration of aminobisphosphonates. They are treated by resection of necrotic bone, and repeated surgical interventions are required. The management is difficult and includes surgical procedures and antibiotic therapy (Eckert et al. 2007).

Bisphosphonates somehow cause cell death in the jawbone, which makes it prone to chronic infection; the reduced resorptive ability of bone due to bisphosphonates hinders the formation of a fresh bone surface for reestablishment of bone cell coverage (Aspenberg 2006).

The clinical symptoms of jaw necrosis are swelling, exudation, loosening of teeth, and pain. The radiographs show persisting tooth sockets after extractions and radiolucency, sequestra, or fracture. Risk factors are as follows:

- Intravenous or long-term bisphosphonate therapy (over three years of oral use, over one year of intravenous use)
- Chemotherapy
- Radiation
- Corticoids
- Age
- Underlying malignant disease
- Oral infection

Bisphosphonate-associated osteonecrosis is characterized by the unexpected appearance of necrotic bone. Osteonecrosis can develop spontaneously or after an invasive surgical procedure such as dental extraction. Symptoms can mimic routine dental problems such as decay or periodontal disease. Risk factors are intravenous bisphosphonate therapy, duration of treatment, age greater than 60 years, myeloma, and history of recent dental extraction (Migliorati et al. 2006).

Before bisphosphonate therapy is started, infections should be treated and risk of injuries to the mucosa should be reduced. Regular dental recall is recommended, for the prevention of infection combined with a follow-up of removable denture for possible ulcerations. Conservative treatment measures are preferred; surgery is carried out nontraumatically using sterile techniques, appropriate oral disinfectant, and antibiotic prophylaxis until the day of suture removal. For patients following bisphosphonate therapy, the indications for dental implants should be very strict; in case of the osteonecrosis, dental implants are contraindicated (Piesold et al. 2006).

Early diagnosis is important; it can make a difference in the outcome of the disease. Technetium 99m-methylene diphosphonate (^{99m}Tc-MDP) three-phase bone scan can be used as a screening test to detect subclinical osteonecrosis. Computed tomography (CT) and magnetic resonance imaging (MRI) are useful in defining the features and extent of lesions. Radiography and CT display osteolytic lesions with the involvement of cortical bone, and MRI shows the edema of soft tissue. ^{99m}Tc-MDP three-phase bone scan is the most sensitive tool to detect necrosis at an early stage (Chiandusi et al. 2006).

The mandible is more commonly affected than the maxilla and 60% of cases are preceded by a dental surgical procedure. Oversuppression of bone turnover is the primary mechanism of necrosis, and there may be comorbid factors. All sites of jaw infection should be eliminated before bisphosphonate therapy in at-risk patients. Conservative debridement, pain control, infection management, use of antimicrobial rinses, and withdrawal of bisphosphonate are preferable to aggressive surgical measures (Woo et al. 2006).

Dental Implants

Bone quality and its presurgical assessment are important for long-term implant prognosis; the implant length and type can also influence bone strain, especially in low-density bone (Tada et al. 2003).

The Process of Osseointegration

In the early bone response to the implant, the first tissue that comes in contact with the implant is the blood clot with platelets and fibrin. During the first days, preosteoblasts and osteoblasts adhere to the implant surface covered by an afibrillar calcified layer to produce osteoid tissue; within a few days, a woven bone and then a reparative trabecular bone are present at the junction between the implant and the bone. Trabecular bone is gradually substituted by a mature lamellar bone, which characterizes osseointegration (Marco et al. 2005).

Osseointegration is a dynamic process: in the establishment phase, there is an interplay between bone resorption in contact regions and bone formation in contact-free areas. During the maintenance phase, osseointegration is secured through continuous remodeling and adaptation to function (Berglundh et al. 2003).

The process of osseointegration is a reliable type of cement-free anchorage for prosthetic tissue substitutes and bone, with a direct contact between living bone and implant (Albrektsson et al. 1981).

It is important to note that senile and postmenopausal osteoporosis have important consequences for the success of endosseous dental implants, for primary stability, biological fixation, and final osseointegration.

Smokers are also at risk. Bone resorption is altered in smokers; there are differences between the amounts of pyridinoline around the teeth of nonsmokers and smokers. Smokers have a higher level of pyridinoline than do nonsmokers in the gingival crevicular fluid of implants, suggesting that smoking may affect implant success (Oates et al. 2004).

Bone-stimulating Factors

A bone differentiation factor can stimulate bone formation in peri-implant bone defects. Bone morphogenetic proteins (recombinant human bone morphogenetic protein-2 [rhBMP-2]) can be used to stimulate bone growth around and onto the surface of endosseous dental implants, placed in sites with extended osseous defects (Cochran et al. 1999). Recombinant human osteogenic protein-1 (rhOP-1) accelerates the healing of extraction defects and the osseointegration of implants. New bone formation can be induced around and adjacent to a dental implant with a recombinantly produced bone inductive protein (Cook et al. 1995).

Enamel matrix derivative (EMD) may contribute to inducing osteoblast growth and differentiation by helping create a favorable osteogenic microenvironment (reducing RANK-L release and enhancing OPG production) (Galli et al. 2006). Amelogenins, EMDs, have a stimulatory effect on mesenchymal cells and tissues and on the regeneration of alveolar bone. They cause an increase in alkaline phosphatase activity and an increased expression of osteocalcin and type I collagen. Researchers found similarities between EMDs and PTH on human osteoblasts (Reseland et al. 2006).

Periodontitis

Patients with aggressive periodontitis share periodontal and hematological characteristics with patients with rheumatoid arthritis or juvenile idiopathic arthritis. Patients with rheumatoid arthritis have a higher percentage of sites with probing depth greater than 4 mm, clinical attachment loss greater than 2 mm, and alveolar bone loss greater than 2 mm. The percentage of sites with clinical attachment loss is correlated with the levels of serum rheumatoid factor (Havemose-Poulsen et al. 2006).

For patients with primary Sjögren syndrome, complications of periodontitis such as bleeding, gingival hypertrophy, and pockets are not improved with better oral hygiene. This phenomenon is associated with high levels of B-cell activating factor (BAFF) in the saliva; the levels of BAFF correlate with the periodontal pocket depth. The known effect of B cells in periodontitis is partly mediated by salivary BAFF in patients with primary Sjögren syndrome (Pers et al. 2005).

Mandibular Osteoporosis

There are relationships between oral bone loss and osteoporosis. There is a positive correlation between systemic bone mass and oral bone mass (Jeffcoat 2005).

Osteoporosis is a systemic disease in which the skeletal condition is characterized by a decreased mass of normally mineralized bone. Alveolar processes provide the bony framework for tooth support; the decline of skeletal mass is correlated with an increased risk of oral bone loss and has a negative effect on tooth stability. Aging and estrogen depletion have a negative influence on tooth retention and residual alveolar crest preservation (Sanfilippo and Bianchi 2003).

Pixel intensity values and fractal dimensions on radiographic panoramic images are useful in detecting changes in the osteoporotic mandibular cancellous bone (Tosoni et al. 2006). The measurement of mandibular alveolar BMD, in postmenopausal women with periodontal disease, shows age-related decrease of alveolar BMD, calcaneus SOS, and vertebral BMD. There are significant correlations between alveolar BMD, calcaneus SOS, and vertebral BMD (Takaishi et al. 2005).

REFERENCES

Albrektsson, T., Branemark, P.I., Hansson, H.A., and Lindstrom, J. (1981). Osseointegrated titanium implants. Requirements for ensuring a long-lasting, direct bone-to-implant anchorage in man. *Acta Orthop. Scand.* 52 (2): 155–170.

Aspenberg, P. (2006). Osteonecrosis: what does it mean? One condition partly caused by bisphosphonates – or another one, preferably treated with them? *Acta Orthop.* 77 (5): 693–694.

Berglundh, T., Abrahamsson, I., Lang, N.P., and Lindhe, J. (2003). De novo alveolar bone formation adjacent to endosseous implants. *Clin. Oral Implants Res.* 14 (3): 251–262.

Chiandusi, S., Biasotto, M., Dore, F. et al. (2006). Clinical and diagnostic imaging of bisphosphonate-associated osteonecrosis of the jaws. *Dentomaxillofac. Radiol.* 35 (4): 236–243.

Cochran, D., Schenk, R., Buser, D. et al. (1999). Recombinant human bone morphogenetic protein-2 stimulation of bone formation around endosseous dental implants. *J. Periodontol.* 70 (2): 139–150.

Cook, S.D., Salkeld, S.L., and Rueger, D.C. (1995). Evaluation of recombinant human osteogenic protein-1 (rhOP-1) placed with dental implants in fresh extraction sites. *J. Oral Implantol.* 21 (4): 281–289.

Crotti, T., Smith, M.D., Hirsch, R. et al. (2003). Receptor activator NF kappaB ligand (RANKL) and osteoprotegerin (OPG) protein expression in periodontitis. *J. Periodontal Res.* 38 (4): 380–387.

Eckert, A.W., Maurer, P., Meyer, L. et al. (2007). Bisphosphonate-related jaw necrosis – severe complication in maxillofacial surgery. *Cancer Treat. Rev.* 33 (1): 58–63.

Galli, C., Macaluso, G.M., Guizzardi, S. et al. (2006). Osteoprotegerin and receptor activator of nuclear factor-kappa B ligand modulation by enamel matrix derivative in human alveolar osteoblasts. *J. Periodontol.* 77 (7): 1223–1228.

Havemose-Poulsen, A., Westergaard, J., Stoltze, K. et al. (2006). Periodontal and hematological characteristics associated with aggressive periodontitis, juvenile idiopathic arthritis, and rheumatoid arthritis. *J. Periodontol.* 77 (2): 280–288.

Haynes, D.R. (2004). Bone lysis and inflammation. *Inflamm. Res.* 53 (11): 596–600.

Hennig, B.J., Parkhill, J.M., Chapple, I.L. et al. (1999). Association of a vitamin D receptor gene polymorphism with localized early-onset periodontal diseases. *J. Periodontol.* 70 (9): 1032–1038.

Jeffcoat, M. (2005). The association between osteoporosis and oral bone loss. *J. Periodontol.* 76 (11 Suppl): 2125–2132.

Liu, D., Xu, J.K., Figliomeni, L. et al. (2003). Expression of RANK-L and OPG mRNA in periodontal disease: possible involvement in bone destruction. *Int. J. Mol. Med.* 11 (1): 17–21.

Marco, F., Milena, F., Gianluca, G., and Vittoria, O. (2005). Peri-implant osteogenesis in health and osteoporosis. *Micron* 36 (7–8): 630–644.

Marieb, E.N. (1998). *Human Anatomy & Physiology*, 4e. Menlo Park, Calif: Benjamin/Cummings Science Publishing.

Migliorati, C.A., Siegel, M.A., and Elting, L.S. (2006). Bisphosphonate-associated osteonecrosis: a long-term complication of bisphosphonate treatment. *Lancet Oncol.* 7 (6): 508–514.

Misch, K.A., Yi, E.S., and Sarment, D.P. (2006). Accuracy of cone beam computed tomography for periodontal defect measurements. *J. Periodontol.* 77 (7): 1261–1266.

Oates, T.W., Caraway, D., and Jones, J. (2004). Relation between smoking and biomarkers of bone resorption associated with dental endosseous implants. *Implant. Dent.* 13 (4): 352–357.

Pers, J.O., d'Arbonneau, F., Devauchelle-Pensec, V. et al. (2005). Is periodontal disease mediated by salivary BAFF in Sjögren's syndrome? *Arthritis Rheum.* 52 (8): 2411–2414.

Piesold, J.U., Al Nawas, B., and Grotz, K.A. (2006). Osteonecrosis of the jaws by long term therapy with bisphosphonates. *Mund Kiefer Gesichtschir.* 10 (5): 287–300.

Reseland, J.E., Reppe, S., Larsen, A.M. et al. (2006). The effect of enamel matrix derivative on gene expression in osteoblasts. *Eur. J. Oral Sci.* 114 (Suppl 1): 205–211.

Sanfilippo, F. and Bianchi, A.E. (2003). Osteoporosis: the effect on maxillary bone resorption and therapeutic possibilities by means of implant prostheses – a literature review and clinical considerations. *Int. J. Periodont. Restor. Dent.* 23 (5): 447–457.

Tada, S., Stegaroiu, R., Kitamura, E. et al. (2003). Influence of implant design and bone quality on stress/strain distribution in bone around implants: a 3-dimensional finite element analysis. *Int. J. Oral Maxillofac. Implants* 18 (3): 357–368.

Takaishi, Y., Okamoto, Y., Ikeo, T. et al. (2005). Correlations between periodontitis and loss of mandibular bone in relation to systemic bone changes in postmenopausal Japanese women. *Osteoporos. Int.* 16 (12): 1875–1882.

Tissandie, E., Gueguen, Y., Lobaccaro, J.M. et al. (2006). Effects of depleted uranium after short-term exposure on vitamin D metabolism in rat. *Arch. Toxicol.* 80 (8): 473–480.

Tortora, G.J. (1989). *Principles of Human Anatomy*, 5e. New York: Harper & Row.

Tosoni, G.M., Lurie, A.G., Cowan, A.E., and Burleson, J.A. (2006). Pixel intensity and fractal analyses: detecting osteoporosis in perimenopausal and postmenopausal women by using digital panoramic images. *Oral Surg. Oral Med. Oral Pathol. Oral Radiol. Endod.* 102 (2): 235–241.

Woo, S.B., Hellstein, J.W., and Kalmar, J.R. (2006). Narrative [corrected] review: bisphosphonates and osteonecrosis of the jaws. *Ann. Intern. Med.* 144 (10): 753–761.

Chapter 3 Anatomy of the Dental/Alveolar Structures and Wound Healing

Albert Price

ANATOMIC REVIEW (EMPHASIS ON VASCULAR SUPPLY)

Knowledge of local anatomy and the physiology of healing tissues is the *sine qua non* of the surgeon's ability to achieve stable results. A practical review of regional and periodontal anatomy at both the macro and micro levels can be applied to a better performance of both periodontal and implant surgical procedures. Following this anatomy review, the basic process, timing and current knowledge of wound healing will be reviewed. Throughout this exploration a few underlying themes are repeated:

1. Understanding the local anatomy of *microvascular patterns* and *local preservation* of them is the key to minimal morbidity. Soft tissue flaps, designed for surgical access, without this understanding can lead to soft tissue necrosis and subsequent underlying bone loss or sequestration.

2. The relative physical dimensions and nutrient demands of the parenchymal and stromal content determine blood vessel volume and its distribution

3. Constant attention to these variations in anatomic microarchitecture allows predictable, biologic manipulation which minimizes risk in surgical procedures.

VASCULAR SUPPLY: MACRO AND MICRO

The external carotid is the major source of arterial supply to the facial structures. After separating from the common carotid at about the level of the thyroid cartilage, the external carotid provides a branch to the superior thyroid and then ascends into the facial structures with major branches in succession being the ascending phayrngeal, lingual, facial, occipital, posterior auricular, and the maxillary artery before distributing into a variety of superficial temporal arteries. Our interests will be focused on the lingual, facial, and maxillary branches.

The Lingual branch of the external carotid ascends from its medial aspect, below the corner of the mandible to supply the tongue and ends in a plexus with the submental branch of the Facial Artery and the terminus of the Mylohyoid artery. This plexus, located to the lingual of the cuspid and lower incisor teeth, serves parts of the sublingual gland and provides branches into the lingual foramina to supply the lingual bone mass of the chin. Injury to this area by perforating through the lingual bone plate during a misplaced or overextended trajectory of dental implant preparation may have fatal repercussions (Bernardi et al. 2017).

The facial artery branches from the carotid just above the lingual artery passing inward beneath the mandibular angle, then courses forward through parts of the submandibular gland after which it curves outward to the facial tissues just in front of the masseter muscle (where its pulse can be felt with light palpation of the area). From its lingual aspect a small submental branch courses medial to join the complex with the lingual and mylohyoid arteries previously noted. The main branch supplies tissues of the face and lips.

The maxillary artery branches inward off the external carotid just below the mandibular condyle. The tributaries of the maxillary artery provide the major supplies to the interior of the facial region. Its regional divisions are three in number: the inferior alveolar (supplying the mandible), the pterygoid (which supplies the major masticatory muscles) and the pterygopalatine (which contains the major supply to the maxillary arch – the posterior superior alveolar) (Woodburne 1965) (Figure 3.1).

1. The inferior alveolar artery: After providing a small, descending mylohyoid branch to the medial, the inferior alveolar artery descends to enter the mandibular foramen and distributes internally to the ramus and body of the mandibular bone, to the posterior teeth, and the periodontal ligaments (PDL) before branching

Practical Advanced Periodontal Surgery, Second Edition. Edited by Serge Dibart.
© 2020 John Wiley & Sons, Inc. Published 2020 by John Wiley & Sons, Inc.
Companion website: www.wiley.com/go/dibart/advanced

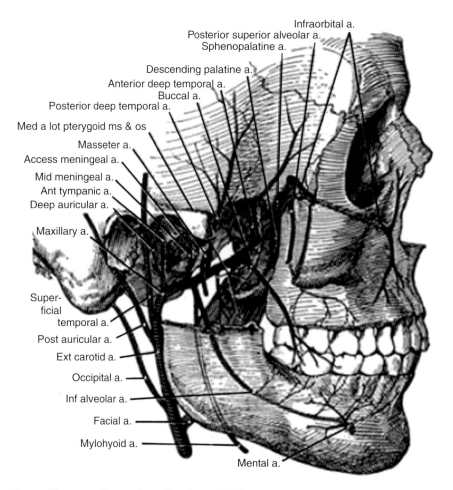

Infraorbital a.
Posterior superior alveolar a.
Sphenopalatine a.
Descending palatine a.
Anterior deep temporal a.
Buccal a.
Posterior deep temporal a.
Med a lot pterygoid ms & os
Masseter a.
Access meningeal a.
Mid meningeal a.
Ant tympanic a.
Deep auricular a.
Maxillary a.
Super-
ficial
temporal a.
Post auricular a.
Ext carotid a.
Occipital a.
Inf alveolar a.
Facial a.
Mylohyoid a.
Mental a.

Figure 3.1 Distribution of the maxillary artery. Source: From Woodburne (1965).

below the mandibular bicuspid area in an upward, reverse curl, to exit through the mental foramen with the mental nerve. The remainder of the inferior alveolar artery continues forward (although there is no clear description of its passage forward) to supply the anterior teeth and a major portion of the chin. A discrete bony canal associated with this incisive branch is seldom seen on a CT Scan. (As noted above the lingual aspect of the chin bone is also supplied through the lingual foramina from the lingual, mylohyoid, and facial submental plexus.)

2. The pterygoid division supplies the major masticatory muscles and the buccinator muscle of the cheek and has secondary branches which complement the facial artery in supplying the cheek mucosa and skin.

3. The pterygopalatine division courses through the pterygopalatine fossa and sends four major branches: posterior superior alveolar, descending palatine, infraorbital, and sphenopalatine.

   a. The posterior superior alveolar enters the distal of the maxillary tuberosity and coursing forward supplies the basal and alveolar bone, the teeth, the gingival margins through the PDL, and (in combination with the infraorbital and sphenopalatine) the tissues of the maxillary sinus (Solar 1999).

   b. The descending palatine exits through the greater palatine foramen apical to the maxillary 2nd molar and courses forward along the inner surface of the palatal vault (Figure 3.2), supplying glands and mucosa before reaching the incisive canal. There it anastomoses with the incisive branch of the sphenopalatine artery.

   c. The infraorbital passes slightly higher and medial through the floor of the orbit with terminal branches to the mid and anterior incisive areas, combines with branches of the posterior superior to supply the maxillary sinus (Solar 1999), and the lacrimal duct and then exits through the infraorbital notch to the soft tissues of the face under the eye.

   d. The sphenopalatine artery ascends higher to the roof of the nose and then distributes forward and down along the lateral nasal wall (common with the medial wall of maxillary sinus) and medially along the vomer groove to the incisive canal, within which it descends to merge with the incisive branch of the greater palatine in the incisal papilla region (Woodburne 1965) (See Figure 3.1).

BLOOD SUPPLY WITHIN THE ALVEOLAR AND BASAL BONE OF THE DENTAL ARCHES

The general pattern or trajectory of blood flow to both hard and soft tissues of the maxillofacial area is from distal to mesial (posterior–anterior). The trabecular bone compartment of the basal and alveolar bone is supplied from within their defining cortical plates (i.e. from inside out) by their major vessels, the posterior superior alveolar and the inferior alveolar. If teeth are present, they are surrounded by a compact woven bone socket that has numerous perforations connecting the vascular net of the marrow spaces with the vascular net of the PDL. This PDL net is also supplied from the apical where dedicated vessels enter the pulp canal of the tooth. The flow of the PDL net is apical–coronal into the marginal attached gingiva where it merges with the investing soft tissue supply of the mucogingival soft tissues (Folkman and Klagsbrun 1987; Folke et al. 1965; Price 1974) (Figure 3.5).

MICROARCHITECTURE OF THE BONE/TOOTH RELATIONSHIP AND THE INTERFACE OF SOFT AND HARD CONNECTIVE TISSUES

Bone has two compartments: a hard mineralized component and a soft, stroma filled inner marrow space. These two compartments are arranged in a variety of shapes and proportions – the *local bony microarchitecture*. The thick mineralized layers that define the bone's outer shape or line the major nerve/vessel channels (inferior alveolar canal, incisive canal, etc.) and tooth sockets (Figures 3.6 and 3.7) are referred to as cortical or compact bone. The inner compartment or marrow space is cross-braced by mineralized struts of various thickness, the *trabeculae*. These trabeculae divide the inner bone space into cells of various sizes and are referred to as *cancellous bone* (Figures 3.2, 3.5–3.7).

The interface between the mineral compartment of the interior trabeculae and the internal soft tissue *(marrow)* is lined by a single cell layer of cells (the liner cells) which is thought to be composed of resting osteoblasts. The interface with the external surfaces of compact or cortical bone and their investing soft tissues is enveloped by a more complex *periosteum,* which varies in configuration dependent on the surrounding connective tissue interfaces (see Figures 3.3, 3.14, and 3.16).

In clinical literature, the word *density* is often misapplied when describing bone structure related to the drilling experience of dental implant placement. Both cortical bone and trabecular bone have a fairly uniform physical, mineral density. What is more relevant to bone surgery is the microarchitecture – the three-dimensional size and arrangement of these compact and cancellous layers within a given site. As can be seen in the representative

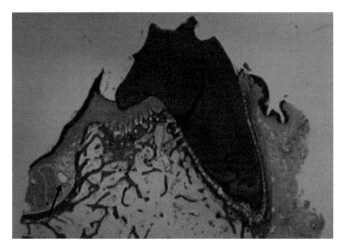

Figure 3.2 Palatal artery extension of greater palatine artery (black *arrow*).

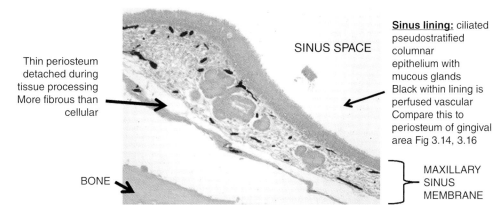

Thin periosteum detached during tissue processing More fibrous than cellular

SINUS SPACE

Sinus lining: ciliated pseudostratified columnar epithelium with mucous glands Black within lining is perfused vascular Compare this to periosteum of gingival area Fig 3.14, 3.16

MAXILLARY SINUS MEMBRANE

BONE

Figure 3.3 Maxillary sinus periosteum (Monkey/vascular-India ink perfused). This is representative of a "lifted" sinus membrane.

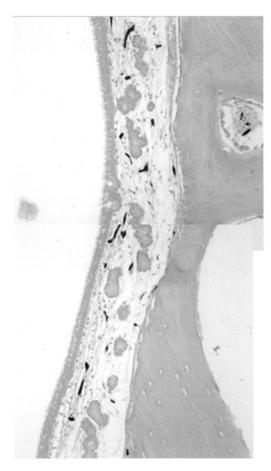

Figure 3.4 Maxillary sinus periosteum (Monkey/vascular-India ink perfused). In contrast to the "lifted" membrane in Figure 3.3, this is representative of an "intact" sinus membrane prior to "lifting." (Compare also to Figures 3.14 and 3.16.)

tissue sections (Figures 3.2, 3.6, and 3.7), the size and distribution of cancellous and cortical layers vary considerably from one tooth location to another. Perhaps a new term, "structural density" would be more appropriate when considering issues related to implant restoration.

Cortical bone may be "without marrow" but it is not "without a vasculature." The cortical layers of bone are densely calcified collagen composites with entrapped live cells *(osteocytes)*. These enclosed cells maintain contact with each other and outside nutritional sources through tiny cytoplasmic extensions within spider web like channels called *canaliculi*. (It should be remembered that the osteocyte functions physiologically in the homeostasis of Ca++ ions for the entire body.) There is a critical distance from the adjacent vasculature to these canaliculi beyond which these cells cannot survive (0.1–0.2 mm) (Ham 1965; Figure 3.9). The latter biologic necessity should be considered when reflecting upon the Branemark/Albrektson clinical findings of the need for at least 1.0 mm circumferential bone for a successful implant and the need to space

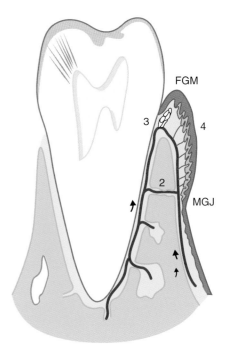

Figure 3.5 Normal dental/alveolar vascular supply. 1, Periosteal supply; 2, vessels from bone; 3, periodontal ligament supply to crest; 4, papillary loops; FGM, Free Gingival Margin; MGJ, Mucogingival Junction.

implants at least 6–7 mm on center especially in the anterior sites (See Figure 3.8).

The spatial position of teeth within the alveolar bone housing requires special consideration in this review because it influences the vascular distribution to and within the adjacent bone mass, especially the buccal aspect of the tooth socket wall. This in turn affects the reaction to periodontal disease, socket grafts, and bone requirements for implant placement. In most cases, the teeth are set toward the buccal limits of their confining bone "house," commonly referred to as the *alveolar bone*. This often results in a very thin, compact/cortical bone plate on the buccal (Figures 3.6b and 3.9), while the palatal often has a thicker wall with marrow between the socket wall and the palatal surface (See Figures 3.6 and 3.7). The vascular supply to these thin compact buccal plates is limited to diffusion externally from the investing buccal mucosal tissues and internally from the PDL. In the interproximal, lingual, and furcal areas, the internal marrow supply supplements the PDL and makes these areas less vulnerable to resorption after surgical interventions.

Additional Issues of Anatomic Interest: the Maxilla vs Mandible

The maxilla and mandible have major differences in their bony microarchitecture, and this is reflected in the pattern of their vascular supply. The maxilla is of lighter, thinner trabecular construction and interfaces with other cranial

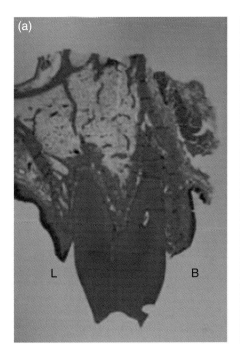
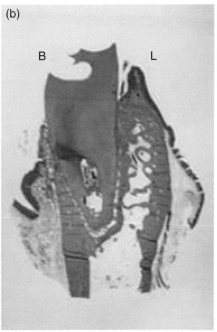

Figure 3.6 Internal microarchitecture. (a) Maxillary bicuspid. (b) Mandibular first bicuspid. Note different cortical and trabecular thicknesses. B, buccal area; L, lingual area.

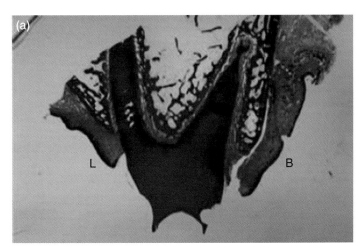
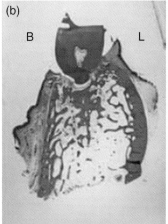

Figure 3.7 Internal microarchitecture of furcation area of first molars. (a) Maxillary first molar. (b) Mandibular first molar. Note differences in cortical and trabecular dimensions at maxillary versus mandibular sites. B, buccal area; L, lingual area.

structures of intramembranous origin with which it shares collateral vascular supplies. In the maxilla, as noted, the major blood supply to bone and teeth comes from the pterygopalatine division of the maxillary artery, the posterior superior alveolar. In the maxillary sinus, the blood flow also has contribution from the infraorbital and sphenopalatine arteries. A major arterial circuit formed from branches of the posterior superior alveolar and the infraorbital coursing from posterior to anterior around the buccal and medial walls of the sinus was reported by Solar et al. (1999). Of interest in performing the lateral window approach to the sinus lift bone graft, the buccal compo-

nent of this encircling anastomosis may be located vertically about 19 mm from the alveolar margin. It may be found within the marrow of the antral wall (if the wall is thick enough) or within the periosteal layer of the sinus lining immediately inside the wall (Figure 3.10). A third variation encountered by the author is illustrated in an ink perfused specimen (Figure 3.11). This latter variation is not always readily apparent on CT scans and may result in significant bleeding during sinus membrane elevation. The sphenopalatine artery also distributes along the lateral nasal wall which is paper thin bone separating the nose and the maxillary sinus (Rosano et al. 2009).

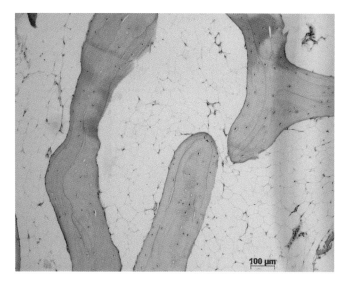

Figure 3.8 Mature resting alveolar bone from core in human maxillary first molar. Note fatty marrow, single layer liner cell layer over mineralized compartment and minimal vascular tissue. Light blue lines in mineralized areas are variously called cement lines, reversal lines, or resting lines and indicate past periods of remodeling.

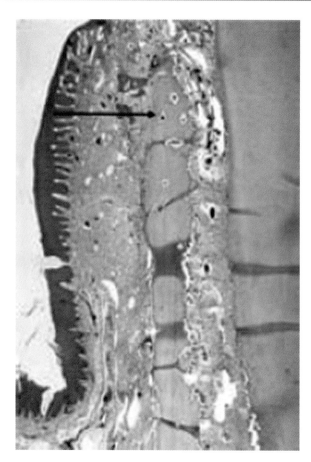

Figure 3.9 Small, India ink perfused vessels in very thin buccal plate (*arrow*). Note: Bone cells cannot live more than 0.1–0.2 mm from the blood supply. Note that resorption is proceeding from the periodontal ligament side of the thin buccal plate, which has had a full-thickness flap reflected and thus had a limited vascular response from the buccal. The surgeon should reflect on the possible effects of disrupting this exterior microanatomy when reflecting access flaps for implant placement and then disrupting the internal bone supply by drilling/extraction prior to placing an endosseous implant.

Because of the previously noted buccal displacement of the teeth within the alveolar housing the external surface of the maxillary alveolar bone is often sculpted with a variety of eminences and depressions. Of particular importance in the maxillary arch are the central incisal eminence and cuspid eminence and the adjacent fossae: the incisal fossa above the lateral incisor and cuspid fossa over the first bicuspid. If typical patterns of resorption occur (Caewood and Howell 1991) and this volume is not recreated by grafting, it forces implant placement to the lingual which in turn affects implant proximity especially in the truncated cone geometry of the maxillary anterior (Lee 2016).

The mandibular bone is a heavy, self-contained structure with a unique embryology (intramembraneous ossification using Meckel's cartilage and the inferior alveolar nerve for patterning). The condyle alone is endochondral in formation. Vascular supply is less diffuse than the maxillary, with one major vessel, the inferior alveolar, entering through a lingual foramen in the mandibular ramus and then spreading internally from within a dense mandibular canal located below the teeth within the basal bone. The flow is from the distal through the marrow, into the periapical and periodontal spaces and outward through the PDL and the mental foramen. Periosteal supplies nourish the external surfaces of the mandibular bone, but there are few interconnections from outside with flow into the bone, and minimal Volkman canal vessels running from inside out through the dense cortical plate. The mandibular lingual surface has the thinnest mucosal cover and thickest compact bone with minimal interconnection between marrow and its external, investing soft tissue (see Figures 3.6b and 3.7b). Interdental and furcal subdivisions of the alveolar bone have a rich marrow supply as noted in Figure 3.12. One deviation from this pattern is noted under lingual artery distribution to lingual of chin.

The buccal has a lesser "washboard effect" in the lower arch but the bucco-lingual thinness of the lower anterior and its resorption patterns post extraction (Caewood and Howell 1991) can lead to significant issues in implant planning. Additional planning constraints are presented by the major lingual concavities beneath the lower cuspid (sublingual gland) and beneath the lower molars (submandibular gland).

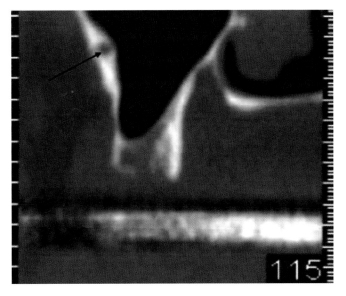

Figure 3.10 CT scan showing artery in buccal wall of sinus (*arrow*).

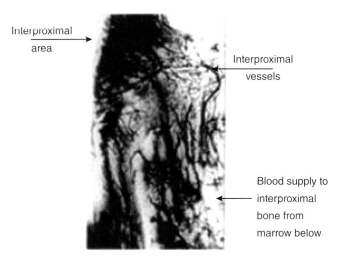

Interproximal area

Interproximal vessels

Blood supply to interproximal bone from marrow below

Figure 3.12 Partial-thickness flap at 14 days showing extensive arborization and density of vessels in interproximal papilla supplied by interdental arteries.

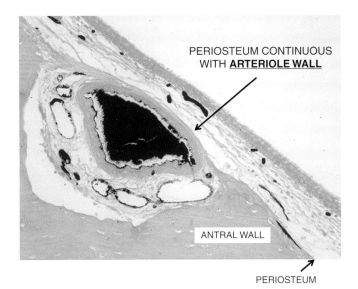

PERIOSTEUM CONTINUOUS WITH **ARTERIOLE WALL**

ANTRAL WALL

PERIOSTEUM

Figure 3.11 (Monkey) Arteriole wall merged with periosteum of antral wall venules surround arteriole. NOTE! sinus elevation hazard.

ANATOMY AND VASCULAR SUPPLY OF THE INVESTING SOFT CONNECTIVE TISSUES

The soft investing tissues of the alveolar/basal bone (the gingiva and mucosa) have internal structural variation, which influences vascular supply. There are three regional patterns to consider: the palatal tissues of the maxilla, the lingual covering of the mandibular teeth, and the buccal mucogingival tissues of both arches.

In the palatal area, the thick, dense collagenous lamina propria of the anterior and bicuspid areas has minimal submucosal thickness with a thin layer of fat content toward the bone. This palatal zone from distal of the cuspid

to mesial first molar is favored as donor site for free gingival grafts and connective tissue grafts. Starting at the mesial–palatal line angle of the first molar region, and moving to distal, the lamina propria layer thins and a thicker layer of submucosa with increased fat and glandular content lies beneath. The main vascular supply is from the greater palatine artery which emanates from the posterior palatine canal just apical to the second molar and courses forward within the submucosa, close to the bone (Figure 3.2). It distributes to the palatal glands and connective tissue stroma and ends with anastomosis to the incisive branch of the sphenopalatine artery at the incisal canal area. This arterial structure is sometimes severed when making deep vertical release incisions in the palatal of cuspid/first bicuspid region.

On the lingual of the mandibular teeth, the thin mucosal connective tissues reflect into the lingual vestibule with loose attachment to the mylohyoid muscle. The lingual artery, complemented by the mylohyoid artery and medial contributions from the submental branch of the facial distribute upward from below the mylohyoid to the muscles, lingual mucosa of the floor, sublingual, and submandibular glands. The mylohyoid nerves also distribute along the inferior surface of the mylohyoid having separated from the inferior alveolar nerve before it enters the mandibular foramen while the lingual nerve distributes above the mylohyoid but tracks to the midline at its distal edge. This lack of extensive vascular or nerve within this thin elastic tissue over the mylohyoid and below the tongue allows for detachment by blunt dissection which adds a few millimeters to tenting expansion over mandibular ridge grafts.

The buccal soft connective tissue over the alveolar bone of both arches is of greater interest from a number of surgical perspectives. As noted several times, the buccal soft

THICK SOFT TISSUE   THIN SOFT TISSUE

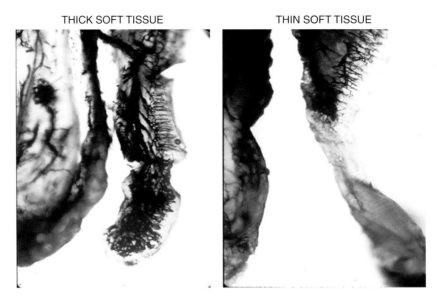

Figure 3.13 Disruption of vascular at mucogingival junction (MGJ) depends on biotype.

tissue is a major blood supply to the very thin cortical plates over the teeth, and therefore the influence of soft tissue biotype is more relevant to surgical disruption (Figure 3.13). This is probably related to Caewood's finding (1991) that the dominant pattern of bone loss after extraction occurs from the buccal (Figures 3.6 and 3.7). In the buccal marginal attached gingiva of both arches, there is no lamina propria. Densely woven collagen bundles are attached into the cementum (supracrestal) between teeth (interdental) and around teeth (circumferential) and apical to this into the underlying marginal bone (Sharpey's fibers) above the mucogingival junction (MGJ) (Figure 3.14).

This heavy fiber insertion into the marginal bone continues to the MGJ and is the "attachment" of the "attached gingiva" (Figure 3.14). The dense, compact structural arrangement of the fiber distribution perpendicular to the bone surface is interlaced with a fine capillary net fed by both the PDL net and a subepithelial plexus of vessels that flows just beneath the rete peg formation. The third source of vascular supply to these tissues is from larger vessels that branch from the thicker mucosal soft tissue corium just below the MGJ (Figures 3.5 and 3.15). The general pattern of external soft tissue flow is from the distal or (posterior) at a slight angle toward the anterior and from apical to coronal through the MGJ.

The arrangement and type of fibers in the periosteal layer of the mucosal zone is quite different. At the transition marked clinically by the MGJ, the dense, tight attachment of fibers through the periosteum of the attached gingiva (Figure 3.14) changes abruptly to a parallel layering of fibers over the bone surface with very little attachment to the bone interface (Figure 3.16). This change in attachment is readily noted during full thickness flap reflection where,

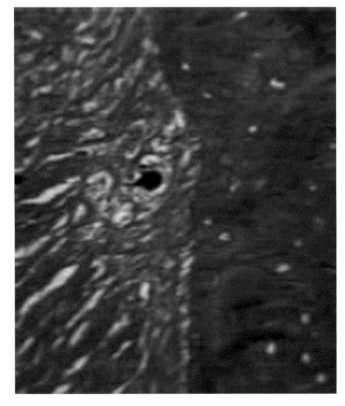

Figure 3.14 Periosteum in attached gingival zone: dense Sharpey's fiber insertion.

after detaching the more resistant tissues of the gingival zone, the remainder of the flap separates easily.

Between the periosteum of the mucosal tissues and the lamina propria in the buccal mucosal zone of both maxillary and mandibular arches there is a less dense submucosa of elastin, fibrillar collagen, and muscle fibers. The

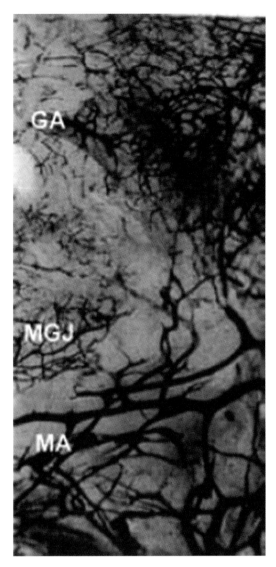

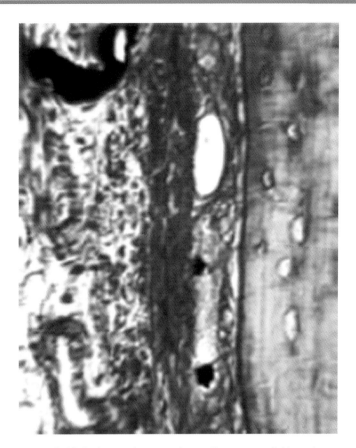

Figure 3.16 Periosteum in mucosal zone: fibers run parallel to surface. Bone surface to right side.

Figure 3.15 India ink perfused cleared specimen full-thickness flap at seven days (seen from the buccal). Note the differences in vessel size and complexity of mucosa (below) versus gingival (above). GA, gingival area; MGJ, mucogingival junction; MA, mucosal area. Compare the relationship of size and distribution to the microarchitecture of the soft tissues seen in Figures 3.14 and 3.16.

internal areolar structure of this submucosa allows for a larger vascular net in the mucosa including arterioles and large veins (Figures 3.15 and 3.17). The elasticity of this submucosal compartment allows for the technique of flap stretching or expansion over bone site augmentations by incision through the confining periosteum, apical to the MGJ, on the inner side of full thickness flaps made in these areas.

Scattered through this submucosal stromal matrix are active mesenchymal and inflammatory cells, which maintain and remodel the matrix; periosteal cells, which may have bone-repair potential; and the cells, platelets, and

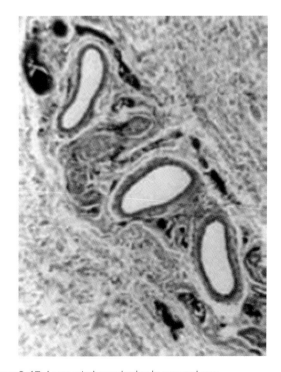

Figure 3.17 Large arteries and veins in mucosal area.

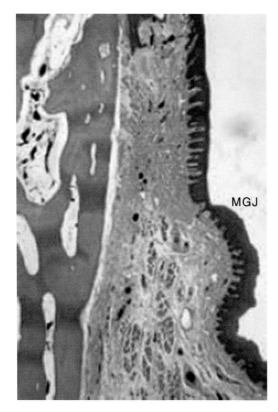

Figure 3.18 Mucogingival junction (MGJ) transition from dense to areolar base tissue.

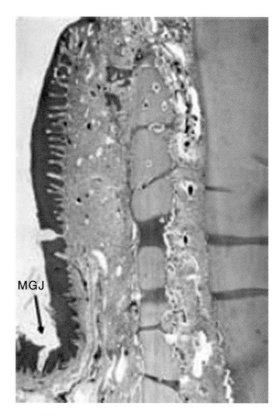

Figure 3.19 Mucogingival junction (MGJ).

soluble biomolecules contained within the vascular channels. As noted before, it is at the MGJ that compaction of the gingival collagen fiber density reaches its most extreme and constricts the corium blood supply most severely (Figures 3.5, 3.18, and 3.19). It should be noted again that the periosteum of the external bone surfaces in the mucosal zones receives nourishment through diffusion from the adjacent connective tissues but rarely from true Volkman canal vessel penetrations from inside the bone outward through the cortical layers (Figures 3.5, 3.7b, 3.20b, and 3.21).

As previously noted, the marginal gingiva of the teeth has several sources of blood flow (Figure 3.5): the PDL, the interdental, the subepithelial, and the deeper mucosal flow. The latter two sources, especially the central flow, become constricted at the MGJ, which is compressed like an hourglass from buccal to lingual and is further limited by the dense fiber arrangement in the gingival tissues (see Figures 3.5 and 3.14). The degree of confinement is influenced by the individual biotype or tissue thickness. In rhesus monkeys, it was observed that when the biotype was thin, there was usually only one artery (45–55 μm) through the MGJ, while in thicker tissue, the arteries were slightly smaller (35–45 μm) but there were more of them (Price 1974). Negotiation of this compact zone while performing a split or partial thickness flap dissection often presents a high level of risk for perforation or vascular embarrassment.

The latter can result in loss of the flap's gingival portion and subsequent bone exposure (see Figure 3.13). This can be reduced by dissection through a vertical from apical upward through the MGJ with a rolling motion toward the bone.

CEMENTUM

The cemental structure at the cemento-enamel junction (CEJ) level is acellular with a tight adhesion at its interface with the underlying dentine. While cellular cementum may persist at more apical layers, its contribution to wound healing is poorly understood. The cemental layer derives its maintenance from the surrounding PDL vessels and cells. Note the PDL net just below the cleared bone surface of buccal cortex in Figure 3.21 and the dense internet with the supracrestal tissue (Figure 3.12). Above the bone margin of the tooth socket, connective tissue fibers from the attached gingiva are embedded into the cemental surface. Below the bone crest, fibers bridge between the cementum and the alveolar socket wall as the principal structure of the PDL. There is no analogous structure for dental implants.

ANTATOMY AND VASCULAR SUPPLY OF THE EPITHELIAL STRUCTURES

Epithelial layers of the oral mucosa are connected by collagen to the underlying soft connective tissues, which in turn are connected to hard tissues such as bone and tooth

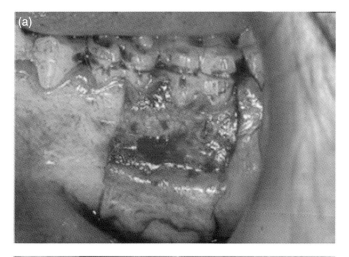

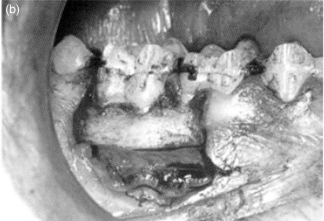

Figure 3.20 (a) Partial-thickness flap. (b) Full-thickness flap. No vessels are exiting bone surface.

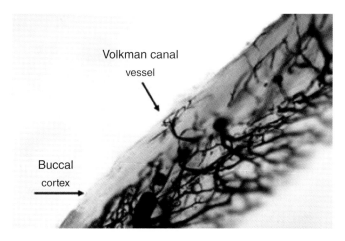

Volkman canal
vessel

Buccal
cortex

Figure 3.21 India ink–perfused specimen.

structure with a variety of collagen. The epithelial attachment is a unique exception to the continuous cover of the external surfaces and its reconnection to the tooth surface/implant abutment form the critical event in the wound-healing process after surgical procedures around teeth and implants. Re-establishment of this seal recreates the barrier between the internal/external environment and isolates/protects the hydrated environment of the vascular and lymphatics below.

At the tooth–enamel interface, the epithelial attachment allows a flow of sulcular or crevicular fluid outward which helps to maintain this dynamic seal around the penetration of the tooth through the body cover. Near the free gingival margin, the epithelial layers thicken into a heavy, multilayered keratinized surface that continues over the buccal and lingual surfaces on both sides of the mandible. At the MGJ, this heavy gingival keratin transitions to a thinner nonkeratinized or poorly keratinized mucosal surface. On the maxillary palatal surfaces, heavy keratin is present throughout and the epithelial enclosure is punctuated by salivary and sebaceous gland openings.

The bond of epithelial tissue to the varied underlying soft connective tissues or lamina propria is composed of a basement membrane of Type IV collagen that may have contributions from epithelium but has collagen loops integrating from the connective tissue side. Because there are no blood vessels penetrating into the epithelial layers, the only source of its nourishment is diffusion through this basement membrane from an extensive subepithelial plexus of capillaries interconnected with the mucosal corium at several levels and at the alveolar socket crest with the vascular net of the PDL (Figures 3.5, 3.12, 3.22–3.24).

Structural differences of the epithelial interface with a titanium implant substitute include an epithelial attachment with a circumferential collagen fiber zone apical to this. There is no supracrestal fiber attachment and vascularity mirrors mucosal supply pattern present below the MGJ (Berglundh et al. 1994).

THE WOUND-HEALING PROCESS

While the wound-healing process in periodontal surgery involves mechanisms common to other areas of the body, most notably, the skin, it has some unique features related to the presence of a tooth. Rates of activity may vary (turnover rate of alveolar bone versus basal bone) (Garant 2003), and microenvironments of local tissue architecture (attached gingiva, PDL, MGJ, etc.) may influence the local microvasculature (Price 1974), but the general pattern and sequence of healing activities seem to be the same as with skin healing. Because vascular disruption and regeneration are central to wound-healing response and we have seen how the microarchitecture of the tissue influences vascular patterns (compare Figures 3.14–3.16), we will review the two compartments – soft tissues of gingiva/mucosa and hard tissues of tooth/bone – separately. As noted in the preceding anatomy review, while there is some interconnection between hard and soft tissue supply at the

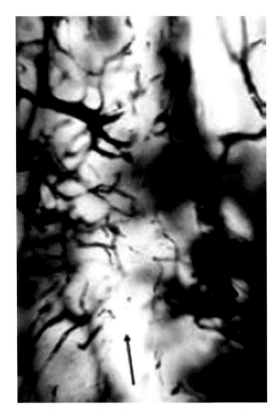

Figure 3.22 Capillary buds at four days begin to cross the incision line of flap (*arrow*).

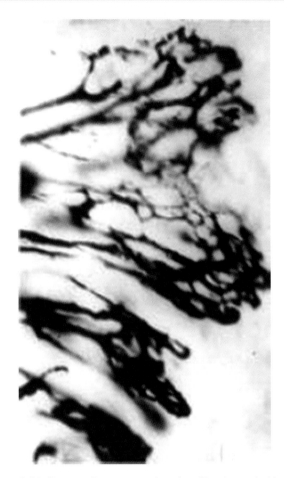

Figure 3.23 Fourteen days: regeneration of papillary loops. At this stage, newly forming connective tissue papillas are supplied by a web of expanded vessels.

gingival margin, the hard tissues receive their vascular supply separately from major arteries inside the bone, while the soft tissues are predominately supplied from outside the bone.

Closure of a soft tissue wound requires epithelialization, fibroplasia, and angiogenesis/vasculogenesis which occur simultaneously but at different rates during the early stages of healing. Immediately following an incision deep enough to injure the vasculature, platelets from within the blood vessels (normal range, 150 000–400 000/µl, produced by megakaryocytes in the bone marrow; Ganong 2001; Schmaier 2003) are exposed to perivascular collagen and begin to adhere to the wound margins. This adherence activates extrusion of granules from inside the platelets, some of which facilitate the transformation of prothrombin to thrombin, which in turn catalyzes soluble fibrinogen to fibrin.

The fibrin net enmeshed with increasing numbers of platelets, red blood cells, circulating polymorphonucleocytes (PMNs), and macrophages contributes to an initial vascular plug or clot, which slows and stops further bleeding. This temporary or provisional matrix of cells and fibers releases a variety of chemical attractants and activators (cytokines). Platelet-derived growth factor (PDGF), vascular endothelial growth factor (VEGF), and transforming growth factor (TGF-ß) stimulate the surrounding tissue

layers and attract more PMNs and macrophages from adjacent leaky venules (6–10 hours) (Clark 1996). The noncollagenous protein vitronectin, which is produced by the liver and circulates in the blood serum, possibly acts as a preliminary substrate for migration of these early scavenger cells.

Epithelial cells adjacent to the wound edge respond almost immediately to injury and begin to migrate across the fibrin clot surface at rates estimated to be 0.5 mm/day. Within 24 hours, adjacent epithelial cells, formerly quiescent, also begin to proliferate and migrate. Meanwhile, the PMNs within the clot begin to phagocytize bacteria, necrotic cells, and platelet debris. Resident macrophages are joined by monocytes migrating out of leaking vascular channels and begin to cleanse the wound of debris and broken degenerating PMNs (PMNs survive 24–48 hours) (Bartold et al. 1998; Garant 2003). At the same time, the macrophages release additional growth factors and cellular fibronectin, which, with fibrin, become the attachment surface for the subsequent wave of migrating cells – the fibroblasts, endothelial, and epithelial cells.

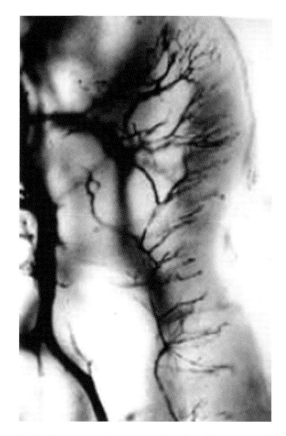

Figure 3.24 Twenty-one–day regeneration of papillary loops: At this stage, web has regressed to single long arching capillaries connected to base by newly forming subpapillary plexus.

The term *fibroplasia* embodies a sequence of shifting priorities within the fibroblast/fibrocyte cell population during which it undergoes several changes in phenotypic expression. Clark in 1993 and later in 1996 described several phases: proliferation, migration, production, and transformation to myofibroblast. The proliferation phase of fibroblasts occurs in the first two to three days in the margins of the wound. These early fibroblasts are said to have vitronectin adhesion capability but not fibronectin connectivity on their membrane surfaces. By days four to seven, the fibroblasts switch to a migrating mode and, aided by their adhesion to fibronectin (two sources: local made by macrophages and another in circulating plasma) and fibrin, invade the space formerly occupied by the provisional matrix. As they migrate, the fibroblasts deposit collagen and matrix molecules externally (Bartold et al. 1998; Clark 1993; Kurkinen et al. 1980).

Angiogenesis parallels this activity with venular endothelium proliferating in place for the first few days forming solid cords of cells. The cell layers thicken, and the outer layer lifts off, forming a space or lumen as the endothelial intracellular cementation breaks down, enabling a migratory phase. This activity at the ends of cut vessels results in an abundance of cord-like arrays and loops that by days

four to five have started to enter the clot space (see Figure 3.22). These early activities are clinically characterized by a red, granular appearance consistent with this rapid vessel and matrix formation – the *granulation tissue*.

This granulation tissue is gradually replaced by mature fibers, matrix, and reconnected blood vessels – the *organization phase*. Extracellular fluids that had previously leaked out into the wound area during the migratory phase are resorbed, and clinical swelling begins to resolve at five to six days. At 7 days, vessels can be found to be patent but leaky, while at 14 days although expanded, the leakage has stopped (see Figure 3.23). The new vascular net is mature by 21–28 days with gradual reduction of vessel size and vessel number and a regression to a regular distribution and flow in the new connective tissue (Price 1974) (compare Figures 3.23 and 3.24).

Collagens and various noncollagen molecules (hyaluron, elastin, fibronectin, etc.) are expressed into the matrix (days 4–10), and this in turn provides further traction and volume for migrating cells (Bartold et al. 1998). Meanwhile the migrating fibroblasts/fibrocytes gradually assume a new phenotype (myofibroblast), which has characteristics of muscle (Bucala et al. 1994; Clark 1996; Mori et al. 2005). The combination of traction and continued migration of these cells pulls the edges of the wound inward in the phenomenon of early wound contraction, which, with continued epithelial reproduction and migration, closes the wound surface to recreate the epithelial seal between internal and external environments (Clark 1996; Kurkinen et al. 1980).

While this contraction phenomenon accommodates closure of puncture wounds and incision closure where margins are replaced, there may be quite different results with more complex procedures such as a bone graft site augmentation. In these cases, underlying volume is expanded, and the release incisions noted in the section on soft connective tissues to allow expansion create two zones of contraction. The total contraction forces may pull the wound margins apart at 7–10 days if the external soft tissue edges of the opening incision were not approximated closely.

Healing in bone follows a different, delayed pathway. An exact chronology is only approximate. Injured bone areas show osteoclast activity as early as 7 days, which persists at 14 days and is coupled at 21 days by osteoblastic presence (Pfeiffer 1965). Osteoclast formation has been shown to be regulated by the RANK/RANK-L/OPG interaction with osteoblasts (Ganong 2001; Schmaier et al. 2003; Boyce and Xing 2007). Since vascular ingrowth always precedes osteogenesis (Albrektsson 1980a, 1980b) it would seem biologically consistent that osteogenesis would not start until the 2nd to 3rd week when vascular stability has occurred (Price 1974; Winet 1996).

Osteoblasts differentiate from mesenchymal precursor cells present within the marrow, from circulating precursor cells and possibly from pericytes around invading blood vessels. Vascular penetration in bone chambers has been demonstrated to move at different rates in cancellous bone (0.5 mm/day) versus cortical bone (0.05 mm/day) (Rhinelander 1974a, b; Winet 1996). With increasingly stable and maturing vascular and matrix formation, the coupled osteoblasts/osteoclasts initiate early clean-up and bone matrix deposition. The maturing collagen/noncollagen matrix then enters a phase where bone healing might begin (10–14 days). This critical period for bone formation at three to five weeks requires mechanical stability of the soft tissue margins.

Epithelial closure, which commences almost immediately because the basal layer is in continuous replacement, is well advanced by seven days. While the epithelial cover is mostly complete with matured layers by 21–28 days, soft connective tissue including its vasculature continues to mature for 35–42 days (5–6 weeks) (see Figures 3.22 through 3.24). Bone healing continues for six to eight weeks, at which time a rapidly formed woven (fibrous pattern seen in stained slides) bone is present. This is gradually remodeled in a slower process, which creates mature lamellar bone with its distinctive reversal/cement lines composed of noncollagenous proteins-ostepontin and bone sialoprotein. All of these events assume a stable environment with no re-injury or mobility of the site.

Intrabony healing after the controlled trauma of implant replacement or bone grafting, is a special situation that places increased demands on basic processes. The initial rates of activity remain the same but there are several secondary responses that need to occur for integration of either implant or graft particle. Mechanical stability of the implant and lack of re-injury is critical in the first four to five weeks of bone healing. In the case of graft particles, it is desirable that the nonvital graft eventually be replaced by new bone (Branemark et al. 1985) to complete the process of implant osseointegration. Observation made in human bone core samples show nonremodeled graft particles at 14–16 months. Observations made clinically suggest that broken or failing implants can be removed by reverse torque within the first year after placement. Subsequent to this first year, implant removal requires removal of integrated circumferential bone.

In the introduction we noted the desire to produce stable and predictable results. In most of our procedures the concept of grafting is inherent. In grafting the need for structural stability is necessary at every tissue level. Whether the grafted unit is a bioactive root form destined to support a dental restoration, a bioactive/biocompatible bone substitute (block or particulate) used to enhance bone volume, or a periodontal/peri-implant soft tissue substitute (gingival, connective tissue) used to stabilize esthetic or hygienic needs, the graft needs to be structurally stabilized to allow the native wound healing process to follow its predictable course.

In the case of the dental implant it was Branemark's flared cylinder stabilized with bicortical engagement which provided the model. In bone grafting the model is provided by a native sheltered space (elevated sinus, intact tooth socket) or Nyman's guided tissue regeneration (GTR) concepts. In the latter techniques an increased space volume can be created by combinations of selective permeable membranes supported with bone or bone substitutes, stabilized with fixation devices and then covered by expansion or stretching of soft tissues (released by blunt mylohyoid detachment or sharp dissection periosteal release) In the case of soft tissue grafts, thinning and fenestration of recipient beds followed by suture stabilization are the most common techniques.

It is hoped that this review of macro- and micro-anatomy followed by the sequence and timing of healing events in different tissue compartments will enhance the reader's ability to understand and perform these and future techniques on the infinite variation of conditions which present during the course of a surgical career. In many ways every case is an N of 1.

REFERENCES

Albrektsson, T. (1980a). The healing of autogenous bone graft after varying degrees of surgical trauma. *J. Bone Joint Surg.* 62B: 403–410.

Albrektsson, T. (1980b). Repair of bone graft. A vital microscopic and histological investigation in the rabbit. *Scand. J. Plast. Reconstr. Surg.* 14: 1–12.

Bartold, P.M. and Narayanan, A.S. (1998). Biology of the Periodontal Connective Tissues. 1. Auflage. Chicago: Quintessence Books.

Berglundh, T., Lindhe, J., Jonsson, K., and Ericsson, I. (1994). The topography of the vascular systems in the periodontal and peri-implant tissues in the dog. *J. Clin. Periodontol.* 21(3): 189–193.

Bernardi, S., Bianchi, S., Continenza, M.A., and Macchiarelli, G. (2017). Frequency and anatomical features of the mandibular lingual foramina: systematic review and meta-analysis. *Surg. Radiol. Anat.* 39: 1349–1357.

Boyce, B.F. and Xing, L. (2007). Biology of RANK, RANK-L, and OPG. *Arthritis Research and Therapy* 9 (suppl 1, S1).

Brånemark, P.I., Zarb, G.A., and Albrektsson, T. (1985). *Tissue-Integrated Prostheses*. Chicago: Quintessence.

Bucala, R., Spiegel, L.A., Chesney, J. et al. (1994). Circulating fibrocytes define a new leukocyte sub-population that mediates tissue repair. *Mol. Med.* 1: 71–81.

Caewood, J.I. and Howell, R.A. (1991). Reconstructive preprosthetic surgery. *Int. J. Oral Maxillofac. Surg.* 20: 75–82.

Clark, R.A.F. (1993). Regulation of fibroplasia in cutaneous wound repair. *Am. J. Med. Sci.* 306 (1): 42–48.

Clark, R.A.F. (1996). *The Molecular and Cellular Biology of Wound Repair*, 2e. New York: Kluwer Academic Publishers, Plenum Press.

Folke, L.E.A. and Stallard, R.E. (1965). Periodontal microcirculation as revealed by plastic microspheres. *J. Periosteal. Res.* 2: 53–63.

Folkman, J. and Klagsbrun, M. (1987). Angiogenic factors. *Science* 23: 442–448.

Ganong, W.F. (2001). *Review of Medical Physiology*, 20e. New York: Lange Medical Books/McGraw-Hill.

Garant, P.R. (2003). *Oral Cells and Tissues*. Chicago: Quintessence.

Ham, A.W. (1965). *Histology*, 5e. Philadelphia: J.B. Lippincott.

Kurkinen, M., Vaheri, A., Roberts, P.J., and Stenman, S. (1980). Sequential appearance of fibronectin and collagen in experimental granulation tissue. *Lab. Investig.* 43: 47–51.

Lee, W. (2016). Space analysis of the maxillary anterior bone geometry to understand anatomical limitation: an implant simulation study using Cone-Beam Computed Tomography (CBCT). MSD thesis. Boston University, Boston.

Lustig, J.P., London, D., Dor, B.L., and Yanko, R. (2003). Ultrasound identification and quantitative measurement of blood supply to the anterior part of the mandible. *Oral Surg. Oral Med. Oral Pathol. Oral Radiol. Endod.* 96: 625–629.

Mordenfeld, A., Andersson, L., and Bergström, B. (1997). Hemorrhage in the floor of the mouth during implant placement in the edentulous mandible: a case report. *JOMI* 12: 558–561.

Mori, L., Bellini, A., Stacey, M.A., Schmidt, M., and Mattoli, S. (2005). Fibrocytes contribute to myofibroblast population in wounded skin and originate from the bone marrow. *Exp. Cell Res.* 30: 81–90.

Pfeiffer, J.S. (1965). The growth of gingival tissue over denuded bone. *J. Periosteal.* 34 (10–16): 1965.

Price, A.M. (1974). Comparison of the microvascular disruption and regeneration following full, partial, and modified partial thickness flaps in the alveolar mucosa of Macaca mulatta. DScD thesis. Boston University, Boston.

Price, A.M., Nunn, M., Oppenheim, F.G., and Van Dyke, T.E. (2011). De novo bone formation after the sinus lift procedure. *J. Periodontol.* 82: 1245–1255.

Rhinelander, F.W. (1974a). The normal circulation of bone and its response to surgical intervention. *J. Biomed. Mater. Res.* 8: 87.

Rhinelander, F.W. (1974b). Tibial blood supply in relation to fracture healing. *Clin. Orthop.* 105: 34.

Rodan, H. (1981). The role of osteoblasts in hormonal control of bone resorption – a hypothesis. *Calcif. Tissue Int.* 33: 349–351.

Rosano, G., Taschieri, S., Gaudy, J.F., and Del Fabbro, M. (2009). Maxillary sinus vascularization: a cadaveric study. *J. Craniofac. Surg.* 20: 940–943.

Schmaier, A.H. and Petruzzelli, L.M. (2003). *Hematology for the Medical Student*. Philadelphia: Lippincott Williams and Wilkins.

Solar, P., Geyerhofer, U., Traxler, H. et al. (1999). Blood supply to the maxillary sinuses relevant to sinus floor elevation procedures. *Clin. Oral Imp. Res.* 10: 34–44.

Winet, H. (1996). The role of microvasculature in normal and perturbed bone healing as revealed by intravital microscopy. *Bone* 19 (Supplement 1): 39S–57S.

Woodburne, A.M. (1965). *Essentials of Human Anatomy*, 3e. New York: Oxford University Press.

Chapter 4 Piezocision™ Assisted Orthodontics in Everyday Practice

Serge Dibart, Elif Keser, and Donald Nelson

INTRODUCTION

What is Piezocision assisted orthodontics? A minimally invasive surgical procedure aimed to accelerate orthodontic tooth movement? A tool given to the orthodontist to control anchorage? A useful complement to treatment with clear aligners? A way to modify/strengthen a patient's thin biotype? Yes indeed, all of the above but further still…it is a way of seeing and treating cases differently. Piezocision has evolved from being initially a minimally invasive surgical alternative to conventional corticotomies to a more sophisticated "intellectual" approach to comprehensive orthodontic and lately multidisciplinary care. It is not just about speed anymore, it is about the possibility for the orthodontist to control selectively the anchorage value of teeth at will, potentially offering a means to successfully treating cases which until now were beyond the scope of conventional orthodontic mechanics. It is also about being an essential part of a multidisciplinary team, providing the necessary space or spacings between teeth for optimal implant placement or prosthetic rehabilitation. Piezocision can be used in a generalized, localized, or sequential manner (Dibart et al. 2015).

THE TECHNIQUE

For a full description of the technique I encourage you to read the chapter on Piezocision in "Practical Osseous Surgery in Periodontics and Implant Dentistry" (Dibart 2011). In brief, Piezocision is performed one week after the placement of orthodontic appliances (fixed or removable). A small vertical incision is made buccally and interproximally. This mid-level incision between the roots of the teeth will allow for the insertion of the piezoelectric knife. Piezocision has a localized and selective effect on the teeth, only the teeth or arch(es) to be moved need to be operated upon. The areas not surgerized have a higher anchorage value, since they are not affected by the demineralization process following Piezocision and can be used as such in the global treatment plan. The tip of the Piezotome (PZ1 insert, Satelec, Acteongroup, Merignac

France) is inserted in the gingival openings previously made and a 3mm deep piezoelectrical corticotomy is done (Figure 4.1). The decortication has to pass the cortical layer and reach the medullary bone to get the full effect of the regional acceleratory phenomenon (RAP). In the areas with thin or little gingiva (recessions) or with thin or no cortical buccal bone (dehiscences, fenestrations) hard and/or soft tissue grafts can be added via a tunneling procedure (Figures 4.2 and 4.3). The patient is seen every one or two weeks post surgery by the orthodontist in order to change aligners or activate wires and take advantage of the temporary demineralization phase created by Piezocision. This results in faster tooth movement and early completion of treatment (Charavet et al. 2016; Dibart et al. 2015) (Figures 4.4 and 4.5).

As mentioned earlier this technique does not have to be used for full orthodontic treatments only. It is versatile enough and it reduces orthodontic treatment time in such a drastic yet friendly manner that it is a great adjunct to multidisciplinary therapy. The patients and the dental team appreciate that allowing teeth to be put in their ideal place, via short orthodontics, prior to restorative procedures is actually beneficial to both parties as it allows for minimally invasive dentistry. Indeed crown preparations for veneers or crowns can be kept to a minimum while creating space for optimal volumes and esthetic outcome.

COMPUTER GUIDED PIEZOCISION ORTHODONTICS

This technique using a surgical guide was first developed and described by Milano et al. in 2014. This was meant as a security measure to avoid injuring the dental roots of the teeth undergoing Piezocision (Milano et al. 2014). Having taken a Cone Beam Computer Tomography, software is being used to place the Piezocision incision (Digital Surgery, S.R.L., Bologna, Italy). This is done in conjunction with the orthodontist as s/he is the one that decides which teeth or group of teeth will be moving. Only the teeth that

Practical Advanced Periodontal Surgery, Second Edition. Edited by Serge Dibart.
© 2020 John Wiley & Sons, Inc. Published 2020 by John Wiley & Sons, Inc.
Companion website: www.wiley.com/go/dibart/advanced

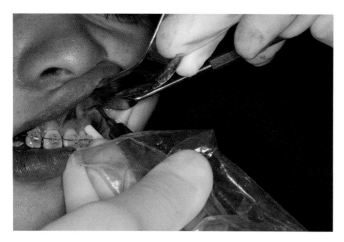

Figure 4.1 Piezocision is done interproximally, making sure to decorticate past the cortex into the medullary bone.

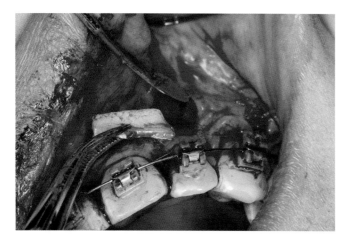

Figure 4.2 Once the interproximal decortication has been done, a tunneling procedure is done and a connective tissue graft is inserted to correct the mucogingival defect on tooth # 11. This is done during the Piezocision assisted orthodontics procedure in order to benefit from the enhanced healing potential coming from the RAP.

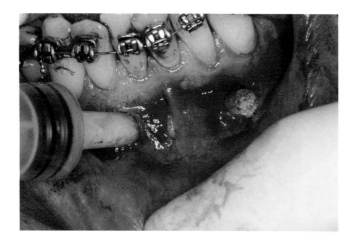

Figure 4.3 Bone grafting at time of Piezocision assisted orthodontics to strengthen or expand buccal alveolar bone.

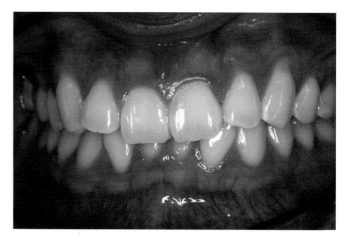

Figure 4.4 Prior to Piezocision assisted orthodontics.

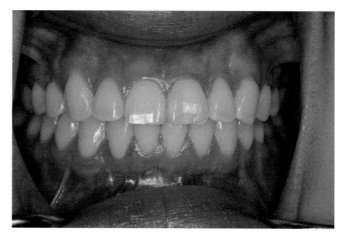

Figure 4.5 Twelve months after starting Piezocision assisted orthodontics. Notice how the recession on tooth # 11 has been treated (see Figure 4.2).

will be moving will get Piezocision (Figure 4.6). This will give the orthodontist the ability to "play" with the anchorage value of the teeth or group of teeth as the demineralization created by the Piezocision procedure is localized and bring a negative anchorage value to the teeth that are "piezocized." As a corollary to this the non piezocized teeth or group of teeth creates a positive anchorage that can be used strategically by the treating orthodontist.

Once the cuts are planned digitally, a digital guide is created (Digital Surgery, S.R.L., Bologna, Italy). Following the finalization of the digital guide (Figure 4.7), a surgical plastic guide is created using a chairside printer (Figure 4.8). The surgical guide is then placed in the mouth of the patient, and is checked for stability. Once that is done, the guide is removed and the patient anesthetized using infiltration anesthesia (Xylocaine 2% with 1/100,000 epinephrine). Following that incisions with a scalpel and blade are made, making sure to cut the periosteum though the

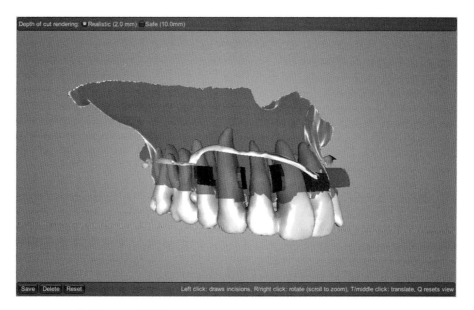

Figure 4.6 The incisions are planned digitally to avoid hitting the roots.

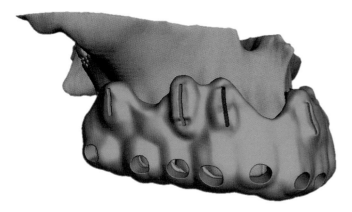

Figure 4.7 A surgical guide is being designed.

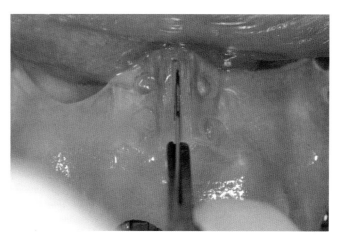

Figure 4.9 The minimal opening provided by the surgical guide allows for precise incisions avoiding the danger of root damage during Piezocision.

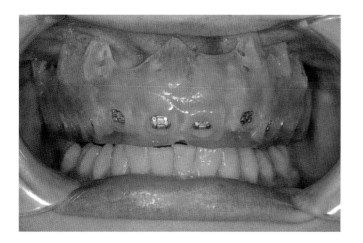

Figure 4.8 This is with the surgical guide in place.

openings (Figure 4.9). This is followed by the corticotomy using the piezotome (Dibart et al. 2009) (PZ1 insert, Acteon, Satelec group, Merignac, France). The surgical guide is then removed (Figure 4.10; Video 1).

DYNAMICALLY GUIDED PIEZOCISION

As technology evolves, we now have access to devices that allow us to do dynamically guided surgeries. Such a device is "Navident" (ClaroNav, Ontario, CA). Originally developed for dental implant surgery, Navident dynamically tracked the implant drill and the patient's jaw, providing real time guidance and visual feedback to ensure the implants were placed according to plan. We used this technology to place the Piezocision cuts and avoid

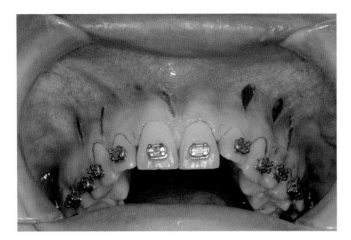

Figure 4.10 The Piezocision is done and the surgical stent is removed.

damaging the roots of the teeth. This allowed us, together with the use of the specific Piezocision inserts (PZ1, PZ2, and PZ3) to deliver the alveolar corticotomy exactly where planned and avoid root damage. One of the added advantages, beside the exquisite precision, is the alleviation of the cooling obstacle that can be represented by the surgical stent (Video 2).

PIEZOCISION ASSISTED ORTHODONTICS WITH CLEAR ALIGNERS

Piezocision can be used advantageously to help accelerate aligner change when patients are undergoing clear aligner orthodontics (Keser and Dibart 2011) (i.e. Invisalign™). Following Piezocision, the tray can be changed every week, every five days or even earlier depending on the orthodontic complexity of the case and the tooth movements. The superimposition of the Clincheck™ images (before and after) will dictate where the Piezocision cuts should take place. Teeth that are not moving should not be touched whereas the teeth that will be moving will receive the Piezocision cuts. The Clincheck superimposition serves as a "roadmap" to plan the surgical cut making the whole treatment planning quite simple for the surgeon.

Typically the patient comes to the surgical appointment one week after wearing the first tray. This will "condition" the cells in the periodontal ligament to respond quickly and extensively to Piezocision. The patient is anesthetized using infiltration anesthesia on the buccal side of the maxilla and/or mandible. The Piezocision cuts are done according to the superimposed Clincheck image. The patient wears the aligners immediately after the procedure and for a minimum of 22 hours per day or more depending on the orthodontist recommendations.

A 25 year old female presented with flared out upper incisors and multiple diastemas, complaining about her smile

(Figure 4.11). Her right posterior occlusion was Class I and left side Class II. The lower incisors were significantly extruded, impinging on the palate. Her main concern was the pushed out and spaced from teeth (Figure 4.12). Aesthetics was her main concern and she wanted to achieve the results very quickly, therefore she chose the treatment option that combined Invisalign with Piezocision. The Clincheck views show the amount of correction of the incisor positions and the amount of lower incisor intrusion that was planned. Figure 4.13 shows the superimposition from the Clincheck, demonstrating the amount of tooth movement that was planned for the upper jaw (blue initial, white final). After receiving the first Invisalign tray, Piezocision was done (Figure 4.14) and the patient started changing the aligners every five days (this was with the old Invisalign protocol where the recommended usage time was two weeks per tray).

At the end of her treatment the patient was very satisfied with her smile as the teeth had been retracted and the diastemas closed (Figures 4.15 and 4.16).

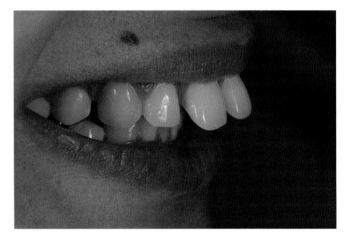

Figure 4.11 Flared anterior teeth and multiple diastemas. Patient unhappy with her smile.

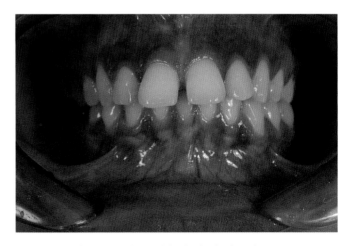

Figure 4.12 Lower anterior teeth impinging in the palate.

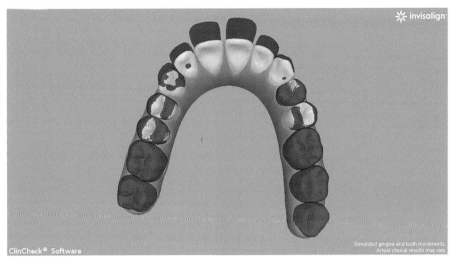

Figure 4.13 Super-imposed before and after Clincheck showing projected teeth movements for the maxilla. Piezocision will be done only around the white teeth as they are the only ones moving.

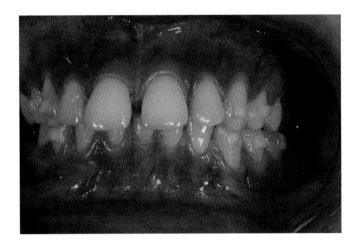

Figure 4.14 Piezocision on the maxilla and mandible is done after Clincheck analysis.

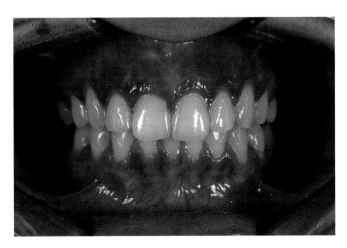

Figure 4.15 Finished treatment.

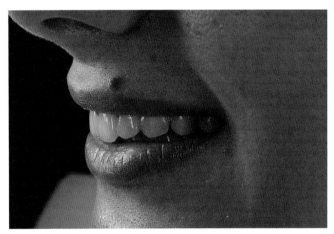

Figure 4.16 Patient has a better smile. The diastemas are closed and the teeth have been retracted to complement her profile.

INCORPORATING PIEZOCISION IN MULTIDISCIPLINARY TREATMENT

A 42 year old woman presented with a Class I malocclusion with anterior crowding. Her main concerns were the crowding and discoloration of her teeth as well as some white dental spots (Figures 4.17–4.19). She was very happy with her present profile and lip support, and did not want any change to the position of her lips. A multidisciplinary treatment plan was devised to address all of her concerns. The first stage of the treatment was the resolution of the maxillary and mandibular crowding and the retraction of the anterior upper teeth to create enough space for the minimally invasive Porcelain Laminate Veneers preparations. When conventional orthodontic therapy was initially suggested to the patient, some resistance was encountered because of the length of treatment. The patient also clearly stated that she

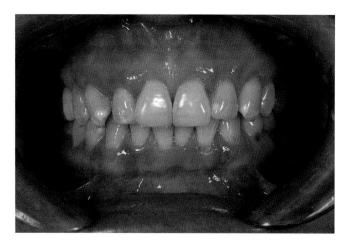

Figure 4.17 Forty two year old female patient intra oral view (notice the discoloration and white spots on the teeth).

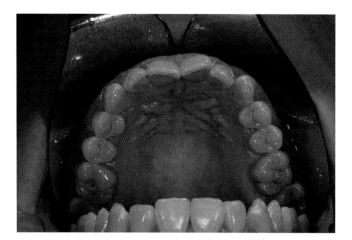

Figure 4.18 Occlusal view of maxilla showing mild crowding.

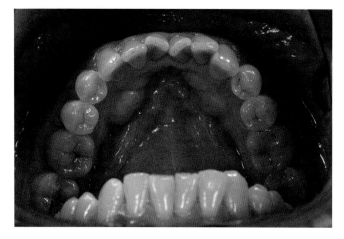

Figure 4.19 Occlusal view of mandible showing mild crowding.

would not wear "braces." An alternative treatment was offered using clear aligners and the issue of time spent in orthodontics was addressed by suggesting Piezocision assisted orthodontics. Piezocision has been shown to cut orthodontic treatment time by approximately half (Charavet et al. 2016; Dibart et al. 2014; Keser and Dibart 2011). Once the teeth were put in an optimal position after short orthodontics, the stage was set for the restorative team to address the problem of teeth discoloration and white spots via prepless/minimally invasive Porcelain Laminate Veneers (PVL). After resolving the crowding, the amount of anterior teeth retraction was limited to 0.5 mm which is approximately the thickness of the PLVs. By doing so, enough space was created to finish the case with minimal preps and without changing the lip support. After a week into wearing the first aligner, Piezocision was done (Figure 4.20). The patient wore the aligner immediately after the procedure and was asked to change her aligners every five days (this was at the time of the old Invisalign protocol when the recommended usage time was changing every two weeks, nowadays with the new Invisalign protocols one can change the aligners even sooner post Piezocision). At the end of her orthodontic treatment crowding was resolved and the anterior teeth had been "over retracted" by 0.5 mm to accommodate the thickness of the restorative material (Figures 4.21–4.23).

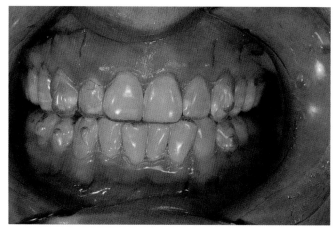

Figure 4.20 The patient wears the aligners after the Piezocision procedure.

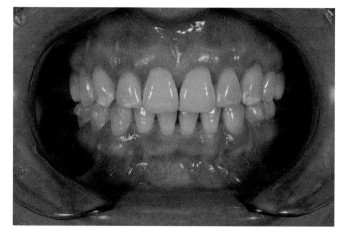

Figure 4.21 At the end of the orthodontic treatment. Treatment time was cut by approximately half after Piezocision.

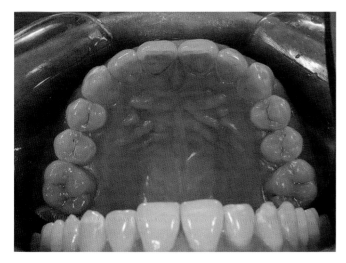

Figure 4.22 Occlusal view of maxilla post treatment.

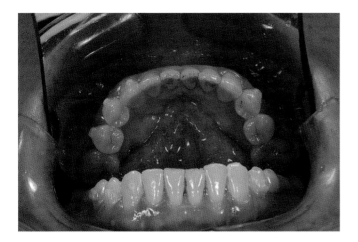

Figure 4.23 Occlusal view of the mandible post treatment.

The patient was then sent to the restorative dentist who pre-pared the teeth for the porcelain veneers (Figures 4.24 and 4.25). Her total treatment time including the restorative work was six months (Figure 4.26). Placing the teeth to be restored in an ideal position prior to prosthetic work using orthodontics allows for the practice of Minimally Invasive dentistry which is most beneficial for the patient.

POST-OPERATIVE CARE

Patients are usually given a short course of analgesic drugs (acetaminophen or ibuprofen). Usually a three days supply will suffice.

Antibiotics are given at the discretion of the operating surgeon.

Chlorhexidine rinses are prescribed twice a day for five days.

Ice packs are given to the patient immediately post sur-gery to control inflammation.

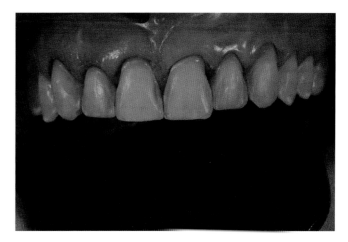

Figure 4.24 The patient is ready to see the restorative specialist for veneer preparations. Because of the use of orthodontics the teeth are in an ideal anatomical position and the removal of tooth structure is kept to a minimum (Prosthetics: Dr. Galip Gurel).

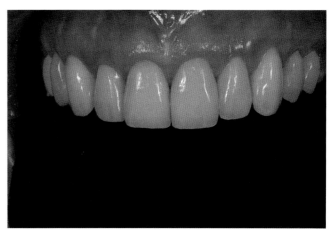

Figure 4.25 Final restoration in place: porcelain laminate veneers (Prosthetics Dr. Galip Gurel).

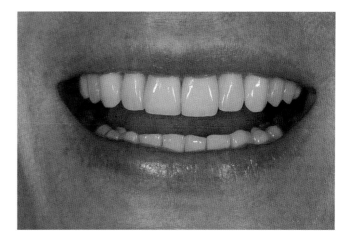

Figure 4.26 The esthetic and functional concerns of the patient have been addressed successfully in a time efficient manner (Prosthetics: Dr. Galip Gurel).

CONTRAINDICATIONS FOR PIEZOCISION

1. Patients on anything that affects bone physiology (i.e. Biphosphonates)

2. Medically compromised patients (specifically bone pathology)

3. Patients on long term anti-inflammatory drugs

4. Untreated periodontal diseases

5. Ankylosed teeth

6. Noncompliant patients

7. Patients/operator with a pacemaker or any other active implants

POTENTIAL COMPLICATIONS

- Root injury
- Infection
- Mucogingival defects

REFERENCES

Charavet, C., Lecloux, G., Bruwier, A. et al. (2016 Aug). Localized piezoelectric alveolar decortication for orthodontic treatment in adults: a randomized controlled trial. *J. Dent. Res.* 95 (9): 1003–1009.

Dibart, S. (2011). Piezocision: minimally invasive periodontally accelerated orthodontic tooth movement procedure. In: *Practical Osseous Surgery in Periodontics and Implant Dentistry* (eds. S. Dibart and J.-P. Dibart). Wiley Publishing.

Dibart, S., Sebaoun, J.D., and Surmenian, J. (2009 Jul-Aug). Piezocision: a minimally invasive, periodontally accelerated orthodontic tooth movement procedure. *Compend. Contin. Educ. Dent.* 30 (6): 342–344.

Dibart, S., Yee, C., Surmenian, J. et al. (2014 Aug). Tissue response during Piezocision-assisted tooth movement: a histological study in rats. *Eur. J. Orthod.* 36 (4): 457–464.

Dibart, S., Keser, E., and Nelson, D. (2015). Piezocision™ assisted orthodontics: past, present and future. *Semin. Orthod.* 21: 170–175.

Keser, E.I. and Dibart, S. (2011 Mar). Piezocision-assisted invisalign treatment. *Compend. Contin. Educ. Dent.* 32 (2): 46–48.

Milano, F., Dibart, S., Montesani, L., and Guerra, L. (2014 Jul-Aug). Computer-guided surgery using the piezocision technique. *Int. J. Periodontics Restorative Dent.* 34 (4): 523–529.

Chapter 5 The Contribution of Periodontics to Endodontic Therapy: The Surgical Management of Periradicular Periodontitis

Mani Moulazadeh

HISTORY AND EVOLUTION

Over the past century, surgical endodontics has been performed for treatment and conservation of teeth with persistent post endodontic treatment infections.

In 1964, with the formation of the American Association of Endodontists and establishment of endodontics as a dental specialty, surgical endodontics began to take on a new face. Early on, much emphasis was placed on development of a root-end filling material that would provide a hermetic seal.

While magnification and the use of a microscope for operations date back to the early 1920s, it was not until 1984 that it was used in conjunction with an apical surgery (Reuben and Apotheker 1984). With the addition of the surgical operating microscope (SOM) to the armamentarium, the technique and outcome for apical surgeries became more conservative and predictable. After all, one cannot treat what one cannot see, and with the magnification of up to ×30 and illumination of up to ×12 with the dental overhead light, the SOM can reveal details previously unseen to the surgeon. The use of the SOM has become the standard of care in all endodontic procedures, and since 1998, all postgraduate programs in endodontics in the United States are required to train their residents to perform procedures under the SOM. As a result, instruments have been either newly designed or modified by scaling them down to a fraction of their original size to be used with the SOM. Ultrasonic tips and micromirrors were developed in the mid-1980s for the purpose of retropreparation and inspection under the SOM. Along with the introduction of new root-end filling material such as ProRoot mineral trioxide aggregate (MTA; Dentsply Tulsa Dental, Tulsa, OK, USA), the art of endodontic surgery has shifted toward endodontic microsurgery and has reached new heights in its levels of precision, predictability, and success.

Today, microsurgical endodontics is considered to be the standard of care. With the advent of SOM, microinstruments,

superior retrofilling material, and more advanced hard and soft tissue management techniques, procedures are more conservative, and outcomes have become more successful. Smaller osteotomy windows are made to conserve cortical bone. Root resection with shorter or no bevel angles, previously impossible due to lack of ultrasonic tips, are now feasible and conserve more root structure in order to preserve a more favorable crown-to-root ratio. The SOM allows for locating and treating isthmuses and extra portals of exit along the root's long axis, ensuring a proper orientation and depth for the placement of a root-end filling. It also enables the surgeon to check for marginal integrity of the apical seal once it is placed. This prevents leaving avenues for leakage, which will prevent the formation of an impermeable seal and may ultimately result in treatment failure. Rubinstein and Kim (1999, 2002) reported the short-term (one year) and long-term (five to seven years) success rates for endodontic microsurgery to be 96.8 and 91.5%, respectively. These results are rather impressive considering that about 60% of the surgeries were performed on premolars or molars.

TOOTH CONSERVATION VERSUS IMPLANTS

With the recent implant paradigm shift in dentistry, some clinicians have made claims as to suggest the placement of immediate load implants is a more logical treatment over treatment of the teeth via endodontics (Ruskin et al. 2005). As clinicians, we must not be easily affected or swept away by advertisements or reading one such article. Rather, our decisions for selecting treatment plans, modalities, and techniques should be made on an evidence-based approach to dentistry and its specialties. Many have attempted to overplay the success of dental implants over nonsurgical and surgical endodontic therapy. However, in a systematic review of the literature (M.K. Iqbal and S. Kim, unpublished data) there were no significant differences between root canal therapy success rates and implants. In fact, comparing the "success" rates of endodontics and implants is sometimes beyond the scope of comparing apples and oranges.

Practical Advanced Periodontal Surgery, Second Edition. Edited by Serge Dibart.
© 2020 John Wiley & Sons, Inc. Published 2020 by John Wiley & Sons, Inc.
Companion website: www.wiley.com/go/dibart/advanced

Endodontically treated teeth are evaluated for success on the basis of clinical and radiographic criteria. An endodontically treated tooth that is asymptomatic while in function and displays no periapical radiolucency is classified as a successful treatment. Implants are often evaluated for their "success" based on their survival rate. This disparity in the evaluation criteria between endodontics and implants immediately changes the "level ground" for comparison. In addition, implant studies often exclude patients who have underlying systemic diseases such as diabetes, smokers, and patients with poor oral hygiene. In certain studies peri-implantitis was not regarded as a criterion for implant failure. Also, at least presently, most implants in these studies are being placed by trained specialists.

Meanwhile, the success of endodontic therapy as evaluated by studies did not abide to the same strict patient exclusion criteria as did the implant studies. Persistent radiographic demineralization was considered to be a sign of failure. Last, the success rate of endodontic therapy as reported by such studies as the Toronto Study is based on treatments performed by dental students, general dentists, and endodontists. In 1999, the American Dental Association reported that only 25% of all endodontic cases were being performed by endodontists (ADA Report 1999).

It is clear that implants have changed the face of dentistry and the way we treatment plan restoring edentulous spaces. They are a great adjunct when treatment is planned properly and when bone quality and esthetics allow for their placement. Implants are clearly not an alternative for periodontally sound and endodontically treatable (nonsurgical or surgical) teeth. Retaining our patients' healthy natural dentition should be our main priority as healthcare providers.

TREATMENT OF FAILED ROOT CANAL THERAPY

When the initial root canal therapy has resulted in a negative outcome, two revisions are possible:

- Nonsurgical retreatment aimed to eliminate bacteria from the canal

- Surgical retreatment aimed to encapsulate bacteria inside the canal

The decision as to which approach to take should be based on the level of evidence and other criteria such as the dentist's training and experience, availability of the necessary armamentarium, and the patient's decision based on informed consent.

Historically, nonsurgical retreatment has enjoyed a higher success rate than the surgical approach. Studies also support that in the event of a surgical approach, prior nonsurgical retreatment will increase the chance of a positive outcome (Zuolo et al. 2000). Therefore, unless nonsurgical retreatment is not feasible due to physical, anatomical, time, or financial hardships, surgical endodontics should not be considered as the treatment of choice.

RATIONALE FOR ENDODONTIC SURGERY

Periapical surgery is performed to eradicate persistent infection/inflammation associated with teeth with previously negative post-treatment outcome from either initial endodontic therapy or retreatment. With advancement in microsurgical endodontics, surgery should not be labeled as a last option, but it should be performed when either initial endodontic treatment or retreatment is not possible or feasibly cannot secure a better outcome. Factors such as inability to properly access the root canal system in order to adequately clean, shape, and obtain an apical seal may warrant surgery as the treatment of choice. The ability of the clinician to properly diagnose which case is suitable for surgery is as important as his or her clinical skills. It was Dr. Irving J. Naidorf who said, "A good surgeon knows how to cut, and an excellent surgeon knows when to cut" (Kim 2002).

INDICATIONS FOR ENDODONTIC SURGERY

Anatomical Challenges

In certain cases, the tooth anatomy renders itself unwilling to proper debridement and obturation, leaving a portion of canal untreated by nonsurgical methods. Teeth with canal blockages due to severe calcification or with severe radicular curvatures fall under such category.

Also, in a few cases when endodontic therapy is performed at a clinically acceptable level, symptoms may continue to persist when the apex of the root may be fenestrating through the facial cortical plate of bone. In these cases, a small surgical procedure to recontour the root end and align it within its bony housing may solve the problem.

Iatrogenic Factors

Previous endodontic "misadventures" account for the need for surgery in cases with persistent symptoms. These include but are not limited to canal blockages, ledges, perforations, separated instruments or posts, underfilled canals, and canals with dental material extruding beyond the biologically tolerant buffer zone around the anatomical apex (Figures 5.1–5.3).

In most of these cases, proper canal debridement is compromised as is the ability to properly obturate the canal and obtain a proper apical seal.

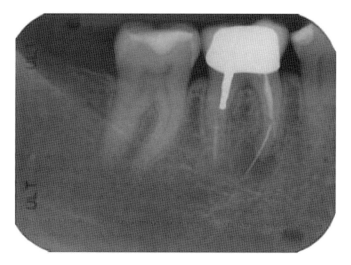

Figure 5.1 Persistent inflammation associated with the mesial root of a mandibular molar with a separated instrument.

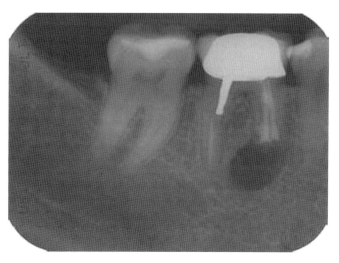

Figure 5.3 Instrument recovery, root resection, and retrograde obturation with MTA.

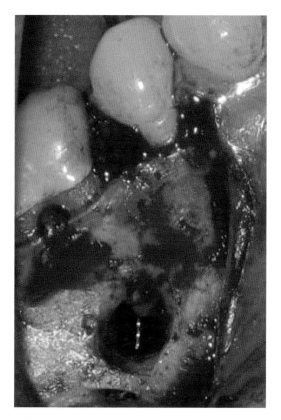

Figure 5.2 Surgery reveals a hand file extending 3–4 mm beyond the root tip.

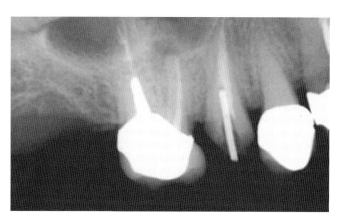

Figure 5.4 Persistent inflammation and symptoms associated with the mesial root of a maxillary molar due to the missed MB-2 canal.

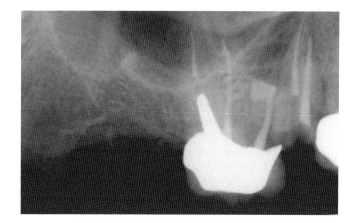

Figure 5.5 Apicoectomy performed in conjunction with finding and obturation of the additional canal and the isthmus between MB-1 and MB-2 canals.

Relentless Inflammation

Previously missed and untreated canals, bifurcations, fins, and extraradicular infections often harbor bacteria and present themselves as chronically and intermittently symptomatic teeth. Apical surgery can be performed to eradicate such factors (Figures 5.4–5.6).

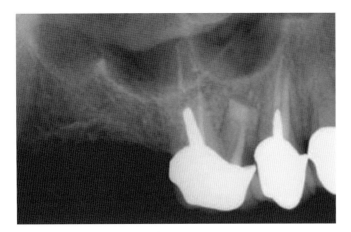

Figure 5.6 A four-year follow-up shows complete healing.

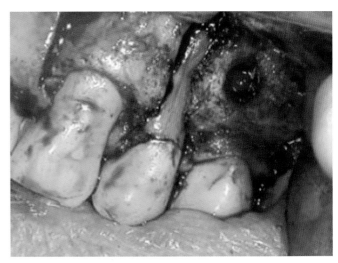

Figure 5.8 An exploratory surgery and staining reveal a vertical root fracture.

CONTRAINDICATIONS FOR ENDODONTIC SURGERY

Medical History

Patients with recent myocardial infarction, with uncontrolled diabetes, patients who are undergoing anticoagulant therapy, patients who received head and neck radiation, or patients with severe neutropenia are not good candidates for surgery. Surgery should be postponed until they are cleared by their treating physician.

Compromised Periodontium

Periodontal pockets and tooth mobility reduce the success of endodontic surgery. High success rates in endodontic microsurgery was achieved in studies where the prospective teeth did not exhibit any pathologic periodontal pocketing or pocketing that either communicated with the apical endodontic component or had completely denuded the buccal or lingual cortical plate of bone resulting in a dehiscence (Rubinstein and Kim 1999).

Skill, Knowledge, and Proper Instruments

General practitioners must be knowledgeable to properly diagnose and refer patients with surgical needs to surgeons who have the specialized training in diagnosing and treating these cases.

Although the skill levels of the surgeons should theoretically be the same, in reality this may not be the case. A study reviewed the outcome of treatment in the oral surgical and endodontics departments of a teaching hospital four years following surgery. Complete healing for cases performed by the endodontic unit was nearly twice as high for those performed in the oral surgery unit.

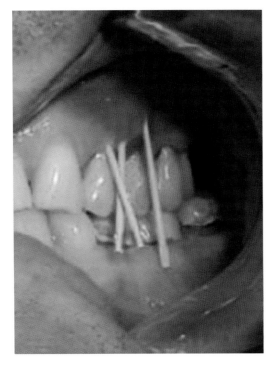

Figure 5.7 Multiple sinus tracts trace to the location of the endodontic lesion.

Exploratory Surgery

In certain cases, it may be difficult to properly diagnose a problem. In cases of root fractures, for example, a small soft tissue flap followed by dying the area in question with methylene blue and inspection under the SOM can quickly reveal a root fracture, which can then prevent unnecessary endodontic treatment to be performed on a nonrestorable tooth (Figures 5.7 and 5.8).

Also, collection of a biopsy specimen may be another indication for performing an exploratory surgery.

The single most important contributing factor was the quality of the procedure, which in turn translated into the surgeon's skill and perhaps level of training and understanding of the problem at hand (Rahbaran et al. 2001).

Despite the surgeon's highest level of clinical competence, proper instrumentation is required for achieving the highest level of technical excellence. It may sound anecdotal, but it is impractical for a world class skier to win any race while skiing on tennis rackets!

Finally, surgeons must keep the welfare of the patient in mind at all times. Case selection for surgery is very important, and indiscriminant use of surgeries to treat endodontic problems is discouraged. Remember, just because you can, does not mean you should (Figures 5.9 and 5.10).

Anatomical Challenges

Proximity to the maxillary sinus, mental nerve, and inferior alveolar canal and the thickness of the buccal bone in the mandibular second molar area due to the external oblique ridge may serve as a contraindication or deterrent for surgery. As long as a properly trained clinician is aware of such hurdles and conceivably knows how to work around them and manage mid-procedure and post-procedure

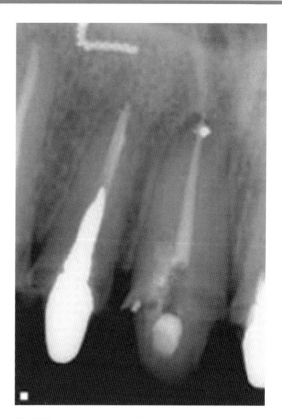

Figure 5.10 Nonsurgical root canal treatment was performed with the aid of the SOM. The tooth was free of symptoms thereafter.

potential complications, these factors may be downgraded to potential risks or contraindications. Extra caution or modifications in the procedure may be required in order to avoid damage to such structures.

As an example, the roots of many maxillary molars and premolars are separated from the maxillary sinus by a thin layer of cortical bone and the Schneiderian membrane. Care must be taken not to violate this space. However, in the event that the sinus is inadvertently perforated, with proper care, the membrane usually heals uneventfully, without any negative effect on the outcome of the apical surgery (Figure 5.11).

Inadequate Root Length

As a critical part of thorough treatment planning, the length of the root before surgery must be estimated. This will allow the clinician to have an understanding whether a favorable crown to root ratio is achievable once the root is resected. If the length of the root after resection is conceived to be inadequate, this may be ground for aborting the surgical procedure and looking for an alternative plan. Although, in select cases where the patient is free of periodontal disease, parafunctional habits, and malocclusion, teeth have been known to survive with as low as 1 : 1 crown-to-root ratio (Figures 5.12–5.14).

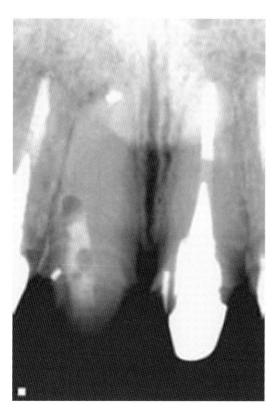

Figure 5.9 Apicoectomy was performed on a "calcified" central incisor without treating the tooth by nonsurgical root canal therapy first.

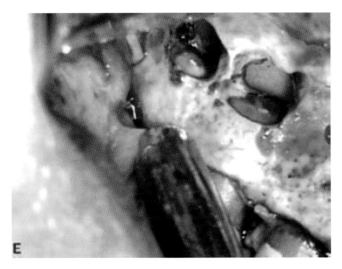

Figure 5.11 Osteotomy and stained resected root ends of a maxillary molar. Note the maxillary sinus and its lining deep to the root tips.

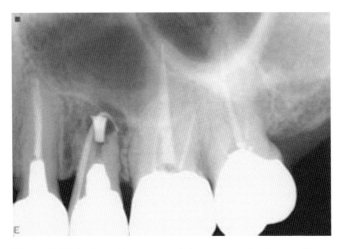

Figure 5.12 Failing apicoectomy and sinus tract tracing in a maxillary second premolar.

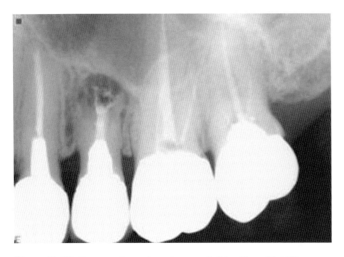

Figure 5.13 Conservative apicoectomy and obturation with MTA was performed despite the unfavorable crown-to-root ratio.

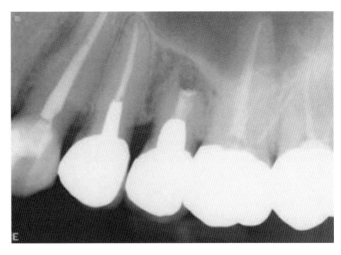

Figure 5.14 Five-year recall revealed complete healing with no signs of the sinus tract or presence of mobility.

TYPES OF ENDODONTIC SURGERY

Incision and Drainage

Incision and drainage is used for treating necrotic teeth with acute apical abscess. After primary drainage through the tooth is established by performing a pulpectomy, a small incision is made at the base of the fluctuant swelling. Blunt dissection with a curved hemostat facing the bone plate is carried out to dissect tissue planes and establish further drainage. A drain must be placed for up to 48 hours to prevent wound closure. Keeping the incision site open will ensure continuous drainage and patient comfort by allowing the pressure to be relieved (Figure 5.15).

In addition, by allowing oxygen to gain access to the site of infection, the anaerobic bacteria are killed, the balance of bacteria colony is disrupted, and the rate of healing may be accelerated.

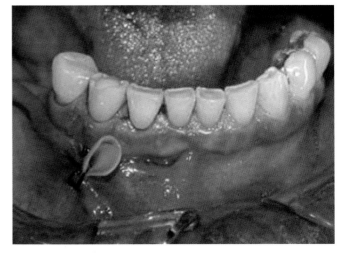

Figure 5.15 Incision and drainage of an intraoral abscess. Note the latex drain was sutured to prevent its premature removal.

Root Amputation and Hemisection

Root amputation and hemisection involve surgical removal and surgical division of roots of multirooted teeth. Although once performed more frequently, with the increased prevalence of dental implants, the frequency is declining. It is preferred that if a tooth is treatment planned for either of these two procedures, the root canal treatment is performed before the surgical phase. It should be noted that with proper case selection, both procedures are viable options for maintaining the natural teeth. As prudent dentists, we must subdue our urges to perform "herodontics" at all cost in order to maintain a tooth in the oral cavity. Teeth that may serve as strategic abutments, exhibit advanced periodontitis or nonrestorable remaining segment, and have fused roots or very low furcations are not good candidates for these types of surgery.

Intentional Replantation

As defined by Dr. Grossman, replantation is "the purposeful removal of a tooth and its almost immediate replacement with the object of obturating the canals apically while the tooth is out of its socket" (Kim et al. 2001a). Intentional replantation is an artificial setting mimicking complete tooth avulsion, and its management as defined by the guidelines of the American Association of Endodontists. However, the circumstancing factors are near ideal. The level of tooth contamination and physical damage is likely to be far less than in the case of an accidental injury. Moreover, the single most important factor in the demise of an avulsed tooth, the extraoral dry time, is not a factor because it is practically nonexistent. During intentional replantation, the tooth is immediately submerged in tissue culture medium, with the tooth out-of-socket times being under 10 minutes.

The procedure dates back to the late 1500s, when Paré replanted three avulsed teeth (Kupfer et al. 1952). Intentional replantation has been performed for over half a century with success rates being reported between 80 and 95% for follow-ups of 2–22 years by Grossman, Kingsbury, and Bender (Kim et al. 2001b). Although many of these teeth exhibited some degree of ankylosis and replacement resorption, they were clinically functional and did not exhibit any signs of periradicular pathosis. With the development of new protocols that call for the use of Hanks balanced salt solution (HBSS) (BioWhittaker, Walkersville, MD, USA) as an intermediate storage and operating medium, and the use of enamel matrix derived protein (Emdogain; Straumann, Waldenburg, Switzerland) along with careful extraction techniques to prevent damage to the cementum and the PDL cells, the chances of resorption can be minimized.

Indications and Case Selection

Intentional replantation should not be the treatment of choice if endodontic retreatment or surgery can be performed with a foreseeable positive outcome. Intentional replantation may be considered to be the treatment of choice for treatment of cases where surgical access to the site is impractical or impossible. Teeth with root perforations in mesial, distal, or furcal regions are great candidates. Teeth with expected elaborate apical anatomy and portals of exit or teeth where the apices are lying deep within the jaw bone and where surgical access is difficult are also good candidates.

Case selection in intentional replantation plays a big role in the success of the treatment. Teeth with conical fused roots are generally good candidates because of their ease of extraction. On the other hand, teeth with periodontal involvement, thick interseptal bone, or dilacerated roots are contraindicated for intentional replantation.

Surgical Technique

After proper case selection and review of the medical history, local anesthesia is administered via block and local infiltration to properly anesthetize the patient. The patient should start to rinse with 10 ml of 0.12% chlorohexidine gluconate twice daily 24 hours before the surgery and continue this regimen for one week following the procedure. Although somewhat of a controversy, some advocate the administration of prophylactic antibiotics 24 hours before and for one week after the procedure. It is also recommended that unless the patient is allergic to NSAIDs, the maximum daily dose of a drug such as ibuprofen should be prescribed and taken 24 hours before and for one week after the procedure. Once the patient is seated and anesthetized, it is crucial to make sure that every step of the procedure is well thought out and ready to be executed. Organization translates into minimized out-of-socket time (less than 10 minutes) and, in turn, maximizes the potential for a successful outcome. After administration of local anesthesia, the tooth can be prepared by working a periotome circumferentially into the gingival sulcus to dissect the fibers. Great care must be taken not to scrape the cementum covering the root surface. Luxation with universal forceps placed only on the anatomical crown is followed. At no time should the beaks of the forceps be making contact with any portion of the tooth apical to the CEJ (cemento-enamel junction) (Figures 5.16 and 5.17).

The use of elevators is contraindicated. It is critical to be extra cautious during this step of the procedure, as a careful and minimally traumatic extraction could be the rate determining step for the outcome. It is not unusual to take as long as 15 minutes to have the tooth fully avulsed. Forcing the extraction could ultimately fracture the tooth or the alveolus and cause its demise. Once the tooth is extracted, the crown may be firmly wrapped with sterile gauze and grabbed tightly with a locking hemostat. Curettage of the socket is not recommended. Making contact with the root

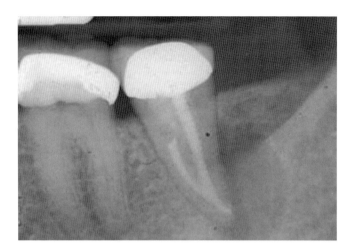

Figure 5.16 Mandibular second molar exhibiting persistent radiolucency even after nonsurgical retreatment.

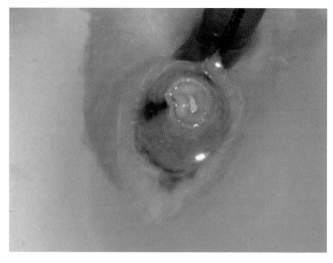

Figure 5.18 Tooth wrapped in sterile gauze and submerged in HBSS. Root resection was carried out by an Impact air 45 high-speed handpiece.

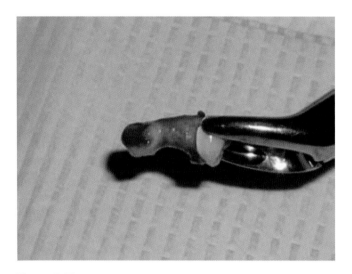

Figure 5.17 Tooth extraction without placing the forceps on root structure. Note the lesion attached at the root's apical third.

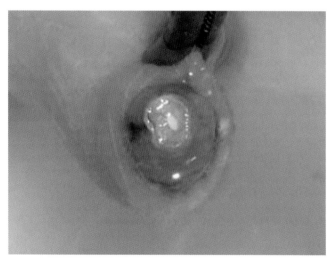

Figure 5.19 White MTA retrofill.

surface should be avoided at all times. The tooth is immediately transferred into a basin which is filled with HBSS and submerged. Root resection is carried out by an impact air handpiece under the microscope and approximately 3 mm of the root is resected (Figure 5.18).

Methylene blue stain is applied to the root end and observed under the microscope with mid-range magnification for cracks, isthmuses, and extra portals of exit. Retropreparation is made by using small pear-shaped carbide burs such as a 330 bur or ultrasonic tips. The canals are then obturated with super ethoxybenzoic acid (Super-EBA; Bosworth, Skokie, IL, USA) or MTA carried in microcarriers and condensed with micropluggers. The root end is then polished or burnished and inspected one last time under the microscope before replantation (Figure 5.19).

The tooth is then reoriented properly and gently placed in its socket. Light apical pressure is applied until the tooth is seated in its correct, most apical position. It is prudent to radiographically confirm the complete seating of the tooth in the socket at this time (Figure 5.20).

The tooth is then splinted by suturing a monofilament suture over the occlusal surface of the tooth. Fishing line and composite bonding can also be used by providing a physiological splint when the treated tooth is splinted to its neighbor on their buccal surfaces. The limitation of this method is that it requires both of the teeth being splinted to have enamel on their buccal surfaces to facilitate bonding. This method excludes teeth with metal or porcelain coronal coverage, which may be a good number of teeth treated by intentional replantation. The patient should be instructed to maintain a maximum intercuspal position at least for the

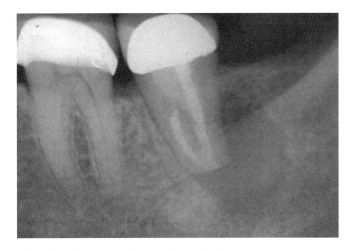

Figure 5.20 Radiograph immediately post reimplantation.

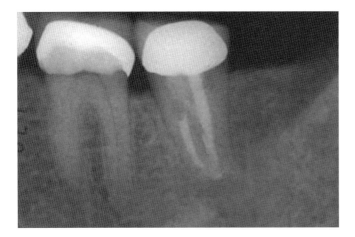

Figure 5.21 Two-year recall exhibits complete healing.

remainder of the day and to chew away from the side for about one week. Postoperative instructions are given, and the patient should be reappointed for follow-up visit in one week, at which time the sutures are removed if still intact. Pain management instructions are given as described earlier. Once regarded as a last resort before extraction, today intentional replantation in selected cases is a viable and logical mode of treatment. With the development of new protocols for intentional replantation, the procedure has become more predictable and should always be considered as a part of possible treatment planning (Figure 5.21).

PERIRADICULAR SURGERY

Periradicular surgeries, otherwise known as apicoectomy, constitute the bulk of endodontic surgeries. By definition, *apicoectomy* involves the reflection of a soft tissue flap, osteotomy of both cortical and cancellous bone, and resection of the root segment, which is suspected to be associated with a persistent inflammatory process. The preparation of a retrocavity and placement of a root-end filling material are not necessary requirements for an apicoectomy, although

they are highly recommended. Apicoectomy is perceived to be technically more difficult than other endodontic surgeries due to difficulties in its accessibility, illumination, and small operating field. This is especially true with the case of posterior teeth, that the access more than the anatomy renders them more difficult to treat (Wang et al. 2004). However, since the addition of the SOM to our armamentarium, we have been able to overcome many of the challenges associated with apicoectomy.

Indications

Apicoectomy is indicated for treatment of teeth with persistent apical or periradicular pathosis due to anatomical challenges, iatrogenic factors, irretrievable dental material inside and outside of the canal, fractures, and repair of resorptions or perforations (Figures 5.22–5.25).

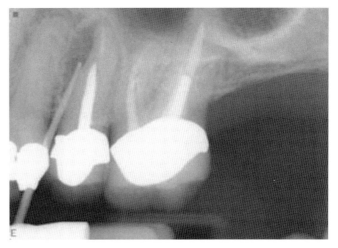

Figure 5.22 Sinus tract tracing and the location of the mid-root radiolucency is suggestive of a post perforation.

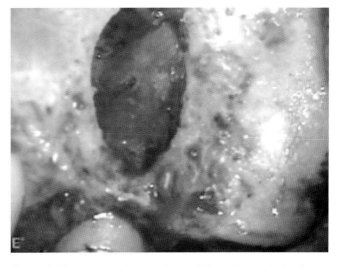

Figure 5.23 Upon the reflection of the soft tissue flap, an isolated endodontic fenestration is visible.

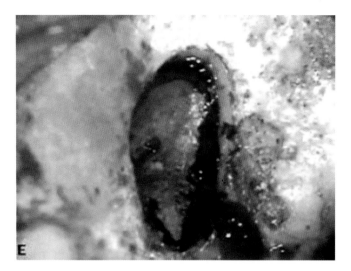

Figure 5.24 Staining reveals a perforation on the mesial aspect of the root. The defect was filled with Super-EBA cement.

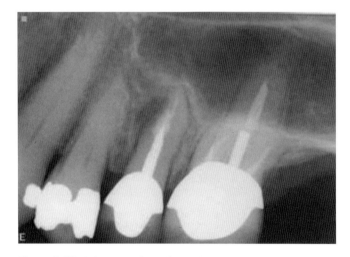

Figure 5.25 A three-month recall revealed partial healing and no signs of the sinus tract.

PHASES OF APICOECTOMY AND SURGICAL TECHNIQUE

Review of Medical History

Once the patient has been selected as a candidate for apical surgery, a complete review of the systemic health of the patient must be performed. High-risk patients as defined by the American Heart Association are to be pretreated prophylactically with oral antibiotics. After consultation with their physician, patients who are on anticoagulant therapy should be taken off of the medication in time before the surgery. Last, patients who have been on oral or intravenous bisphosphonates should be informed about the potential risks and complications that may arise after the surgery as sequelae of the drug therapy.

Intraoral Examination

A thorough intraoral examination is crucial in postulating and designing the appropriate approach for treatment via surgery. Intraorally, the surgical site should be investigated for any type of periodontal defect by careful probing. Evaluation of periodontal recession, width of attached gingiva, and the patient's gingival biotype may ultimately determine the type of incision used during the surgery. Any sinus tracts, swellings, or areas sensitive to palpation should be noted. Evaluation of muscle attachments and patient's opening are critical in determining accessibility to the prospective surgical site.

Radiographic Examination

Exposure of two periapical radiographs is the minimum requirement before commencement of surgery. The first radiograph should be exposed using a paralleling technique and the second should be deviated in its horizontal component by 20° to the mesial or distal. The radiograph should be studied for root length, number of roots, root curvature, size of the potential lesion, and proximity of the osteotomy to neurovascular bundles, maxillary sinus, and neighboring teeth. It is strongly recommended that, when possible, a panoramic radiograph is obtained, especially when treating mandibular posterior teeth.

Presurgical Preparation

Preoperatively, unless contraindicated, the patient should take 600–800 mg of ibuprofen just before surgery. The patient should continue to take this regimen of anti-inflammatory every eight hours for up to three days after the surgery.

In addition, the patient should commence rinsing with 10 ml of 0.12% chlorohexidine gluconate twice daily, 24 hours before surgery. This oral rinse should be used before surgery to reduce the quantity of the microorganisms in the mouth and decrease the chance of a postsurgical flap infection.

Local Anesthesia (Pain Control and Hemostasis)

Choosing and administering the appropriate localanesthetic has a trifold effect. First, it provides pain control during the surgery. Second, it provides hemostasis. Third, by administering a long-lasting anesthetic, postoperatively, the cycle of pain is broken. This is in part due to prevention in amplification of responses from the peripheral nerves, which could ultimately lead to central sensitization.

Typically, local anesthesia is administered via nerve blocks and local infiltrations. Nerve blocks are aimed at achieving profound pain control but must be supplemented by local infiltrations and papillary injections on both the buccal and lingual aspects of the teeth for additional pain control and hemostasis.

Unless contraindicated, 2% lidocaine with 1 : 50 000 epinephrine is the anesthetic of choice because of its high concentration of epinephrine, which is suitable for hemostasis. Although this high concentration of epinephrine may cause a transient tachycardia in the patient, the effects are generally short lived. It should be noted that some clinicians prefer 3% marcaine with epinephrine for nerve block because of its long duration of action.

In addition to the administration of one cartridge of anesthetic for the appropriate nerve block when working on maxillary or mandibular teeth, local infiltration into oral tissue for hemostasis is required. Generally, up to two cartridges of anesthetic should be infiltrated locally around two or three teeth on either side of the surgical site. Because most of the receptors in the masticatory mucosa are of α–adrenergic type, once bound to epinephrine, they produce a desired vasoconstrictive effect. In contrast, because the majority of the receptors in skeletal muscles are of the β_2–adrenergic variety and their binding to epinephrine causes vasodilation, care must be taken to prevent injecting deep into these tissues.

Soft Tissue Flap Design

Proper flap design not only should provide easy access to the location of the pathosis but should also consider and provide postsurgical aesthetics of the periodontium and the gingiva, especially preserving marginal gingiva and papillary heights. With the evolution of periodontal surgery and introduction of new techniques, some older techniques have been phased out.

Periodontal condition of the failing tooth and its neighboring teeth play an important role in the design of the soft tissue flap; as does the prosthetic state of the surgical site. When working on teeth with crowns or areas near the pontic of a fixed partial denture, modifications to the incision line may be needed to facilitate suturing and ensure soft tissue esthetics in the long term. Also of importance are anatomical factors, such as the mental foramen, which may ultimately play a role in the selection of the location for the placement of the vertical release incision.

In endodontic surgery, incisions are made to facilitate elevation and reflection of a full-thickness flap. Generally, a horizontal component and two vertical release incisions are used to provide easy access without pulling and tearing the corners of the flap. Once the tissue is reflected, great care must be taken to prevent the placement of the retractors on soft tissue. Many manufacturers have developed contour specific retractors that provide good ergonomic

retraction of the flap in different locations of the mouth. In some cases, slipping of the retractor can be prevented by placing a notch or a groove superficially on the cortical bone and subsequently placing the retractor in this groove.

The following is a list of flaps that are associated with endodontic surgery:

Semilunar Incision

Although once frequently used by endodontists and oral surgeons for performing apicoectomies, semilunar incisions are an inferior and obsolete technique. Typically, they provide poor access to the site and do not allow for addressing or treating periodontal–endodontic involvements. They often result in unsightly scars as the incision line is made in unattached, mobile oral mucosa, and over the osteotomy where healing by primary intention is impractical, if not impossible.

Today, semilunar incisions are performed only during emergency incision and drainage.

Full-Thickness Intrasulcular Incision

In this technique, the horizontal incision commences at the base of the gingival sulcus and is carried through to the crest of the bone by dissecting the periodontal ligament fibers. Generally, the horizontal component should be extended by the width of two teeth on either side of the tooth being treated. Interproximally, the incision should be made with a sharp 15C or a CK-2 microblade (Sybron Endo, Orange, CA, USA) lingually while following the contour of the teeth. The complete dissection of the interdental papilla before elevation is desired to prevent recession and formation of "black triangles" postoperatively.

Two variations of the full-thickness intrasulcular flap exist:

- The triangular flap, which uses one vertical releasing incision in the more medial aspect of the flap, typically requires a longer horizontal incision. The releasing incision should begin perpendicular to the line of the free gingival margin for a short distance of approximately 2–3mm. It is then rounded off at the corner and transitioned into the vertical component of the releasing incision. It is not unusual to extend the release incision up to the mucobuccal fold and up to two times the length of release incisions in periodontal surgery in order to access the root apex easily. Triangular flaps are commonly used in surgeries of the posterior region (Figures 5.26–5.28), or in the anterior region when treating teeth with cervical resorptions or perforations.

- The rectangular flap is similar to the triangular flap, except it uses two vertical releasing incisions and as a result, the horizontal incision may be shorter. This flap provides better access to the apex of anterior teeth than the triangular flap.

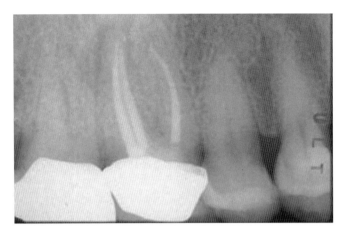

Figure 5.26 Maxillary first molar exhibiting persistent symptoms despite the radiographically acceptable appearance of the nonsurgical root canal therapy.

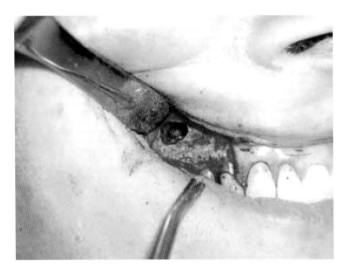

Figure 5.27 Triangular full-thickness flap provides access to the surgical site.

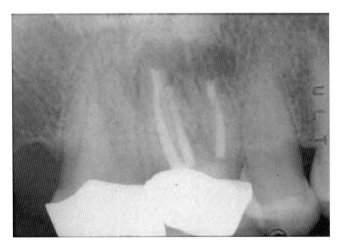

Figure 5.28 Apicoectomy and retrofill with MTA was performed on all three roots via a buccal approach.

Full-Thickness Submarginal Incision

Also known as the mucogingival flap, it is indicated primarily in anterior surgeries to treat teeth with crowns and where esthetics of the crown margin is of great importance. The beveled scalloped horizontal component of the incision is placed in attached gingiva and is terminated by rounding off and transitioning into the placement of two parallel vertical releasing incisions at either end. The scalloping aids in exact repositioning of the flap postsurgically to ensure healing by primary intention. It is critical to have a 2-mm band of healthy attached gingiva coronal and apical to the horizontal incision line (Figures 5.29 and 5.30).

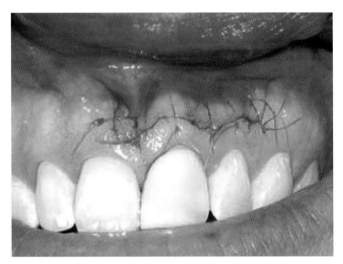

Figure 5.29 Submarginal incision and suturing with 6-0 Vicryl sutures in the esthetic zone.

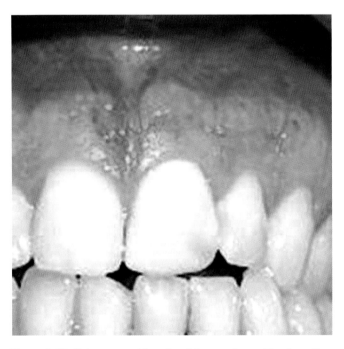

Figure 5.30 Suture removal four days later reveals great healing with minimal scar formation.

Lack of such attachment especially coronal to the incision may critically undermine the blood supply and result in disastrous postsurgical recession. Needless to say, acquiring accurate preoperative periodontal probing depths is critical.

This flap differs from the Luebke-Ochsenbein flap in that it is not wider at the base because the two vertical releasing incisions are made parallel to each other.

Papillary-based Incision

This technique has been developed in recent years with the purpose of maintaining the height of the interdental papilla. The incision is similar to the full-thickness intrasulcular incision. However, in the region of the interdental papilla, instead of the incision including and dissecting the papilla, it is placed at the base of the papilla. This incision is a curved incision that connects the sulcus of one tooth at its mesial line angle to the sulcus of the more anterior tooth at its distal line angle. This incision is carried out by a microblade first to a depth of 1.5 mm. A second incision is directed toward the osseous crest and retraces the initial superficial incision.

Upon completion of the surgery, proper suturing is important to guarantee optimal results. Generally, the use of 7-0 or smaller monofilament nonresorbable sutures has been recommended for closure of the papillary-based incision. A minimum of two single interrupted sutures are placed to ensure primary closure at the papillary base. Sutures are to be removed within three to five days (Velvart and Peters 2005).

Osteotomy and Curettage

Once the flap is reflected and stabilized without causing trauma to the soft tissue, the hard tissue management phase of the surgery may begin. The root tip location must be approximated from a pre-operative radiograph, presence of pathology, cortical bone fenestration, or a root prominence underlying the cortical bone. In some cases sounding the bone quality over the root apex with a sharp endodontic DG16 explorer (Hu-Friedy, Chicago, IL, USA) may give information about the location and the extent of the underlying lesion (Figures 5.31 and 5.32).

Once the location for the osteotomy is determined, using an Impact Air 45 (Palisades Dental, Englewood, NJ, USA) high-speed handpiece and Lindemann H 161 (Brasseler USA, Savannah, GA, USA) bone-cutting carbide bur, the osteotomy is made under low magnification with copious irrigation with sterile saline to cool the surgical site. This is done by brushing away at the bone until the root apex is visualized (Figure 5.33).

With the advent of modern microsurgical instruments, the ideal osteotomy can now be only 5 mm in diameter.

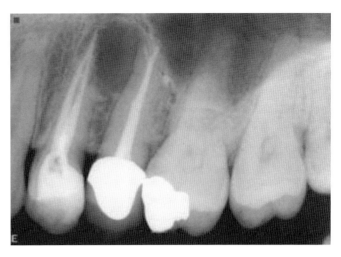

Figure 5.31 Failing root canal treatment on maxillary first and second premolars.

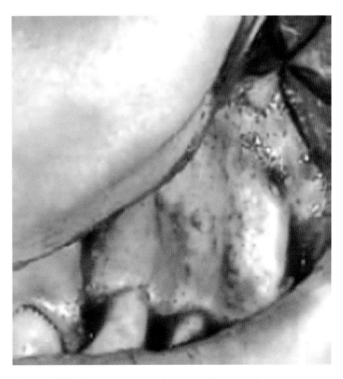

Figure 5.32 Flap elevation reveals fenestrations over the root prominences identifying the location of the defects.

Any soft tissue lesion attached to the root tip must be curettaged before root resection. This is achieved by the back-action use of long shank spoon excavators or bone curettes to detach the lesion from its bony housing in total. This tissue must be submitted for biopsy. Any remnants still attached to the root can be removed via a 34/35 Jaquette scaler or a 13/14 periodontal curette (Hu- Friedy). Excessive curettage of the bony crypt may cause excessive bleeding, which may in turn complicate and compromise the stages of root-end resection, retropreparation, and

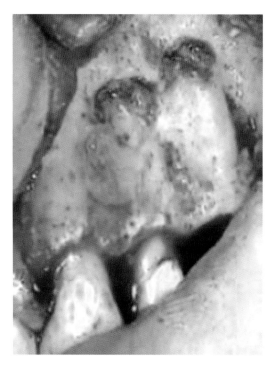

Figure 5.33 Osteotomy is initiated by slow removal of the buccal cortical bone until the root tips are visible.

retrofilling. Therefore, it may be more strategic to leave small amounts of granulation tissue behind and clean it after the root-end filling is placed.

The Impact Air 45 high-speed handpiece is designed in such way that only a water coolant is sprayed out from the front onto the bur. The air jet is contained within a closed circuit and ejected from the rear of the handpiece. This innovation allows for a much cleaner operation due to the lack of splatter previously caused by the air stream forced out of the head of conventional handpieces. Most important, it creates a safer operation by eliminating the air that may be forced into the open vessels of the surgical site and potentially cause an air emphysema.

Root Resection

The logic behind root resection and its extent is derived from the models developed by Hess. A 3-mm reduction in the root end will decrease the incidence of lateral canals by 93% and apical ramifications by 98%. Therefore statistically, a 3-mm apicoectomy will markedly favor the elimination of persistent bacteria and undebrided tissue in the apical root canal portion (Kim et al. 2001b). This will also enable the surgeon to remove and eliminate iatrogenic factors more prevalent to the last 2–3 mm of the root canal system. Once the root is resected, access to the canal is possible for evaluation and formation of an impervious retroseal.

Up until the early 1990s, the practice was to resect the root end with a 45° buccolingual bevel. This was practiced because it was impossible to form a cavity preparation into the canal even with the smallest handpiece. Presently, with the development of microsurgical instruments, and, more specifically, ultrasonic tips, micromirrors, and pluggers, the recommended root-end resection bevel angle is between 0 and 10°. This modification in technique has its many advantages. It conserves root and buccal cortical bone and reduces the chance of incomplete resection and perhaps missing lingual anatomy. By reducing the cavity preparation, cavosurface margin, and number of exposed dentinal tubules, the risk of microleakage is reduced (Kim 2002).

This phase of the procedure should be carried out under mid-range magnification using the Impact Air 45 handpiece and Lindemann H 161 bur with sterile saline irrigation (Figures 5.34 and 5.35).

Staining and Inspection

Once the root end is perceived as being completely resected, it is time to switch the magnification to the high range for root-end inspection. The root end should be stained with sterile methylene blue dye (American Regent Inc., Shirley, NY, USA) and rinsed away with sterile saline or water. The dye will stain the PDL circumferentially, revealing a circle or an ovoid blue perimeter. This is a sign that the root resection was completely carried out through the lingual aspect. The blue dye will also penetrate into any

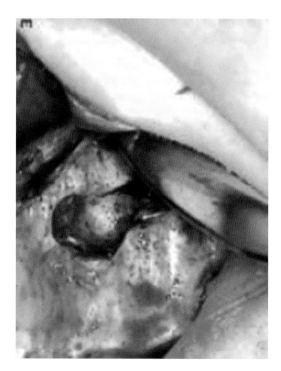

Figure 5.34 Endodontic lesion is enucleated in whole and the root tips are resected with almost a zero bevel angle.

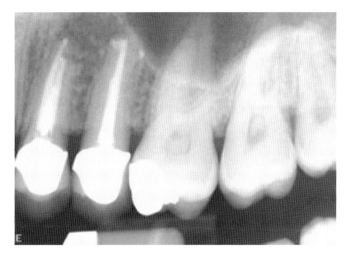

Figure 5.35 One-year follow-up demonstrates complete healing of both teeth.

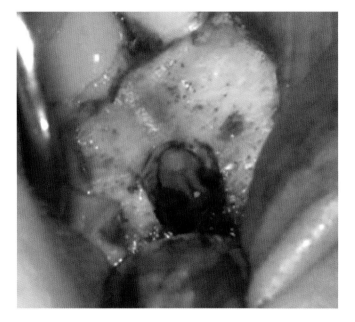

Figure 5.36 The resected and stained mesial root of a mandibular molar reveals an unfilled MB canal and the isthmus connecting the MB and ML canals.

canal, isthmus, portal of exit, or fracture and reveal areas that need to be prepared with the ultrasonic tips (Figure 5.36).

Prior to the use of ultrasonic tips, a CX-1 microexplorer (Sybron EndoA) may be used to probe into these areas. Sometimes it is helpful to scribe the preparation outline with the CX-1 onto the root-end surface before the use of ultrasonic tips.

Retropreparation

After the areas to be retroprepared have been identified, ultrasonic tips with the appropriate angulations can be used to create the cavity preparation along the long axis of the root. This step should also be carried out under high magnification and constant irrigation. Incorporating the isthmus between two canals or a fin to the side of a canal into the preparation is just as critical as preparing the canals themselves (Figures 5.37–5.39).

Any tissue left in the isthmus could be a source for a potential failure. The preparation is carried out to a depth of 3–4mm. The preparation should be inspected under the microscope in order to ensure that no gutta percha remains on the prepared portion of the canal walls. A microplugger/condenser can be used to compact any residual gutta percha coronally and away from the root tip.

Some surgeons prefer to treat the root end with 2% chlorohexidine gluconate (Ultradent, South Jordan, UT, USA). This antibacterial agent has proved to be effective against

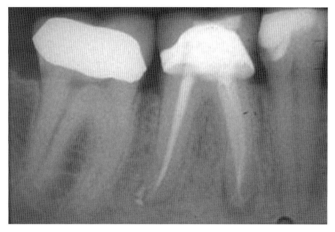

Figure 5.37 Mandibular first molar exhibiting persistent pathology of the mesial root.

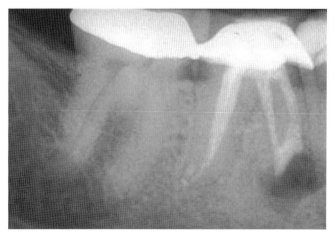

Figure 5.38 Apicoectomy, retropreparation, and retrofill of the MB and ML canals and the isthmus connecting them.

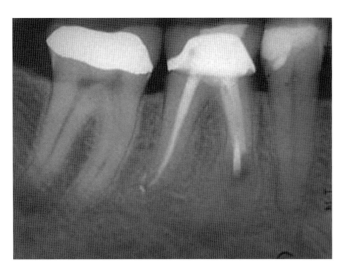

Figure 5.39 Near-complete healing is noted at six-month recall appointment.

Enterococcus faecalis, the persistent bacteria species in many endodontic failures.

Moisture Control

The bone crypt must be dry before the placement of the retrofill material. If bleeding is present, it may be controlled by the application of topical hemostatic agents. Racellet #3 (Pascal Co., Bellevue, WA, USA) epinephrine pellets are usually effective in controlling the bleeding in most osteotomy sites. They contain racemic epinephrine, which aid in hemostasis. These pellets are packed into the osteotomy site with moderate pressure maintained on them for a few minutes. Once hemostasis is achieved, all but the last of the pellets are removed. The last pellet is deliberately left in the crypt to maintain the hemostasis. Aspiration into the crypt once hemostasis has been achieved should be prevented, because it may draw blood out of the capillaries and initiate bleeding again. It is important to keep track of the number of pellets placed, so at the end of the procedure, pellets are not forgotten and left behind.

For more persistent bleeding in larger osteotomies, ferric sulfate solution such as Cut-Trol (Ichthys Inc., Mobile, AL, USA) may be used. Ferric sulfate has been shown to delay postoperative healing (Lemon et al. 1993). Therefore, it should only be used sparingly and currettaged and rinsed thoroughly at the end of the surgery before suturing.

Calcium sulfate such as Surgiplast (ClassImplant, Rome, Italy) can also be used as a mechanical barrier to promote hemostasis in large osteotomies. Calcium sulfate is an osteoinductive resorbable agent that may act as a barrier against the more rapid mobilization of soft tissue cells toward the osteotomy site and, therefore, promote bone formation.

Retrofill

Once the moisture is controlled, it is time for sealing the root end. The root end must be irrigated and air dried with a Stropko irrigator/drier with a microtip (Sybron Endo).

Although amalgam was once the root-end filling of choice, today it is no longer the standard of care to place amalgam as a retrograde filling. Today's materials provide a better seal, do not tattoo the gingiva, do not corrode, and are more bio-compatible than amalgam. Although an array of materials are presently available, MTA and Super-EBA are the most promising and most widely used.

MTA exhibits many of the desired characteristics of a retrofill material. MTA is radiopaque and gentle to the periapical tissue, induces cementogenesis, has great sealing ability, and is tolerant to moisture. In fact, MTA requires moisture to harden and set. Unfortunately, it is difficult to handle. MTA is mixed with sterile water to form a wet sand–like granular mixture. The easiest way to place it into the root-end preparation is with the MAP System (Roydent, Johnson City, TN, USA) or the MTA pellet forming block (G. Hartzell & Son, Concord, CA, USA). Once placed, MTA takes a long time to set and should not be rinsed out. The crypt may be cleaned with a moist cotton pellet.

Super-EBA, on the other hand, is difficult to mix but easier to handle. It is mixed into a hard, dull, dough-like mixture by incorporating powder into liquid with a thick spatula over a glass slab. Once ready, time is limited to place it because it sets quickly, especially in the presence of heat and humidity. Super-EBA is rolled into a small cone and picked up in small segments with an instrument such as a Hollenbeck or the back side of a spoon excavator. It is then placed into the root end, compacted gently with a microplugger, and finally burnished with a microball burnisher. After the material is fully set, it may be polished with a composite finishing bur using a high-speed handpiece with irrigation.

Once the retrofill material is placed, it is a good practice to radiographically verify the density and the depth of the fill before suturing the flap. If any modifications need to be made, this is a good time for it.

After the quality of the filling is confirmed to be satisfactory, the crypt must be curettaged to remove any residual material or coagulum and to induce bleeding. The surgical site should be rinsed with sterile saline to wash off any particles or loose debris and also to rehydrate the flap and the cortical bone, which may have been drying under the intense illumination from the SOM.

Suturing and Suture Removal

The flap needs to be reapproximated passively before suturing. Best results are obtained when the flap margins approximate without the use of force or under tension. For this purpose, a wet 2×2 gauze is compressed gently over the flap and cortical bone until tissue margins assume their preferred position.

As for suture material, monofilament nonresorbable Prolene (Ethicon Inc., Somerville, NJ, USA) sutures in sizes of 6-0 or smaller provide the optimal results. The advantage of these types of sutures is that their size causes the least amount of trauma and that they are nonresorbable, which minimizes the inflammation typically associated with suture materials. When suturing the apical margins of the vertical release incision near the mucobuccal fold, however, it is advantageous to use a resorbable suture such as a coated Vicryl or Monocryl (Ethicon Inc.). Sutures in this region sometimes have a tendency to become imbedded into the wound closure and may be difficult to remove.

In terms of suturing technique, single interrupted and vertical mattress sutures are the most commonly used. Vertical mattress sutures are preferred when suturing mobilized interdental papillae in the anterior esthetic zone. Sling sutures in the posterior region can be used in place of two single interrupted sutures. When suturing the vertical releasing incision, a continuous interlocking suture can be used to expedite suturing by eliminating the need for multiple knots.

Whatever the suturing technique, care must be taken that the suture and the knots are free of any tension. Tissue margins may be torn when sutures are tight and act as a guillotine. In addition, the underlying tissue may become deprived of blood perfusion and ultimately necrose in presence of over-tight knots.

Postsurgically, sutures should be removed within 3–5 days, although some studies advocate suture removal by 48 hours.

Postoperative Instructions

Postoperative instructions should be directed toward ensuring patient's comfort, control of bleeding and swelling, and prevention of infections.

Patient reassurance is an important part of postoperative instructions. It is better for the patient to know about potential pain, swelling, or bruising ahead of time rather than being caught by surprise.

Pain following endodontic surgery is usually mild. For this reason, non-narcotic analgesics are more than adequate in controlling patient's pain. Just before the start of the procedure, 1000 mg of acetaminophen or 800 mg of ibuprofen should be taken by the patient as a preemptive strike against pain when the local anesthetic slowly wears off. Postsurgically, ibuprofen 800 mg three times daily should be prescribed and taken by the patient for three to five days. This regimen should be followed regardless of the level of patient's comfort as an anti-inflammatory medication. For those patients who are allergic to ibuprofen, 1000 mg acetaminophen can be taken four times daily. Some more recent studies suggest combination therapy with ibuprofen and acetaminophen will achieve more effective levels of analgesia (Menhinick et al. 2004).

Applying an ice pack to the face over the region of surgery with moderate pressure for 20 minutes on and 20 minutes off is very important in controlling inflammation, swelling, and ecchymosis. This regimen is most effective if followed up to eight hours postsurgically. Moist heat application is recommended for 24–48 hours after surgery.

Rinsing with 10 ml of 0.12% chlorohexidine gluconate solution twice daily should begin 24 hours before surgery and continue for up to 2 days after suture removal. Gentle brushing with a soft bristle toothbrush should be limited to the areas away from the surgical site and to the occlusal surfaces of teeth proximal to the incision line.

Patients should be informed that in the event of a suture becoming untied, they should not pull on the loose end as they may detach the flap from the underlying bone.

Consumption of a normal diet is recommended, although a soft diet is preferred for the first 48 hours. In addition, hot liquids should be avoided because they may promote bleeding and cause pain if they come in contact with exposed tissue or bone. Smoking and consumption of alcohol should be avoided until sutures are removed and proper healing is confirmed.

Patients should avoid physical activities that can increase their heart rate and increase bleeding. In addition, patients should be discouraged to manipulate the areas of the face or mouth, which may pull on the sutures and ultimately extricate them.

Complications

Serious complications after endodontic surgery are infrequent. Most cases of pain, swelling, and bleeding are easily managed. In some rare cases, patients may have serious infection or paresthesia. Immediate attention is required for such incidences.

Although paresthesia is often transient and is not due to the complete severing of a nerve bundle, it may cause some concern in the patient. Patients should be reassured that the sensation will often return, and it could simply be the result of inflammation and nerve compression. Only in rare occasions is paresthesia irreversible. The patient must be re-evaluated at the office, and the affected area must be mapped intraorally by the use of a sharp dental instrument. A diagram of this area must be drawn in the patient's dental record and compared to subsequent examinations to check for signs of improvement. If no improvement is noted, the patient should be referred to a specialist for further care and monitoring.

Infections after endodontic surgery are uncommon. Routine prescription of oral antibiotics is not supported by studies and therefore not recommended. The antibiotic of choice for treating endodontic infections is 500 mg penicillin VK every six hours for one week. If this initial therapy does not provide the desired pharmaceutical result, it can be supplemented with 500 mg metronidazole every six hours for one week. Also, the patient can be taken off of the Penicillin VK and placed on 300 mg clindamycin every eight hours for one week. In those rare cases where the patient is severely swollen, febrile, and may have difficulty breathing or swallowing, immediate referral to the hospital and administration of intravenous antibiotics is indicated.

Last, during maxillary posterior surgeries where the maxillary sinus and the Schneiderian membrane have been involved, the patient must be placed on a prophylactic dose of 875 mg of Augmentin twice daily for one week to prevent invasion and infection of the sinus by normal oral flora. The patient should also be advised not to blow the nose and to take over-the-counter nasal decongestants. A one-week follow-up visit is recommended to ensure no complications have arisen. Maxillary sinus involvements, if treated in a timely manner, will often heal uneventfully.

RECALL

Patient's healing must be monitored periodically. Because the average healing time for surgical cases has been reported to be seven months, it makes sense to recall the patient within one year post-treatment. Earlier follow-up appointments may not indicate any healing, although healing may be in progress.

For cases in which a timely secondary intervention would be imperative in case of a failure, a three- to four-month recall schedule is justified and perhaps more beneficial.

REFERENCES

ADA (1999). Survey of Dental Services Rendered. ADA Report: September 2002.

Kim, S. (2002). Endodontic microsurgery. In: *Pathways of the Pulp*, 8e (eds. S. Cohen and R.C. Burns), 683–725. St Louis: Mosby.

Kim, S., Pecora, G., and Rubinstein, R. (2001a). *Color Atlas of Microsurgery in Endodontics*, 125. Philadelphia: WB Saunders.

Kim, S., Pecora, G., and Rubinstein, R. (2001b). *Color Atlas of Microsurgery in Endodontics*, 85–94. Philadelphia: WB Saunders.

Kupfer, I.J., Sidney, R., and Kupfer, B.S. (1952). Tooth replantation following avulsion. *N.Y. State Dent. J.* 19: 80.

Lemon, R.R., Steele, P.J., and Jeansonne, B.G. (1993). Ferric sulfate hemostasis: effect on osseous wound healing. Left in-situ for maximum exposure. *J. Endod.* 19: 170–173.

Menhinick, K., Gutmann, J.L., Regan, J.D. et al. (2004). The efficacy of pain control following nonsurgical root canal treatment using ibuprofen or a combination of ibuprofen and acetaminophen in a randomized, double-blind, placebo-controlled study. *Int. J. Endod.* 37: 531–541.

Rahbaran, S., Gilthorpe, M.S., Harrison, S.D., and Gulabivala, K. (2001). Comparison of clinical outcome of periapical surgery in endodontic and oral surgery units of a teaching dental hospital: a retrospective study. *Oral Surg. Oral Med. Oral Pathol. Oral Radiol. Endod.* 91: 700–709.

Reuben, H. and Apotheker, H. (1984). Apical surgery with the dental microscope. *Oral Surg. Oral Med. Oral Pathol.* 57: 433–435.

Rubinstein, F.A. and Kim, S. (1999). Short-term observation of the results of endodontic surgery with the use of a surgical operation microscope and Super-EBA as root-end filling material. *J. Endod.* 25: 43–48.

Rubinstein, F.A. and Kim, S. (2002). Long-term follow-up of cases considered healed one year after apical microsurgery. *J. Endod.* 28: 378–383.

Ruskin, J.D., Morton, D., Karayazgan, B., and Amir, J. (2005). Failed root canals: the case for extraction and immediate implant placement. *J. Oral Maxillofac. Surg.* 63: 829–831.

Velvart, P. and Peters, C.I. (2005). Soft tissue management in endodontic surgery. *J. Endod.* 31: 4–16.

Wang, N., Knight, K., Dao, T., and Friedman, S. (2004). Treatment outcome in endodontics – the Toronto study. Phase I and II: apical surgery. *J. Endod.* 30: 751–761.

Zuolo, M.L., Ferreira, M.O.F., and Gutmann, J.L. (2000). Prognosis in periradicular surgery: a clinical prospective study. *Int. Endod. J.* 33: 91–98.

Chapter 6 The Contribution of Periodontics to Prosthodontics: Treatment Planning of Patients Requiring Combined Periodontal and Prosthodontic Care

Haneen N. Bokhadoor, Nawaf J. Al-Dousari, and Steven Morgano

INTRODUCTION

Treatment planning for patients with complex dental needs involves multidisciplinary collaboration with the prosthodontist, periodontist/oral surgeon, orthodontist, endodontist, and patient. It is a carefully sequenced process and is designed to eliminate or control etiologic factors, repair existing damage, and create a functional, maintainable oral environment. Successful treatment depends on a thorough evaluation of all available information, a definitive diagnosis, and a thorough integration of all necessary procedures prescribed for the patient. The treatment process is composed of a series of phases: a diagnostic phase, a treatment-planning phase, a treatment phase, and a maintenance phase.

DIAGNOSTIC PHASE (DATA COLLECTION)

Diagnosis involves the collection of data obtained from a comprehensive patient history (medical and dental), a patient interview (chief complaint), a clinical examination (inspection, palpation, and percussion), a critical evaluation of mounted diagnostic casts, and a radiologic interpretation.

Patient History

Patient's Social and Environmental History

The patient's social and environmental history are important adjuncts to diagnosis and treatment planning and can often determine the entire course of treatment. Examples include a patient's age, gender, occupation, alcohol intake, tobacco use, and illicit drug use.

Medical History

The importance of an accurate comprehensive medical history cannot be overstated. The medical history reveals systemic conditions that could be contributing factors related to the existing dental disease or that could affect the prognosis of dental treatment. A thorough medical history and interview should reveal any previous systemic diseases, injuries, surgical procedures, allergies, adverse drug reactions, and medications. An example of a systemic disease affecting oral health is diabetes mellitus. Patients with diabetes mellitus are more likely to develop periodontal disease compared with patients without diabetes, and periodontal disease is often considered the sixth complication of diabetes mellitus. Patients with uncontrolled diabetes are especially at risk (Mealey and Oates 2006).

The medical history can also alert the dentist to other disorders, such as a prosthetic cardiac valve that requires antibiotic prophylaxis (Davies 1993). The presence of a pacemaker contraindicates the use of electrosurgery (Flocken 1980). Previous radiation therapy for neoplastic diseases of the head and neck region can have a profound effect on the oral cavity (AAP position paper 1997). Medications causing xerostomia can lead to cervical dental caries and periodontal disease, and can contribute to early failure of fixed restorations (Thomson et al. 2006). Osteonecrosis of the jaw has been observed in cancer patients who have undergone invasive dental procedures, such as dental implant surgery or tooth extractions, while receiving treatment with intravenous bisphosphonates. Invasive dental procedures should be avoided for these patients whenever possible (Soileau 2006; Wooltorton 2005).

Dental History

The dental history serves as a companion to the medical history. It establishes information on the patient's involvement in previous dental treatment, when and why missing teeth were removed, previous problems with dental treatment, para-functional habits, and oral hygiene habits.

Chief Complaint

The chief complaint can establish the need for additional diagnostic tests to assist in determining the cause of the dental problems. It is important that any recommended treatment addresses this chief complaint and that the patient's expectations with regard to the outcome of treatment are realistic.

Practical Advanced Periodontal Surgery, Second Edition. Edited by Serge Dibart.
© 2020 John Wiley & Sons, Inc. Published 2020 by John Wiley & Sons, Inc.
Companion website: www.wiley.com/go/dibart/advanced

Clinical Examination

Extraoral Examination

A thorough examination should include an evaluation of the size, shape, and symmetry of the head and neck including the patient's profile (retrognathic, mesiognathic, prognathic). Normal and abnormal clinical findings should be noted in detail as a permanent component of the patient's record.

Intraoral Examination

The intraoral examination includes screening for malignancies, an evaluation of the patient's overall caries activity, a general overview of the periodontal status, and the quality and quantity of saliva. The dentist should then thoroughly examine the existing restorations and their status, the presence of dental caries, and missing teeth. A complete periodontal assessment is an important component of a comprehensive oral examination. It includes an evaluation of the oral hygiene, a description of the color, form, and texture of the gingiva, a recording of probing depths, an assessment of bleeding on probing, a determination of tooth mobility, a mucogingival evaluation, and an evaluation of furcations.

Occlusal Examination and Analysis

One of the most critical factors with regard to treatment planning is an evaluation of the patient's occlusion. Alterations and deviations in the occlusal plane can result in a dysfunctional maximal intercuspal position (MIP), attrition, bruxism, widened periodontal ligament spaces (trauma from occlusion), and impaired mastication. Mounted diagnostic casts represent an important diagnostic aid for the thorough evaluation of a patient's occlusion (Morgano et al. 1989).

Radiographic Examination

Basic knowledge of normal radiographic appearances is essential. The minimal examination requirements for a comprehensive treatment plan include a panoramic radiograph and a complete-mouth radiographic series. The presence of dental caries, loss of tooth-supporting bone, furcation invasions, and any other abnormalities should be carefully noted and recorded in the patient's record.

Diagnostic Casts and Diagnostic Waxing

Diagnostic casts are made from impressions of the dental arches. Irreversible hydrocolloid (alginate) material is usually used in stock metal trays. The trays should allow a uniform thickness of 3–5 mm of impression material. These trays should be large enough to cover the retromolar pads in the mandible and the hamular (pterygomaxillary) notches in the maxillary arch. The impressions should be poured immediately with cast (Type III) stone. Once the casts are retrieved, small nodules are removed. The casts are mounted in a semiadjustable articulator with a face-bow transfer. Duplicate diagnostic casts are also made and mounted. A diagnostic waxing of the proposed treatment plan is then made. Diagnostic casts and the diagnostic waxing represent the guide or "blue-print" for the restorative plan that assists the dentist and laboratory technician in coordinating the reconstruction of esthetics, phonetics, and function (Morgano et al. 1989).

Prognosis

The prognosis is a forecast of the probable course and outcome of a disorder. The overall prognosis is concerned with the entire dentition. Criteria used to assign a prognosis to individual teeth are subjective and are usually based on clinical and radiographic findings. A favorable, questionable (guarded), unfavorable (poor), or hopeless prognosis is assigned to each tooth depending on available bone support, probing depths, furcation exposure, mobility, crown-to-root ratio, root proximity, occlusal relationships, extent of tooth damage, abutment status, endodontic status, remaining tooth structure (restorability), caries susceptibility, quality and quantity of saliva, and parafunctional habits.

Making the decision to retain or extract a compromised tooth requires a thorough evaluation of all factors, including the expense and discomfort involved in maintaining the tooth, the overall strategic value of the tooth, available literature from clinical studies on the probability of success of the treatment required to retain the tooth, the prognosis of an artificial replacement for the tooth, and the patient's desires, expectations, and needs. Extraction of one or more teeth may be prescribed based on the presence of one or more of the following factors: greater than 75% bone loss, Miller Class III mobility (greater than 1-mm buccolingually, or a vertical mobility) (Miller 1950), Glickman advanced Grade II or Grade III/IV (through-and-through defect) furcation invasion (Glickman 1958), recalcitrant probing depth(s) greater than 8 mm, unfavorable crown-to-root ratio, and a history of recurrent periodontal abscesses. A tooth can also be extracted for esthetic reasons or to improve the results of orthodontic treatment. When a surgical crown-lengthening procedure will lead to compromised esthetics, furcation invasion, and/or poor crown-to-root ratio, extraction is commonly advised (Becker et al. 1984; Chase Jr. and Low 1993).

Diagnosis

Diagnosis is a determination of any variations from what is considered normal. The dentist should be sensitive to the signs and symptoms presented and note any variations from normal. The dental diagnosis commonly includes a determination of the periodontal health, occlusal relationships, function of the temporomandibular joints (TMJs) and muscles of mastication, condition of edentulous areas, anatomic abnormalities, serviceability of existing prostheses and restorations, and status of the remaining dentition.

TREATMENT-PLANNING PHASE

Sequencing of the treatment plan involves the process of scheduling the necessary procedures into a time frame. Effective sequencing is critical to the success of any treatment plan. Some treatment procedures must follow others in a logical order, while other treatment procedures can or must occur concurrently. Thus, thoughtful coordination is mandatory. Complex treatment plans are commonly sequenced into phases, including a control phase, an evaluative phase, a definitive phase, and a maintenance phase.

Control Phase

The control phase is divided into two parts: an initial periodontal phase and a provisional phase. This phase is intended to remove the etiologic factors, stabilize the patient's oral health, eliminate any active periodontal disease, and resolve inflammation. In this phase, often only a tentative treatment plan can be presented to the patient. Changes commonly occur relative to the prognosis of individual teeth at the termination of this phase. The initial periodontal phase includes extraction of hopeless teeth, periodontal debridement and scaling, oral hygiene instructions, and any indicated occlusal adjustments. The provisional phase then strives to remove conditions preventing effective maintenance, beginning the preventive dentistry component of the treatment. This phase includes caries control to determine restorability of teeth, replacement or repair of defective restorations, minor tooth changes, and an endodontic evaluation of all remaining teeth.

Evaluative Phase

The evaluative phase occurs between the control and the definitive phase. It allows for resolution of inflammation and time for healing. Home-care habits are reinforced, motivation for further treatment is assessed, and all preliminary treatment is re-evaluated before definitive care is initiated.

Definitive Phase

After completing the control and the evaluative phase, the patient can enter the definitive phase. This phase begins with presenting the definitive treatment plan to the patient, including a wax replica of the proposed treatment plan. This phase is also divided into two parts: a preprosthetic phase and a prosthetic phase. The preprosthetic phase includes preprosthetic periodontal, oral surgical, endodontic, or orthodontic procedures. If implant surgery is proposed, then a computed tomographic (CT) scan is prescribed to evaluate the width and height of available bone as well as the location of vital structures, such as the inferior alveolar nerve, artery, and vein (inferior alveolar canal and mental foramen). The definitive phase is completed with the prosthetic phase for the fabrication and delivery of prostheses.

Some of the considerations and suggestions a dentist should follow when providing fixed prosthodontic treatment include the following (Morgano et al. 1989):

- A physiologic plane of occlusion
- A physiologic vertical dimension of occlusion (VDO)
- Simultaneous contacts of all anterior and posterior teeth in MIP
- A functional anterior guidance free of posterior interceptive occlusal contacts
- An unlocked arrangement of cusps and fossae that will allow comfortable jaw function
- Axial loading of posterior teeth
- The use of a material that will not unduly abrade the opposing dentition
- Narrowed occlusal tables, especially with implant-supported restorations, to minimize unfavorable leverage and bending moments

Maintenance Phase

This phase includes regular recall examinations that may reveal the need for adjustments to prevent future breakdown and provides an opportunity to reinforce home care. The frequency of this phase depends on the patient's risk for developing new dental disease. Maintenance visits are usually at three- to six-month intervals.

FINAL PROGNOSIS

The prognosis can be divided into a short- and long-term prediction, based on an educated forecast of the response to the planned treatment. It must take into account existing dental and periodontal support, vulnerability to expected disease, host resistance, the patient's adaptability, the dentist's capabilities, and expectations with regard to the patient's compliance with prescribed measures. When determining a prognosis, it should be tailored to the specific clinical situations. The prognosis can be (i) favorable, (ii) guarded (questionable), (iii) unfavorable (poor), or (iv) hopeless. The dentist should provide a treatment plan that offers a favorable prognosis (McGuire 1991).

A *favorable prognosis* implies a high probability of success based on the best available evidence. A *guarded* or *questionable prognosis* suggests that one or more mitigating factors are present that are known to adversely affect the outcome of care. As an example, an endodontically treated tooth restored with a post-and-core and crown but lacking a ferrule would have a questionable prognosis (Morgano and Brackett 1999). An *unfavorable (poor) prognosis* implies a high probability of failure. A molar with a Glickman

Grade III or IV furcation invasion will usually have a poor prognosis. Teeth with a *hopeless prognosis* cannot be treated with current materials and methods and must be extracted. An example is a pulpless tooth with a longitudinal root fracture that extends deeply into the alveolar bone.

Patients

Throughout this chapter, the Universal Numbering System has been used to designate individual teeth. Figure 6.1 summarizes and illustrates this numbering system.

Patient I

A 43-year-old woman presented to the clinic with a chief complaint of, "I don't like my smile" (Figures 6.2 and 6.3).

Diagnostic Phase

The patient's medical history was noncontributory. She did not have any known drug or food allergies. She did not smoke and drank alcohol only occasionally. Her dental history included orthodontic treatment that was performed many years previously to move the maxillary canines into the positions of the lateral incisors. She brushed twice per day and did not use dental floss. Extraoral examination revealed no cervical or submandibular lymphadenopathy and no signs of temporomandibular disorders (TMD) or reports of muscle pain.

The intraoral and radiographic examinations noted the following (Figures 6.4 and 6.5):

• Missing Nos. 1, 5, 16, 17, and 32 and congenitally missing Nos. 7, 10, 20, and 19

• Maxillary canines in the position of the lateral incisors and restored with metal-ceramic crowns to mimic lateral incisors

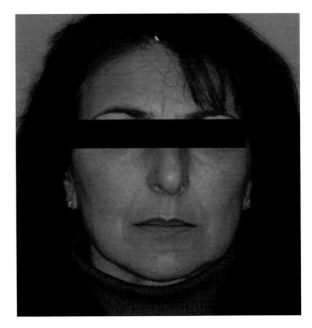

Figure 6.2 Full-face frontal view of patient.

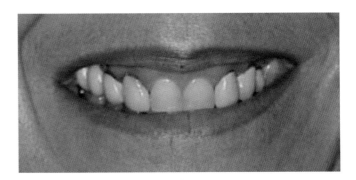

Figure 6.3 Smile line.

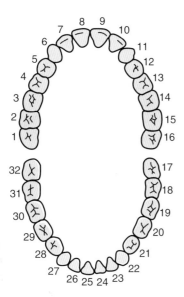

Figure 6.1 Numbering system used in this chapter.

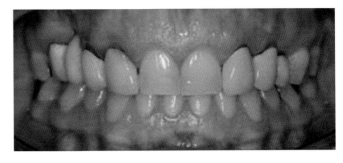

Figure 6.4 Intraoral view.

• MO silver amalgam restorations, Nos. 2, 15, 30, and 31

• Metal-ceramic fixed partial dentures (FPDs), Nos. 3-x-5-6, and splinted crowns, Nos. 12-13-14

• MOD silver amalgam restoration, No. 16

• Defective MO silver amalgam restoration, No. 18

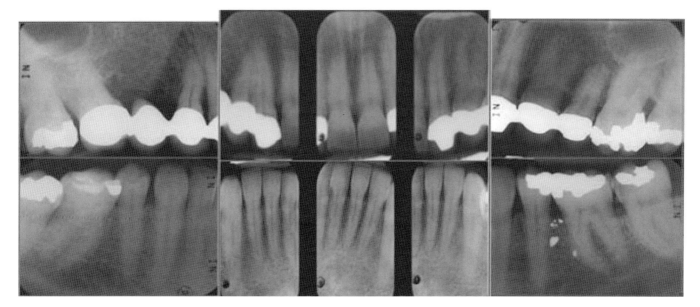

Figure 6.5 Complete-mouth radiographs.

- DO silver amalgam restoration, No. 20

- Occlusal silver amalgam restoration, No. 30

- Generalized inflammation with supragingival calculus in the mandibular anterior

- Bony defect, site No. 4 (extraction site)

- Probing depths within normal range for most teeth with the exception of teeth No. 3 (distal 5 mm) and No. 14 (distal 5 mm) (Figure 6.6)

- Rotated tooth, No. 12

- Absence of hypermobility or furcation invasion

The diagnosis for this patient was as follows:

- Generalized chronic mild gingivitis

- Localized chronic moderate periodontitis

- Partial edentulism

- Multiple defective dental restorations

Treatment-Planning Phases

The objectives of therapy for this patient were elimination of the etiologic factors (open margins and defective restorations), control and resolution of periodontal inflammation,

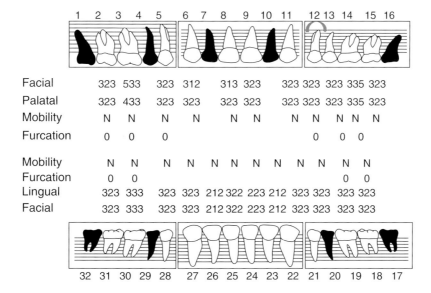

Figure 6.6 Periodontal charting.

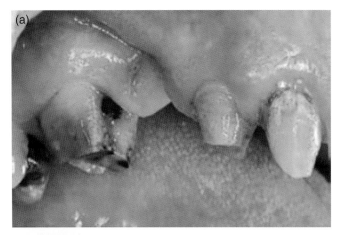

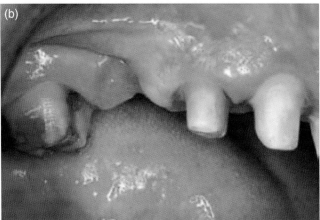

Figure 6.7 (a) Teeth Nos. 3, 5, and 6 after removal of defective restorations. (b) Teeth after repreparation.

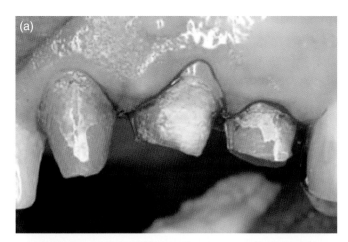

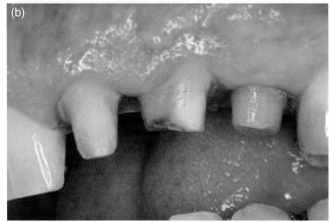

Figure 6.8 (a) Teeth Nos. 11, 12, and 13 after removal of defective restorations. (b) Teeth after repreparation.

and restoration of esthetics and function. Initially, only a tentative treatment plan was presented to the patient. This plan included the removal of artificial crowns, evaluation of the restorability of teeth, and plaque control measures.

Initial Periodontal Phase

This phase included scaling and root planing on the distal surfaces of Nos. 3 and 14, oral hygiene instructions, and reevaluation of any pocket reduction and oral hygiene.

Provisional Phase

In the provisional phase, the defective fixed restorations were removed (Figures 6.7 and 6.8) and replaced with physiologically and esthetically acceptable provisional restorations.

In evaluating the gingival line in the maxillae, a gingival line discrepancy was noted that was caused by the pontic

in the area of No. 4. This discrepancy compromised the overall esthetic appearance and contributed to plaque accumulation. There was also a gingival line discrepancy between the central incisors and the lateral incisors because the lateral incisors were originally canines that were orthodontically repositioned.

In addition, there was a gingival line discrepancy between Nos. 11, 12, and 13 (Figure 6.9). Based on these findings, a definitive treatment plan was presented to the patient. This plan was (Figure 6.10) as follows:

- Soft tissue augmentation, area No. 4
- Microsurgical crown lengthening procedure, Nos. 8 and 9 for esthetic purposes
- Surgical crown-lengthening procedure, No. 13 for esthetic purposes
- Metal-ceramic FPD, No. 3-x-5

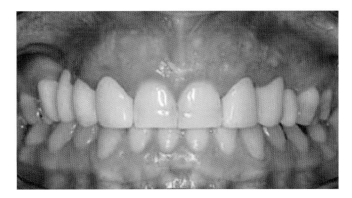

Figure 6.9 Provisional restorations, Nos. 3-x-5, 6, 11, 12, and 13. Note the gingival line discrepancies at sites Nos. 3-x-5, 8-9, and 11-12-13.

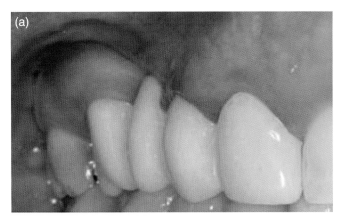

(a)

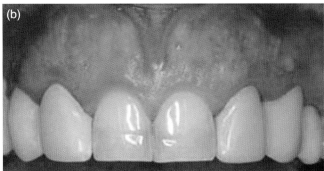

(b)

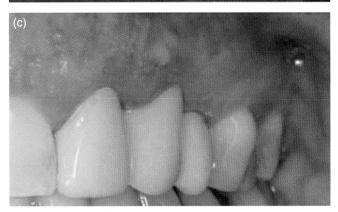

(c)

Figure 6.10 Preprosthetic treatment plan: (a) Soft tissue augmentation, area No. 4. (b) Microsurgical crown-lengthening procedure, Nos. 8 and 9, for esthetic purposes. (c) Crown-lengthening procedure, No. 13, for esthetic purposes.

- Ceramic crowns, Nos. 6 and 11

- Porcelain laminate veneers, Nos. 8 and 9

- Metal-ceramic crowns, Nos. 12 and 13

Preprosthetic Periodontal Phase

Soft tissue inlay graft, site No. 4. A split-thickness flap was elevated. Soft tissue augmentation for site No. 4 was accomplished by using an autogenous connective tissue inlay graft obtained from the patient's palate. The graft was sutured and secured to the periosteum. The flap was positioned and sutured without tension. The tissue surface of the pontic was relieved in the area of the surgical site to prevent tissue impingement. The pontic was relined eight weeks after surgery with autopolymerizing acrylic resin (Coldpac; the Motloid Co., Chicago, IL, USA) to allow gentle pressure on the graft to contour the soft tissue at the pontic site and develop an esthetic gingival line. The pontic was relined again one week later to allow for additional contouring of the gingival line (Figure 6.11).

Surgical crown lengthening, No. 13. A submarginal incision was made at the anticipated gingival line and a full-thickness flap was elevated. Ostectomy was performed to allow a 3-mm distance between the anticipated gingival line and the crest of the alveolar bone (Rosenberg et al. 1980). The flap was repositioned and sutured with 4-0 chromic gut sutures (Figure 6.12).

Surgical crown lengthening, Nos. 8 and 9. Surgical crown lengthening was required for esthetic reasons on the facial surfaces of Nos. 8 and 9 only (Figure 6.13).

To preserve the papillae and the soft tissue around Nos. 7 and 10, a microsurgical crown-lengthening procedure was performed. There are many advantages of this technique when compared with conventional surgical crown-lengthening procedures (Dibart and Karima 2006). This procedure:

- Is less invasive

- Requires smaller incisions

- Allows greater precision when closing wounds

- Is less traumatic

- Is less painful postoperatively

- Allows faster healing and vascularization

- Produces more predictable results in areas with very thin gingiva or in the "esthetic zone"

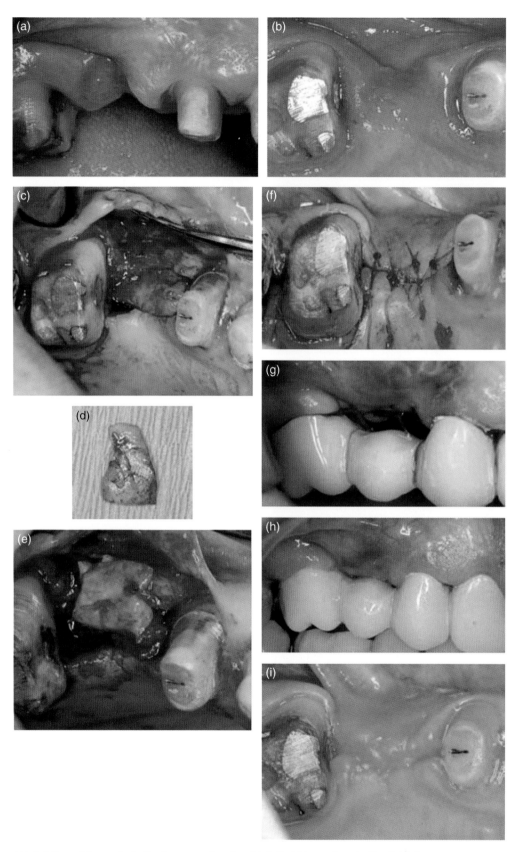

Figure 6.11 (a and b) Soft tissue inlay graft site No. 4, preoperative view. (c) Split-thickness flap site No. 4. (d) Connective tissue graft obtained from the patient's palate. (e) Graft sutured to the periosteum with chromic gut sutures. (f and g) Flap sutured without tension. (h) One week after surgery. (i) Two months after surgery.

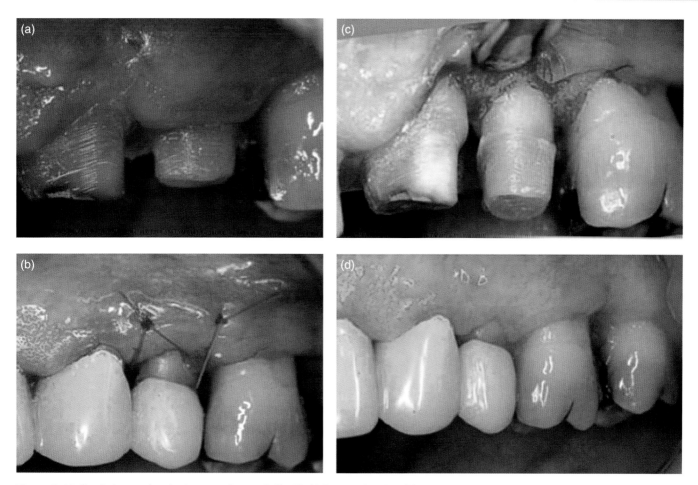

Figure 6.12 Surgical crown lengthening procedure tooth No. 13. (a) Preoperative view. (b) 3-mm distance allowed between anticipated finish line of crown preparation and alveolar crest. (c) Site sutured with vertical mattress technique and 4–0 chromic gut sutures. (d) Two weeks after surgery.

Prosthetic Phase

Figure 6.14 is a wax replica of the proposed treatment plan.

Two months after completion of all periodontal surgical procedures, the margins for all crown preparations were finalized, and Nos. 8 and 9 were prepared for porcelain laminate veneers (Figure 6.15).

New provisional restorations were fabricated, relined, and cemented with temporary cement (Temp Bond; Kerr, Romulus, MI, USA) (Figure 6.16).

One week later, a final impression was made with polyether impression material (Permadyne Penta L and Impregum Penta; 3M ESPE, Seefeld, Germany) (Figure 6.17).

A face-bow record was made and jaw relation records at MIP were made. A definitive cast was fabricated, along with a cast of the provisional restorations, and these casts were mounted in an articulator (Mark II Denar; Water Pik Technologies, Fort Collins, CO, USA). The shade was

selected (Vita B1) (VITAPAN Classical Shade Guide; H Rauter GmbH & Co., Sackinggen, Germany). Porcelain laminate veneers for Nos. 8 and 9, zirconia copings for Nos. 6 and 11, metal copings for No. 12 and 13, and a metal framework for No. 3-x-5 were made. All copings and castings were tried in the mouth, and the fit was verified with black and white silicone disclosing material (Fit Checker; GC Corporation, Tokyo, Japan) (Figure 6.18).

The veneers were luted with resin cement (Variolink II, Ivoclar Vitadent, Amherst, NY, USA). The provisional restorations for Nos. 3-x-5, 12, and 13 were recemented with Temp Bond cement. Because the resin luting agent requires an average of two weeks for the shade to mature beneath the veneers, the final shade selection for the remaining restorations was delayed. The final determination after two weeks was Vita A2 (Figure 6.19).

At that stage, the application of porcelain to the remainder of the restorations was accomplished with Vita A2 porcelain. Restorations were glazed and the metal was polished. At the day of final delivery, provisional restorations were removed.

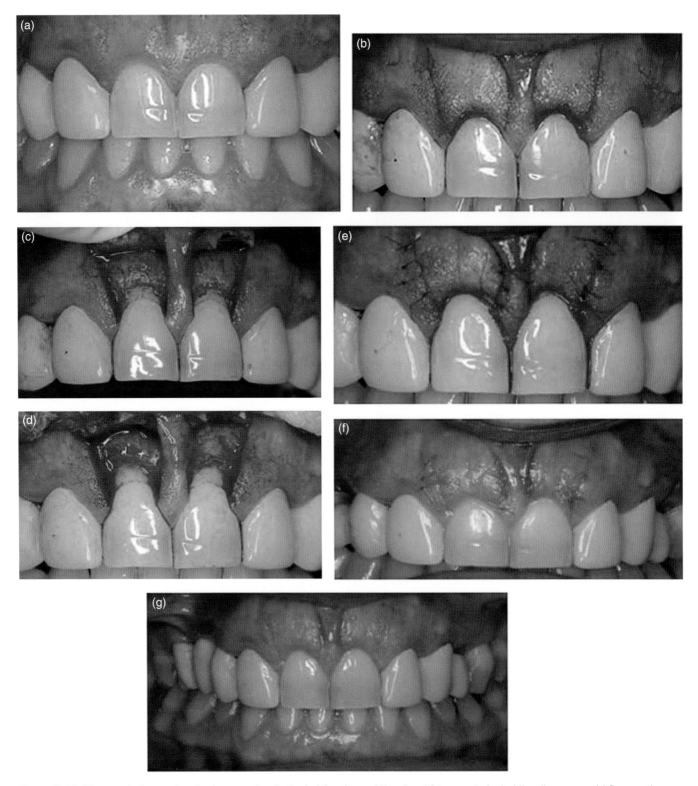

Figure 6.13 Microsurgical crown-lengthening procedure for the facial surfaces of Nos. 8 and 9 to correct gingival line discrepancy. (a) Preoperative view. (b) Vertical incisions at the line angles of Nos. 8 and 9 by using a microsurgical blade. (c) Full-thickness flap elevated. (d) Ostectomy completed. (e) Flaps sutured with 7-0 Vicryl sutures. (f) One week after surgery. (g) Two weeks after surgery.

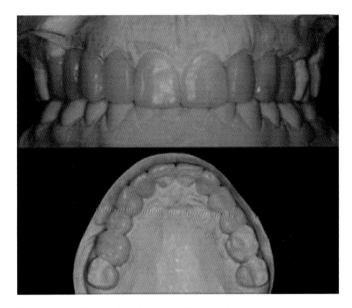

Figure 6.14 Wax replica of proposed treatment plan.

A cleaning solution (Cavidry; Parkell, Farmingdale, NY, USA) was applied to all preparations to remove any oily residue, and clinical try-in of all restorations was completed. A resin-modified glass ionomer cement (Rely-X Luting; 3M ESPE) was used for final cementation of all restorations (Figures 6.20–6.23) two months after completion of all periodontal surgical procedures.

Maintenance Phase

The maintenance phase included recall visits every four months.

Prognosis

The overall prognosis for the treatment provided (short and long term) is favorable.

Patient II

A 70-year-old man presented to the clinic with a chief complaint of, "I need some implants for my lower jaw. My other dentist just finished all my upper teeth last year, and he sent me to you for the implants" (Figure 0.24).

Diagnostic Phase

The patient's medical history was noncontributory. He did not have any known drug or food allergies. He had a previous history of smoking for 30 years, but for the past 3 years he has been using a nicotine patch and nicotine supplement gum. He had been smoke-free since then. He drank alcohol occasionally. His dental history included multiple extractions and fixed restorations. Extraoral examination revealed no cervical or submandibular lymphadenopathy and no signs of TMD or reports of muscle pain.

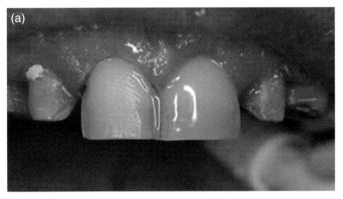

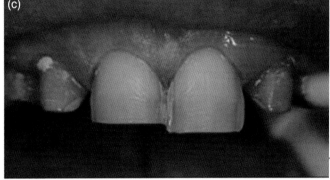

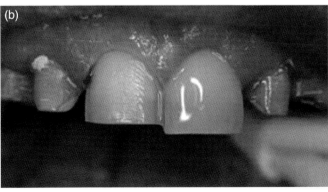

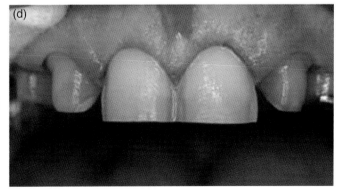

Figure 6.15 Preparations for veneers, Nos. 8 and 9.

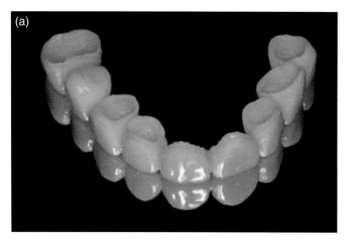 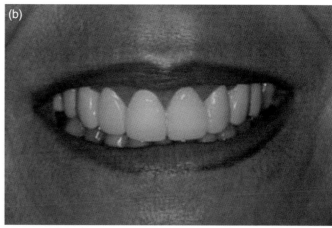

Figure 6.16 Provisional restoration, Nos. 3-x-5-6-8-9-11-12-13. (a) After contouring. (b) In the mouth.

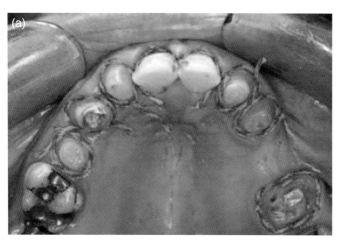 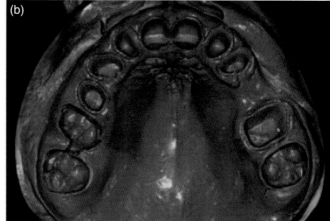

Figure 6.17 (a) Gingival displacement cord in place. (b) Final impression with polyether impression material.

The intraoral and radiographic examinations revealed the following (Figures 6.25 and 6.26):

- Missing, Nos. 1, 2, 3, 5, 14, 15, 16, 17, 19, 21, 23, 24, 25, 26, 29, 30, and 32

- Metal-ceramic FPD, Nos. 4-x-6

- Metal-ceramic crowns, Nos. 7, 8, 9, 10, 11, 12, and 13

- Defective metal-ceramic FPD, 22-x-x-x-x-27-28

- MOD silver amalgam restorations, Nos. 18 and 31

- Inadequate endodontic therapy, No. 20 with defective restoration

- Normal probing depths (between 2 and 3 mm), without bleeding upon probing, except for No. 18 where the probing depths were 6 mm on the mesial surface and 5 mm on the distal surface

- No hypermobility of the teeth or furcation invasions, except for No. 18, which had Class II hypermobility and Grade III furcation invasion

Maxillary and mandibular alginate impressions were made, along with a face-bow transfer and centric jaw relation record. The diagnostic casts were mounted in a semi-adjustable articulator.

The diagnosis for this patient was as follows:

- Generalized mild gingivitis with localized moderate periodontitis, No. 18

- Partial edentulism

- Recurrent dental caries

- Defective dental restorations

- Inadequate endodontic treatment

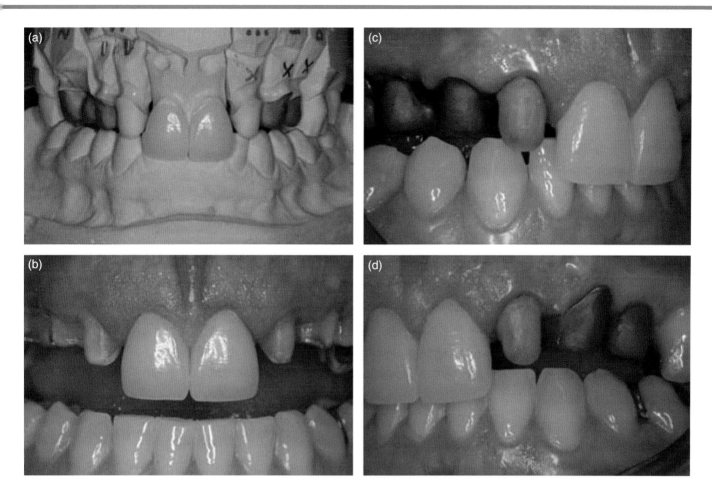

Figure 6.18 Porcelain laminate veneers, Nos. 8 and 9, on cast (a) and bonded (b). (c) Cast framework for FPD, Nos. 3-x-5, and zirconia coping, No. 6. (d) Zirconia coping, No. 11, and castings for crowns, Nos. 12 and 13.

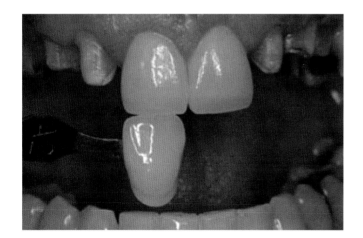

Figure 6.19 Two weeks after cementation of veneers, shade was selected (Vita A2).

Treatment-Planning Phases

The treatment plan for this patient included the following:

- Extraction of Nos. 18, 20, and 31

- Implant-supported metal-ceramic crowns, sites Nos. 19-20-21 (immediate implant placement for No. 20), and 29

- Replacement of the defective metal-ceramic FPD, Nos. 22-x-x-x-x-27-28, to restore esthetics and function

Initial Periodontal Phase

The initial periodontal phase included complete-mouth prophylaxis and oral hygiene instructions.

Preprosthetic Periodontal Phase

For the preprosthetic periodontal phase, a CT scan was prescribed and the proposed implant sites (Nos. 19, 20, 21, and 29) were evaluated (Figure 6.27).

Tooth No. 20 was extracted, and implants were placed at sites Nos. 19, 20 (immediate implant placement, No. 20), 21, and 29 (Figure 6.28). Implants were uncovered four months after placement, and healing abutments were placed (Figure 6.29).

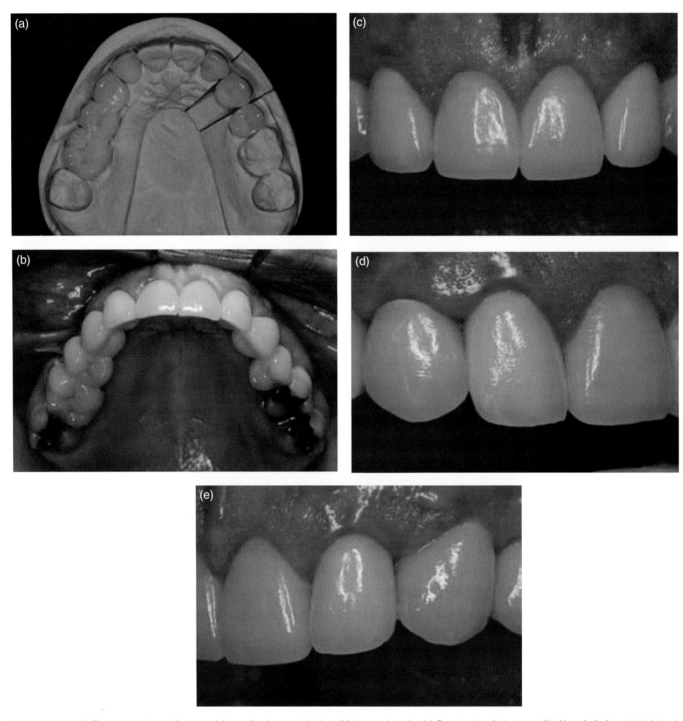

Figure 6.20 (a) Final restorations after porcelain application and glazing. (b) Intraoral try-in. (c) Corrected soft tissue profile Nos. 6, 8, 9, and 11. (d and e) All-ceramic crowns Nos. 6 and 11 with the clinical appearance of missing Nos. 7 and 10.

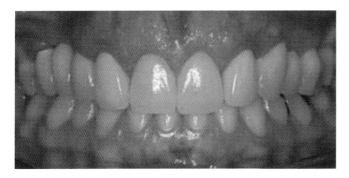

Figure 6.21 Intraoral view of final restorations.

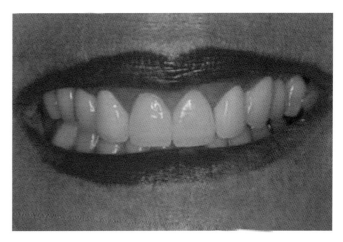

Figure 6.22 Postoperative view of the new smile line.

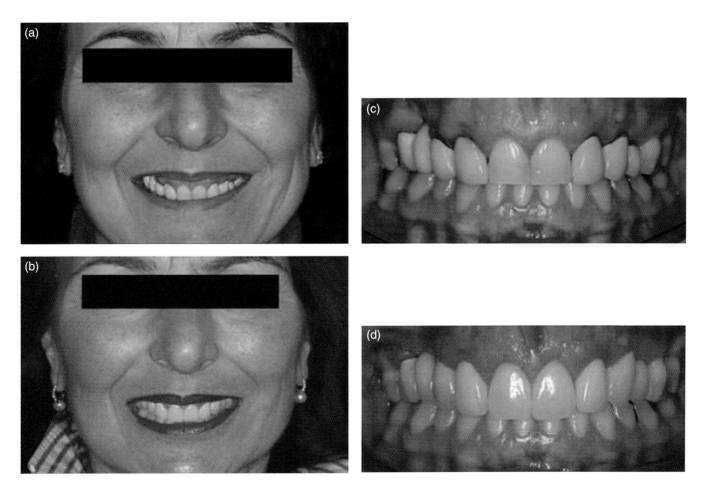

Figure 6.23 Before (a) and after (b) (full-face view). Before (c) and after (d) (close-up view).

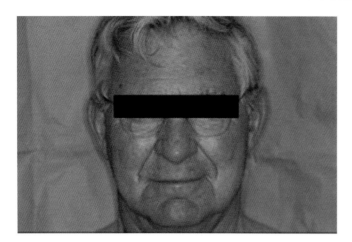

Figure 6.24 Full-face frontal view of patient.

Provisional Phase

The defective metal-ceramic FPD Nos. 22-x-x-x-x-27-28 was removed (Figure 6.30).

After removal, it was discovered that No. 22 had a horizontal coronal fracture. Endodontic therapy was completed. A custom-cast post-and-core was made for No. 22 and cemented with zinc phosphate cement (Zinc Cement; Patterson Brand, Saint Paul, MN, USA) (Figure 6.31).

An impression of the mandibular arch (implants Nos. 19, 20, 21, and 29 and all natural teeth) was made with polyether impression material (Permadyne Pental L and Impregum Penta) (Figure 6.32).

Alginate impression material (Jeltrate; Dentsply, Melford, DE, USA) was used for the maxillary arch. A face-bow transfer was made, and a centric jaw relation record was made for the fabrication of the provisional restorations (Figure 6.33).

The surgical mounts for the dental implants were prepared to be used as provisional abutments (Figure 6.34).

A wax replica of the proposed treatment plan was prepared, and the wax pattern was invested and heat processed to produce an acrylic resin (Namilon; Justi, Oxnard, CA, USA) provisional restoration (Figure 6.35).

The provisional FPD was cemented with Temp Bond cement (Figure 6.36).

Prosthetic Phase

Two weeks later, the patient presented for definitive impressions with polyether impression material (Permadyne Pental L and Impregum Penta) (Figure 6.37).

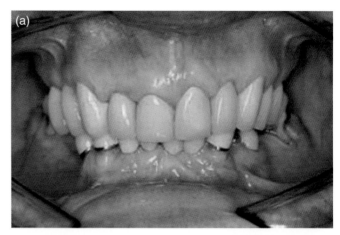

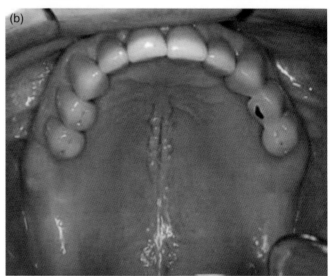

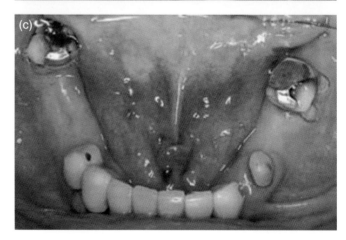

Figure 6.25 Intraoral views. (a) MIP. (b) Maxillary arch. (c) Mandibular arch.

A centric jaw relation record was completed, and the mandibular cast was mounted. An alginate impression (Jeltrate) of the mandibular provisional restorations was made for the dental laboratory technician to use as a guide in the fabrication of the final restorations (Figure 6.38).

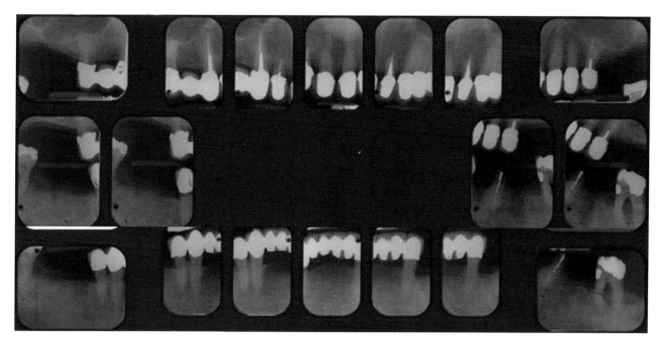

Figure 6.26 Complete-mouth radiographs.

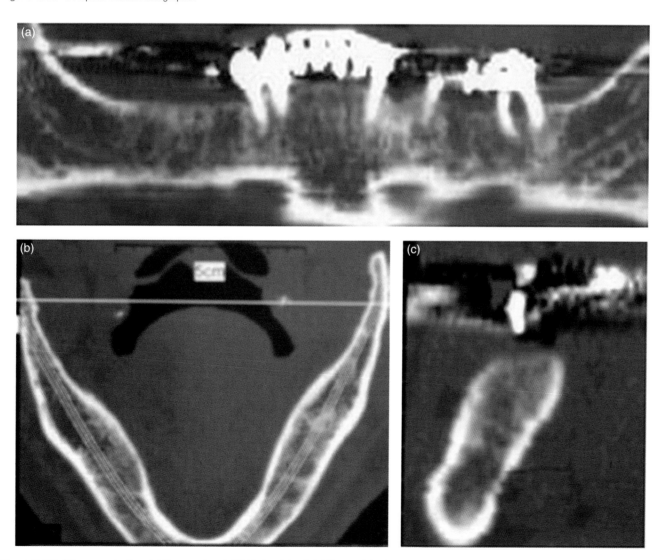

Figure 6.27 CT scan evaluation. (a) Panoramic cut. (b) Horizontal cut. (c) Segmental cut.

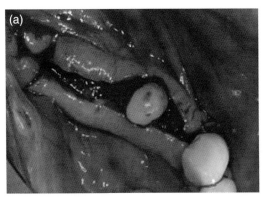
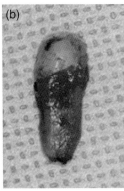
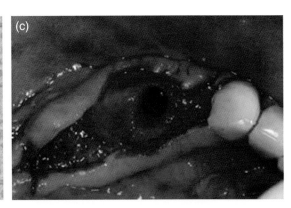

Figure 6.28 Preprosthetic phase. Tooth No. 20 was extracted atraumatically. (a) Incision. (b) Extracted tooth. (c) Undamaged socket (then implants were placed, Nos. 19, 20, 21, and 29).

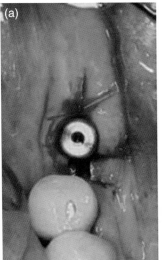
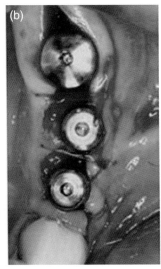

Figure 6.29 Implants were uncovered four months later. (a) Right side. (b) Left side.

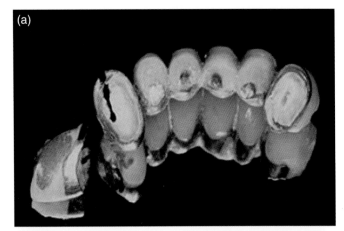
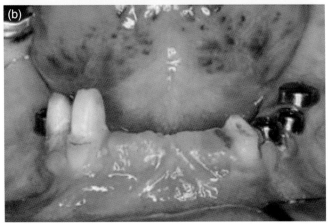

Figure 6.30 (a) Removal of defective FPD Nos. 22-x-x-x-27-28. (b) Horizontal tooth fracture No. 22 was noted.

A clear plastic, vacuum-formed shell of the mandibular provisional restoration was also provided to the dental laboratory technician as a three-dimensional guide for the fabrication of the custom abutments (Figure 6.39).

Metal castings and frameworks were fabricated. The fit of all metal castings was verified with silicone disclosing material (Fit Checker). The selected shade was Vita A2 (Figure 6.40).

Metal castings and frameworks were returned to the dental laboratory for porcelain application (Figure 6.41). Canine guidance was established for the dynamic occlusal scheme (Figure 6.42). Final delivery of the fixed prostheses was completed by using zinc phosphate cement (Zinc Cement) for the cementation of the tooth-supported FPD and by using Temp Bond cement

for the cementation of implant-supported restorations (Figures 6.43–6.45).

Maintenance Phase

The maintenance phase included recall visits every three to four months.

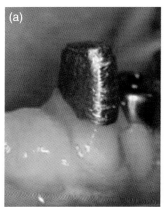
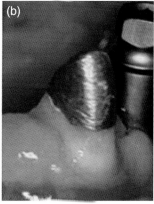

Figure 6.31 Cast post-and-core. (a) Try-in. (b) Delivery.

Prognosis

The overall prognosis for the treatment provided (short- and long-term) is favorable.

Patient III

A 40-year-old woman presented to the clinic with a chief complaint of, "I need new crowns, and I want a better smile" (Figure 6.46).

Diagnostic Phase

The patient's medical history was noncontributory. She did not have any known drug or food allergies. She did not smoke or drink alcohol. Her dental history included multiple extractions and multiple restorations performed outside of the United States in 2001. She brushed twice per day and did not use dental floss. Extraoral examination revealed no cervical or submandibular lymphadenopathy and no signs of TMD or reports of muscle pain.

The intraoral and radiographic examinations noted the following (Figures 6.47 and 6.48):

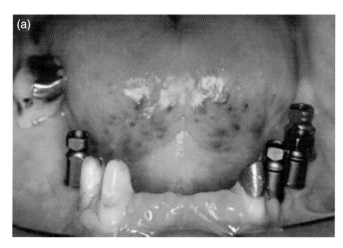
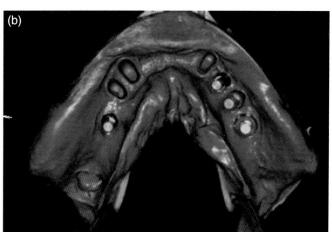

Figure 6.32 Impression was made for fabrication of provisional restorations. (a) Impression copings in place. (b) Impression.

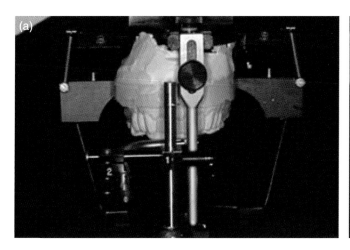
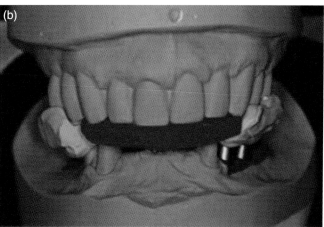
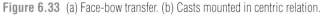

Figure 6.33 (a) Face-bow transfer. (b) Casts mounted in centric relation.

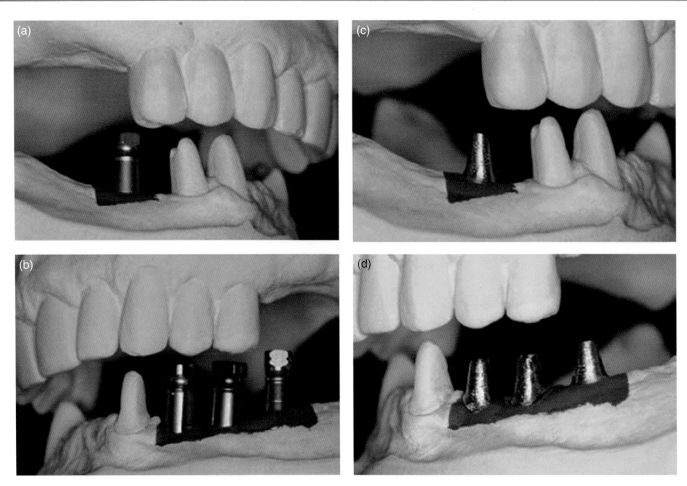

Figure 6.34 Surgical mounts (a and b) of the dental implants were prepared to be used as temporary abutments (c and d).

- Generalized redness, edema, and glazing of the gingiva, especially in the maxillary anterior sextant
- Missing, Nos. 1, 3, 5, 9, 13, 14, 17, 18, 19, 28, 30, and 32
- Multiple defective restorations, Nos. 2-x-4-x-6, Nos. 7-8-x-10, and Nos. x-29-x-31
- Endodontic therapy, Nos. 4, 7, 11, 29, and 31
- Periapical radiolucency, No. 29
- Inadequate endodontic therapy, No. 31
- Occlusal silver amalgam restoration, No. 16 with mesial and distobuccal carious lesions
- Mesial drift, Nos. 15 and 16
- Defective restorations, dental caries, and inadequate endodontic therapy, Nos. 20 and 21

- Distal carious lesions, Nos. 22 and 27
- Probing depths within the normal range (2–3 mm), except for teeth Nos. 4, 6, 10, 11, and 15, where probing depths ranged between 4 and 5 mm (Figure 6.49)
- Generalized bleeding upon probing
- No hypermobility or furcation invasions (Figure 6.49)
- Multiple defective FPDs
- Multiple teeth with inadequate endodontic therapy
- Localized bone loss (10–15%), distal surface of No. 15 and the mesial surface of No. 10 (Figure 6.48)

Impressions were made with alginate (Jeltrate). Her diagnostic casts were mounted in centric relation in a semi-adjustable articulator with a face-bow record (Figure 6.50).

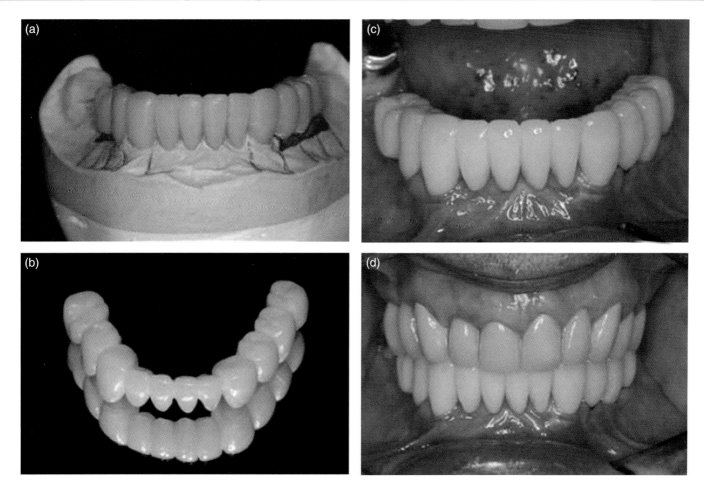

Figure 6.35 (a) Wax replica of the mandibular arch. (b) Heat processed provisional restoration. (c and d) Provisional restoration after reline and temporary cementation.

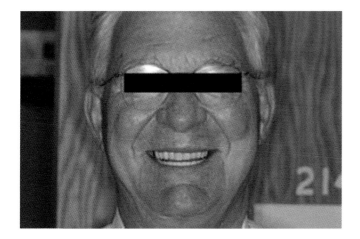

Figure 6.36 Patient's smile after provisional restorations were placed.

The diagnosis for this patient was as follows:

- Generalized moderate chronic gingivitis
- Localized moderate chronic periodontitis, No. 15
- Partial edentulism
- Defective dental restorations
- Carious lesions
- Chronic periradicular periodontitis, No. 29

The etiologic factors contributing to this diagnosis were bacterial plaque as the primary factor and previous dentistry and patient neglect as secondary factors.

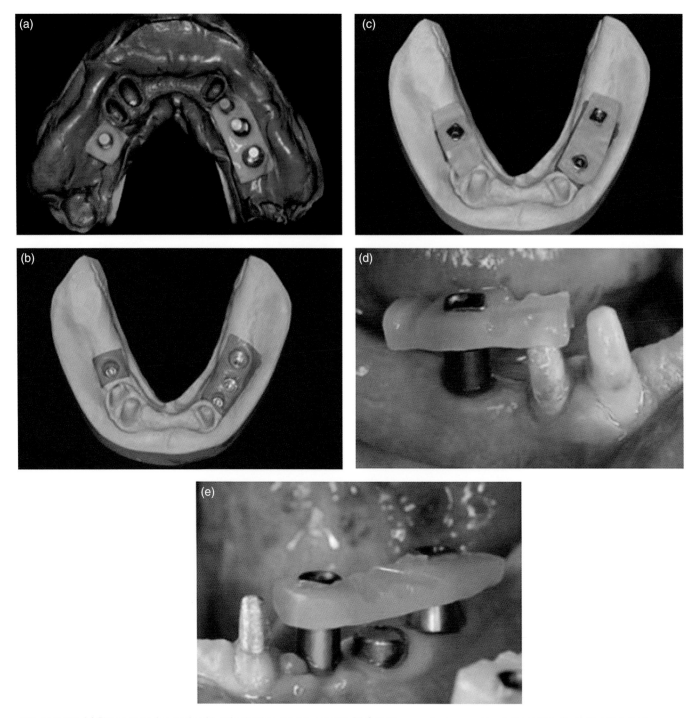

Figure 6.37 (a) Final impression made with polyether impression material. (b) Soft tissue replicas around implant analogs. (c–e) Fixed bilateral mandibular record bases for centric relation record.

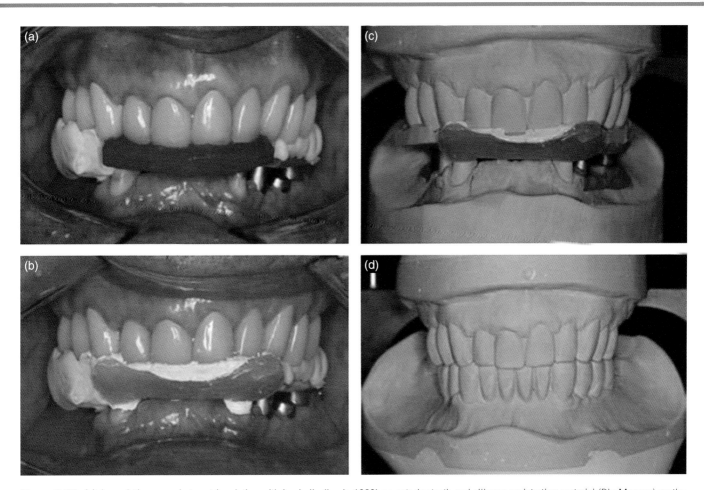

Figure 6.38 (a) Jaw relation record at centric relation with Lucia jig (Lucia 1983) on anterior teeth and silicone registration material (Blu Mousse) on the posterior teeth. (b) Lucia jig was then replaced with hard wax and relined with Temp Bond cement for stability of the casts during the mounting. (c) Casts mounted. (d) Diagnostic cast of existing mandibular provisional restoration was also mounted.

Treatment-Planning Phase

The objectives of therapy for this patient were elimination of the etiologic factors (open margins, overcontoured artificial crowns, inadequate endodontic therapy, and dental caries), control and resolution of periodontal inflammation, and restoration of esthetics and function.

Initially, only a tentative treatment plan could be presented to the patient. This plan, according to the diagnostic waxing, included the following (Figure 6.51):

• Removal of artificial crowns to evaluate the restorability of the teeth and to eliminate plaque retentive factors

• Extraction of No. 16

• Metal-ceramic FPDs, Nos. 2-x-4-x-6, 12-x-15, 27-x-29-x-31, and 8-x-10

• Metal-ceramic crowns, Nos. 7, 11, 20, and 21

• Endodontic retreatment, cast posts-and-cores, and metal-ceramic crowns, Nos. 7, 20, 21, 29, and 31

Initial Periodontal Phase

This phase included complete-mouth dental prophylaxis with scaling and root planing on the distal surface of No. 15, oral hygiene instructions, re-evaluation of oral hygiene and pocket reduction, three to four weeks after the initial therapy.

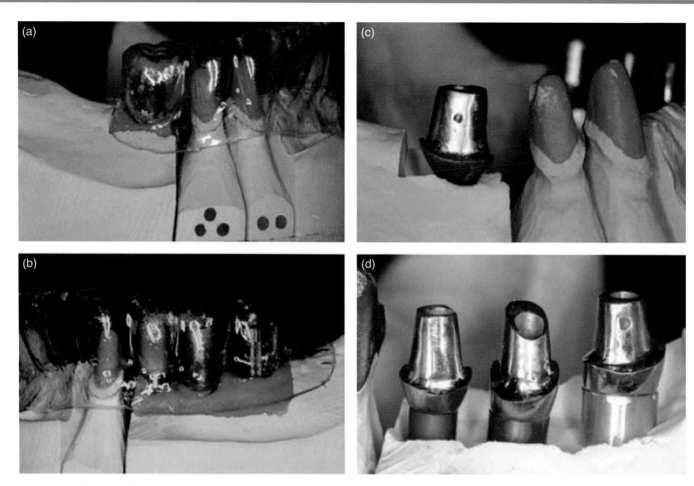

Figure 6.39 (a and b) Clear vacuum-formed shell of duplicate cast of patient's provisional restoration to be used as a three-dimensional guide for fabrication of custom abutments. (c and d) Milled custom abutments.

Provisional Phase

The purpose of the provisional phase was the elimination of the etiologic factors and the maintenance of the health of the treated periodontium. The defective fixed restorations were removed, and caries control was completed to evaluate the remaining teeth and determine their restorability and prognosis. At this stage, it was determined that all of her abutment teeth were restorable except for No. 4. Tooth No. 4 was compromised because of limited remaining tooth structure and deep subgingival margins (Figure 6.52).

A crown-lengthening procedure would lead to furcation exposure and an unfavorable crown-to-root ratio. The recommended treatment was extraction of No. 4 and replacement with an implant-supported metal-ceramic crown. Caries control and temporization for teeth Nos. 20 and 21 were completed. Evaluation of the abutments indicated that surgical crown lengthening was required in the interproximal area between Nos. 20 and 21 (Figure 6.53).

As a result of meticulous oral hygiene and replacement of the defective fixed restorations with physiologically and esthetically acceptable provisional restorations, the tissue health improved within two weeks, and the patient was satisfied with her appearance (Figure 6.54). A gingival line discrepancy was noted between Nos. 8 and 9 (Figure 6.55).

At this stage, the definitive treatment plan was presented to the patient (Figures 6.56 and 6.57).

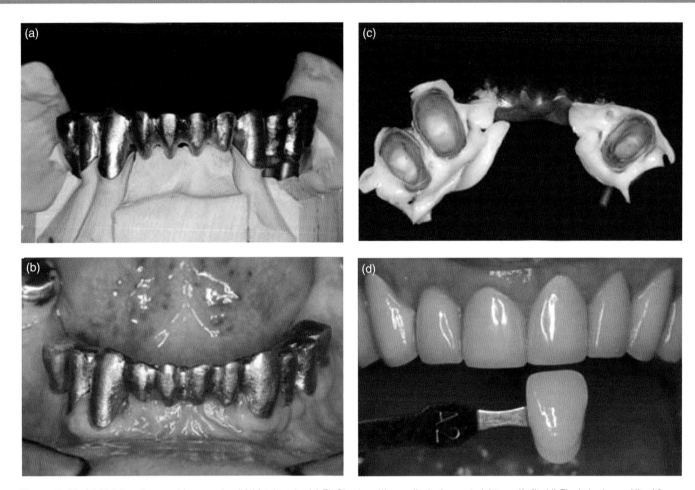

Figure 6.40 (a) Metal castings and frameworks. (b) Metal try-in. (c) Fit Checker silicone disclosing material to verify fit. (d) Final shade was Vita A2.

The treatment plan consisted of the following:

- Extraction of No. 16

- Metal-ceramic FPD, Nos. 8-x-10, 12-x-15

- Metal-ceramic crowns, Nos. 2, 6, 11, 20, 21, and 27

- Implant-supported metal-ceramic crowns, Nos. 3-4-5, 18-19, 28, and 31

- Surgical crown-lengthening procedure, Nos. 6–11

- Endodontic retreatment, cast posts-and-cores, and metal-ceramic crowns, Nos. 7, 20, 21, 29, and 31

The patient accepted the proposed treatment plan for the maxillae, but because of financial constraints, she accepted an alternative treatment plan for the mandible that included the following:

- Endodontic retreatment, Nos. 20, 21, 29, and 31

- Metal-ceramic crowns, Nos. 20 and 21

- Metal-ceramic FPD, Nos. 27-x-29-x-31

Preprosthetic Periodontal Phase

After the definitive treatment plan was presented to the patient, the patient entered phase III of the treatment, which was the preprosthetic periodontal phase. This phase began with surgical crown lengthening in the anterior sextant to obtain more crown length and to improve esthetics. A surgical guide was used (Figure 6.58).

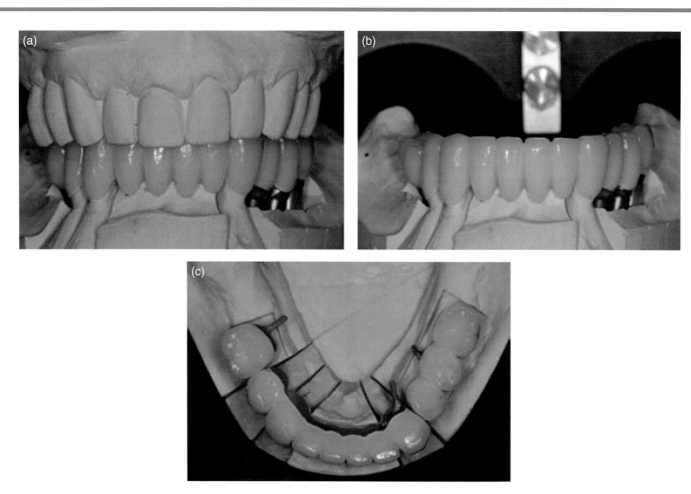

Figure 6.41 Restorations after porcelain application. (a) In occlusion. (b) Frontal view. (c) Occlusal view.

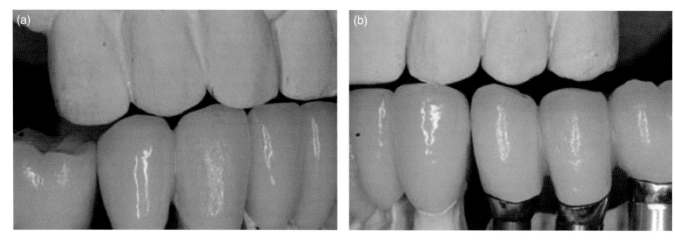

Figure 6.42 Canine guidance. (a) Right side. (b) Left side.

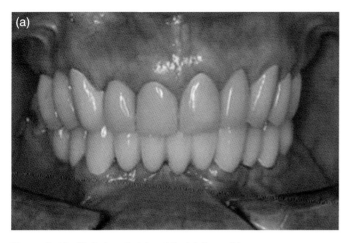

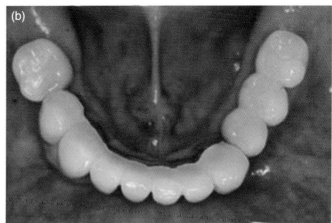

Figure 6.43 Clinical try-in (a) and final delivery (b).

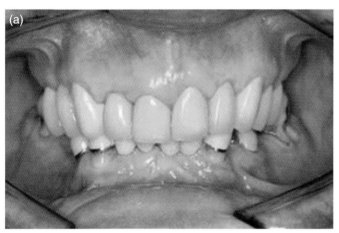

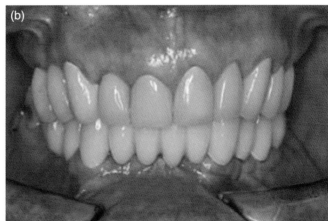

Figure 6.44 Intraoral view before (a) and after (b) treatment.

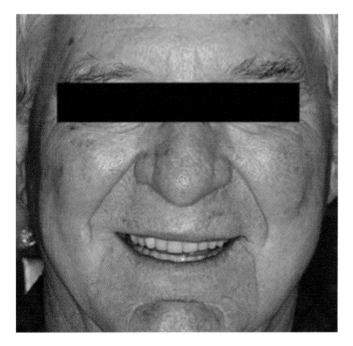

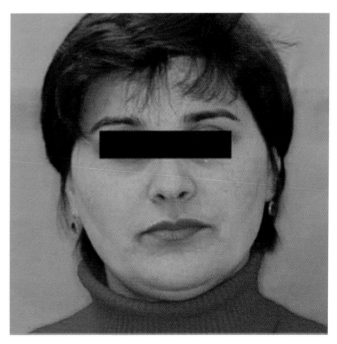

Figure 6.45 Patient's smile after treatment.

Figure 6.46 Full-face frontal view of patient.

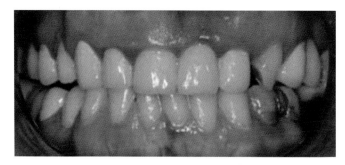

Figure 6.47 Intraoral view.

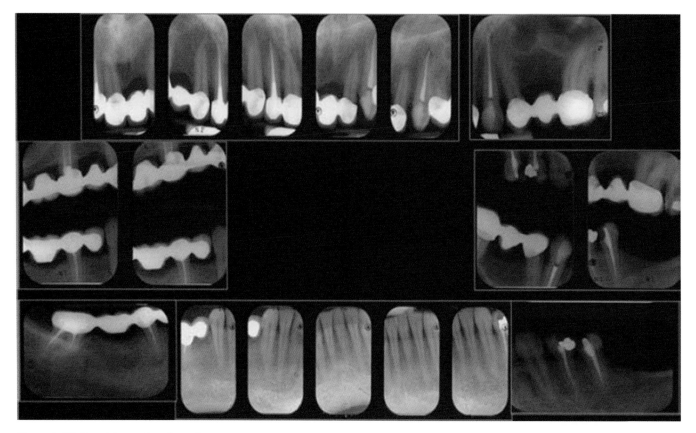

Figure 6.48 Complete-mouth radiographs.

A full-thickness flap was elevated and ostectomy was performed to obtain a 3-mm distance between the anticipated gingival line Pas displayed in the template and the osseous crest, allowing space for the supracrestal gingival tissues. The flap was placed at the desired position and sutured with a vertical mattress technique by using 4-0 chromic gut sutures (Figure 6.59).

After crown-lengthening procedures, a minimal healing period of six weeks was required before repreparation of the teeth and relining of the provisional restorations because 12 days are required for the junctional epithelium to form, but the lamina propria is not completely formed until six weeks (Listgarten 1972a, 1972b) (Figure 6.60). This patient also required a surgical crown lengthening

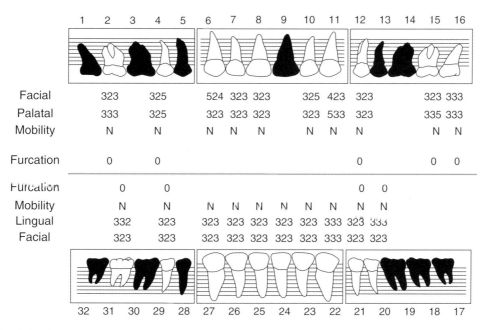

	1	2	3	4	5	6	7	8	9	10	11	12	13	14	15	16
Facial		323		325		524	323	323		325	423	323			323	333
Palatal		333		325		323	323	323		323	533	323			335	333
Mobility		N		N		N	N	N		N	N	N			N	N
Furcation		0		0								0			0	0

	32	31	30	29	28	27	26	25	24	23	22	21	20	19	18	17
Furcation		0		0								0	0			
Mobility		N		N		N	N	N	N	N	N	N	N			
Lingual		332		323		323	323	323	323	323	333	323	333			
Facial		323		323		323	323	323	323	323	333	323	323			

Figure 6.49 Periodontal charting.

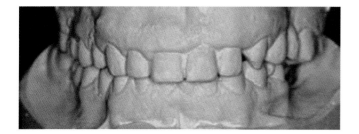

Figure 6.50 Diagnostic casts.

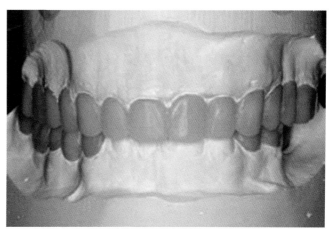

Figure 6.51 Wax replica of tentative treatment plan.

procedure for Nos. 20 and 21. This procedure was required primarily in the interproximal area to ensure sufficient height of tooth structure to develop an acceptable ferrule effect. After flap elevation, ostectomy was completed, and the area was sutured with a vertical mattress technique and 4-0 chromic gut sutures (Figure 6.61).

The last phase of the preprosthetic periodontal phase was the implant phase for sites Nos. 3, 4, and 5. For this phase, the patient was referred for a CT scan with a dual-purpose template (Figure 6.62).

The CT scan was evaluated for the selection of the size of the implants (Figure 6.63).

For site No. 3, the available bone width was 5 mm and the height was 4 mm. The implant size planned for this site was 4 × 11.5 mm. Because of the location of the maxillary sinus and the width of the bone, the treatment plan for this site included a sinus floor elevation along with buccal augmentation of the residual alveolar bone with demineralized freeze-dried bone allograft (DFDBA; ACE Surgical, Brockton, MA, USA) and bovine bone (Bio-Oss; Osteohealth, Shirley, VA, USA).

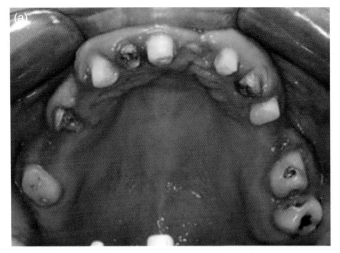

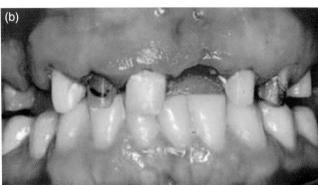

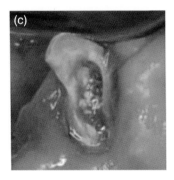

Figure 6.52 (a and b) Defective fixed restorations were removed. Note the compromised remaining tooth structure on No. 4 (c).

For site No. 5, the available bone width was 5 mm and the height was 15 mm. The implant size planned for this site was 3.75 × 13 mm. Placing this implant according to the surgical guide would result in a thin buccal plate that is primarily composed of cortical bone; therefore, the recommended treatment included buccal augmentation with DFDBA (ACE surgical) and bovine bone (Bio-Oss).

A full-thickness flap was elevated, and tooth No. 4 was extracted. In evaluating the ridge at sites Nos. 3 and 5, Seibert's Class I ridge defect was noted (a defect in the buccolingual direction) (Seibert 1983) (Figure 6.64).

Sinus floor elevation for the site was accomplished by using the lateral window approach. The sinus membrane was elevated to receive an implant 11.5 mm in length. The sinus was grafted with DFDBA (Ace Surgical), bovine bone (Bio-Oss), and autogenous bone obtained from the palatal aspect of the surgical site. After the sinus was elevated and grafted, guided bone regeneration for sites Nos. 3, 4, and 5 was completed. The first step in accomplishing guided bone regeneration was decortication of the site with a No. 1 round carbide bur to increase the blood supply to the graft material. After decortication (Buser et al. 1990, 1996), the site was grafted with DFDBA (ACE surgical) and bovine bone (Bio-Oss). A resorbable membrane (Osteohealth) was used to protect and contain the graft material (Figure 6.65).

The surgical area was closed without tension, and the pontic of the provisional FPD was trimmed away from the tissue to avoid irritation and facilitate plaque control. Another CT scan was made nine months after surgery to determine the bone width and height in preparation for implant placement after the sinus elevation and grafting procedure (Figure 6.66).

A full-thickness flap was elevated. The patient's provisional restoration was used as a surgical guide to place the implants. The flap was repositioned and sutured with 4-0 chromic gut sutures (Figure 6.67).

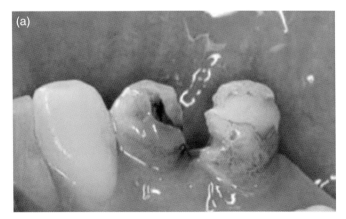
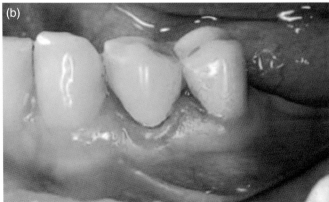

Figure 6.53 Caries control and temporization, teeth Nos. 20 and 21. (a) Facial view. (b) Lingual view.

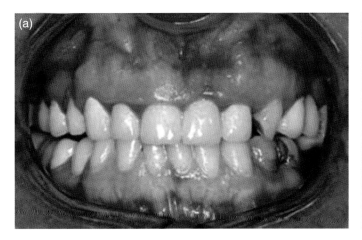

Figure 6.54 Intraoral views before (a) and after (b) provisional restorations were placed. Note improved oral hygiene in (b)

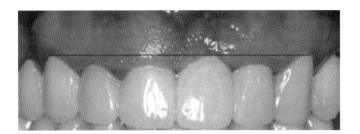

Figure 6.55 Gingival line discrepancy.

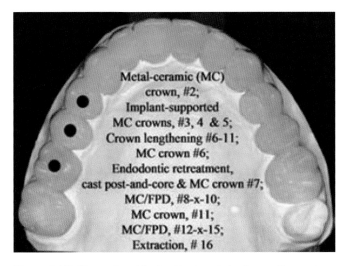

Figure 6.56 Wax replica of finalized treatment plan for maxillary arch.

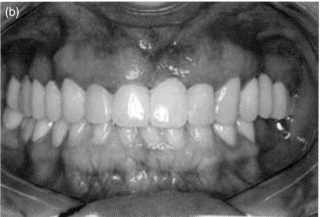

Figure 6.57 Wax replica of finalized treatment plan for mandibular arch.

Prosthetic Phase

The implants were uncovered six months after placement (Figure 6.68). The provisional restoration was relined over the healing abutments four weeks after uncovering (Figure 6.69).

Four weeks later, final impressions of all teeth and implants were made with polyether impression material (Permadyne Penta L and Impregum Penta) and plastic stock trays (Coe Spacer Trays, Disposable Plastic Trays: GC America Inc., Alsip, IL, USA) (Fig. 6.70). A face-bow transfer and centric

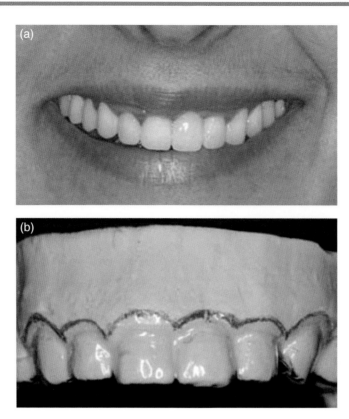

Figure 6.58 Crown lengthening for the anterior sextant to gain crown length and for esthetic purposes (a) with the use of a surgical guide template to assist the periodontist (b).

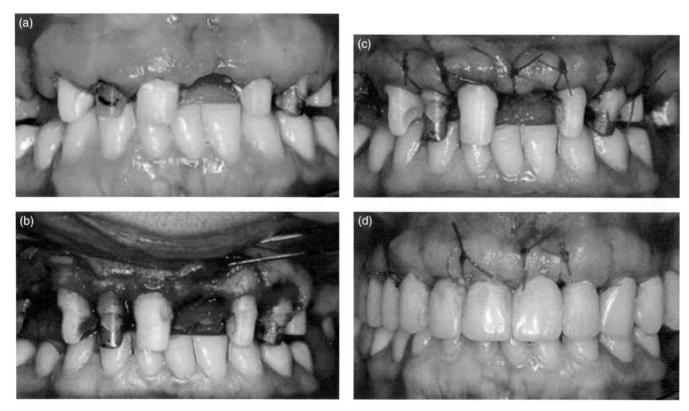

Figure 6.59 Crown-lengthening procedure for teeth Nos. 6–11. (a) Preoperative view. (b) Full-thickness flap elevated and ostectomy performed. (c) Closure with 4-0 chromic gut sutures. (d) One week after surgery.

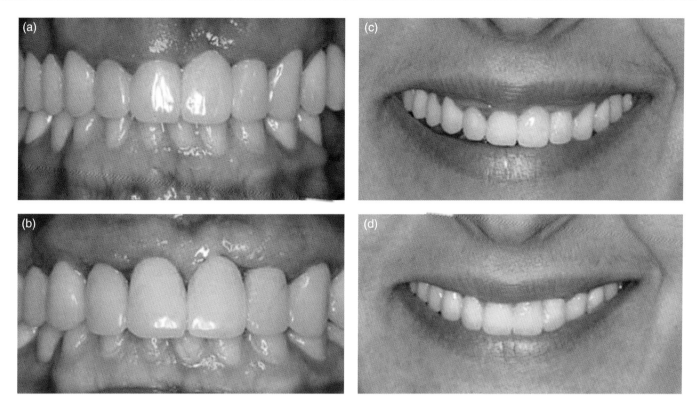

Figure 6.60 Intraoral view before (a) and after (b) surgery. Smile before (c) and after (d) surgery.

jaw relation record were made for the mounting of the definitive cast and for the cross mounting with the cast of the provisional restorations. A jig described by Lucia (Lucia 1983) was used as an anterior stop and extra-hard baseplate wax (Tru Wax; Dentsply, York, PA, USA) was used to make the record on the posterior teeth (Figure 6.71). The definitive cast and the cast of the provisional restorations were mounted and cross-mounted (Figure 6.72).

Die relief was placed on the dies (Die Spacer; Patterson Brand), and an artificial acrylic resin tooth (Pilkington Turner 30° tooth, 230 LS; Dentsply) was arranged to replace No. 19 at a height equal to half the height of the retromolar pad (Figure 6.73). A putty (Exaflex Putty; GC America Inc.) index of the provisional restorations was made to provide a three-dimensional view of the available space to the dental laboratory technician for the fabrication of the custom abutments (Figure 6.74).

A clinical try-in was accomplished to verify the position of the custom abutments by using a verification jig fabricated from light polymerizing urethane dimethacrylate resin (Triad Tru Tray VLC Custom Impression Tray Material; Dentsply) on the definitive cast (Figure 6.75). At try in, it was noted that the custom abutment for No. 4 was rotated on the cast. The verification jig was relieved in the area of No. 4, and auto-polymerizing resin material (Pattern resin LS: GC America Inc.) was used to reline and re-register the position of the custom abutment in the mouth. This relationship was then transferred to the definitive cast by altering the cast (Figure 6.76).

Metal castings and frameworks were fabricated. The castings were tried in the mouth, and the fit was verified with a silicone disclosing material (Fit Checker). The framework was sectioned between Nos. 3–4 and 4–5 and then soldered (Figure 6.77). The soldered casting for Nos. 3-4-5 was tried again in the mouth, and the fit was verified.

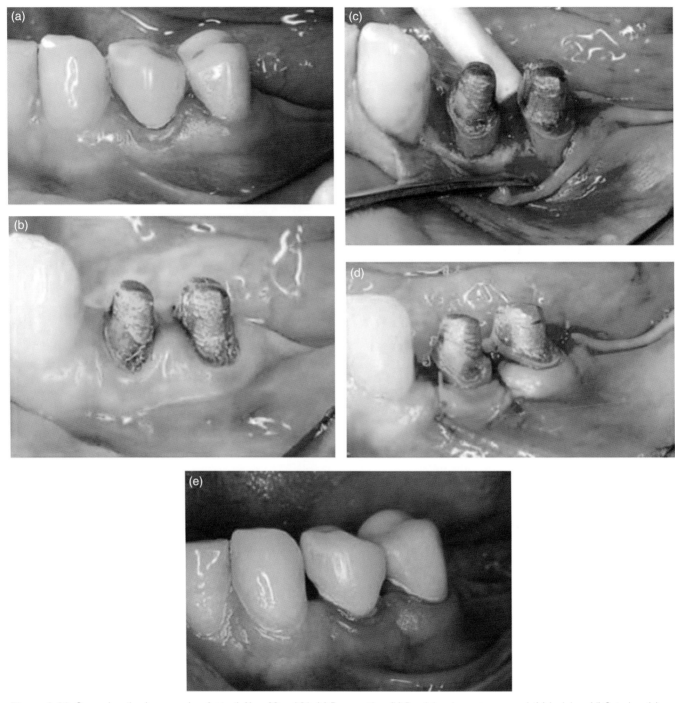

Figure 6.61 Crown-lengthening procedure for teeth Nos. 20 and 21. (a) Preoperative. (b) Provisional crowns removed. (c) Incision. (d) Suturing. (e) After suture removal.

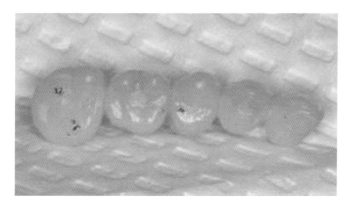

Figure 6.62 Dual-purpose template for implants Nos. 3, 4, and 5.

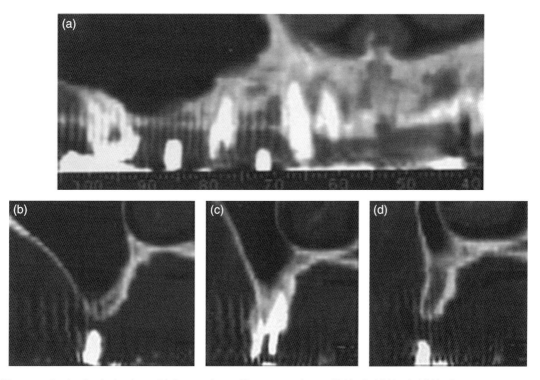

Figure 6.63 CT scan evaluation for the implants. (a) Panoramic cut. The segmental cuts. (b) No. 3. (c) No. 4. (d) No. 5.

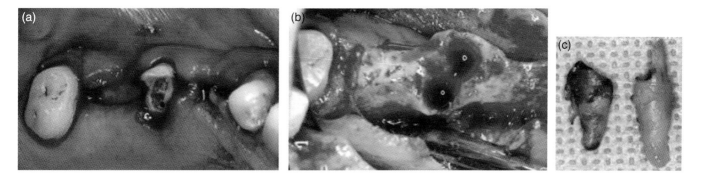

Figure 6.64 Extraction of tooth No. 4. Note the Seibert's Class I ridge defect. (a) Incision. (b) Socket. (c) Tooth sectioned and removed in two pieces.

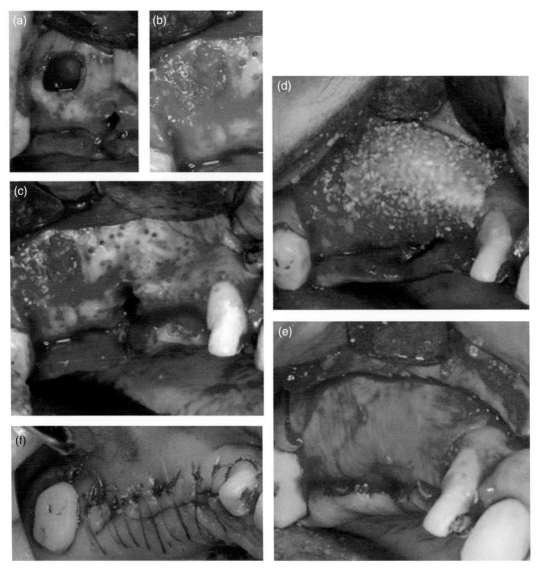

Figure 6.65 Sinus floor elevation and guided bone regeneration. (a) Lateral window approach performed and sinus membrane elevated. (b) Sinus augmented with DFDB, Bio-Oss bovine bone, and autogenous bone. (c) Decortication of buccal plate for ridge augmentation. (d) Site grafted with DFDBA and Bio-Oss bovine bone. (e) Resorbable membrane placed. (f) Closure with 4-0 Vicryl sutures.

A second jaw relation record was made at the desired VDO with the use of a Lucia jig as an anterior stop and extra-hard baseplate wax (Tru Wax; Dentsply) on the posterior teeth. A pick-up impression was made of the metal castings with the use of polyether impression material (Permadyne Penta L and Impregum Penta). The casts were mounted and sent to the dental laboratory for porce-

lain application (Figure 6.78). The shade selected was Vita B1, as per the patient's request.

At the porcelain bisque try-in, modifications to proximal and occlusal contacts were made. Some adjustments were made also to the contours of the restorations. Canine guidance was established. The restorations

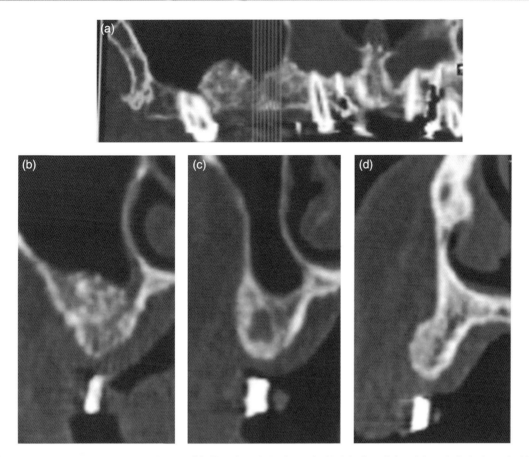

Figure 6.66 CT scan evaluation after sinus floor elevation (a). Note the gain in the vertical height (b and c) and the gain in horizontal width (d).

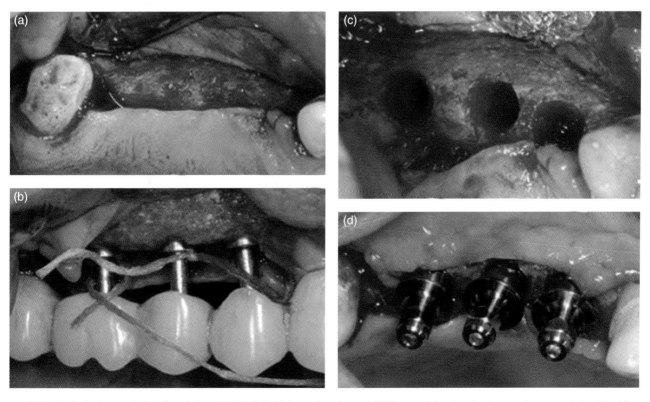

Figure 6.67 Implant placement sites Nos. 3, 4, and 5. (a) Full-thickness flap elevated. (b) The provisional restoration used as a surgical guide. (c) Osteotomy sites. (d) Implants placed.

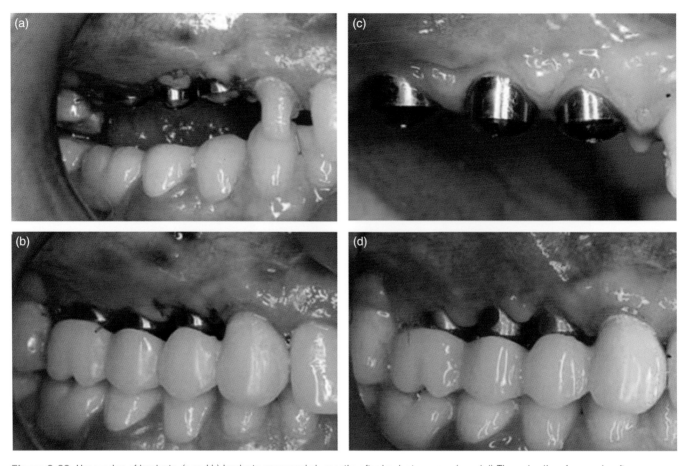

Figure 6.68 Uncovering of implants. (a and b) Implants uncovered six months after implant surgery. (c and d) Tissue healing, four weeks after uncovering. Note formation of papillae.

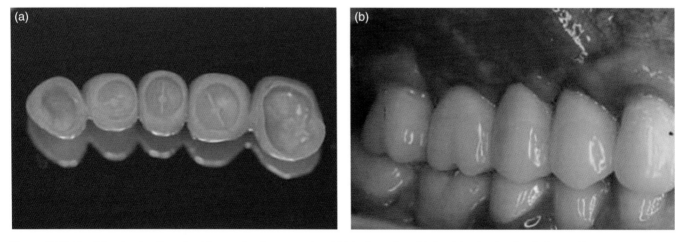

Figure 6.69 Provisional restoration relined four weeks after uncovering. (a) Intaglio surface. (b) Provisional restoration in the mouth.

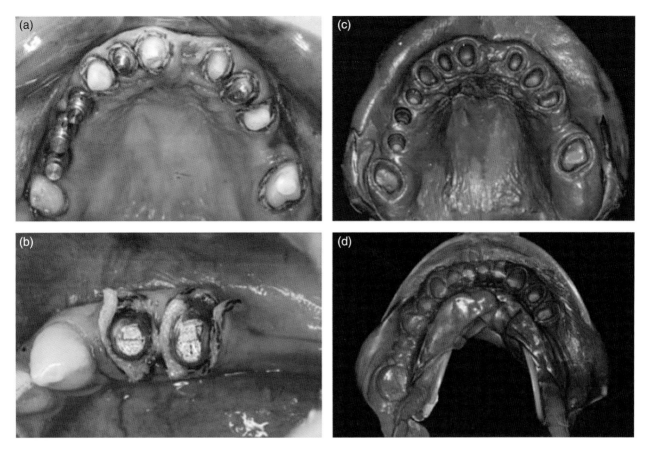

Figure 6.70 Final impression of all teeth and implants. (a and b) Gingival displacement cords. (c and d) Impressions.

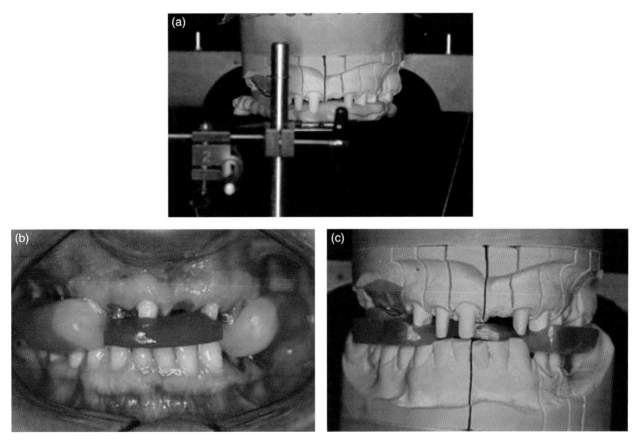

Figure 6.71 Face-bow transfer (a) and centric jaw relation record (b and c) by using a Lucia jig on the anterior teeth and extra-hard baseplate wax on the posterior teeth.

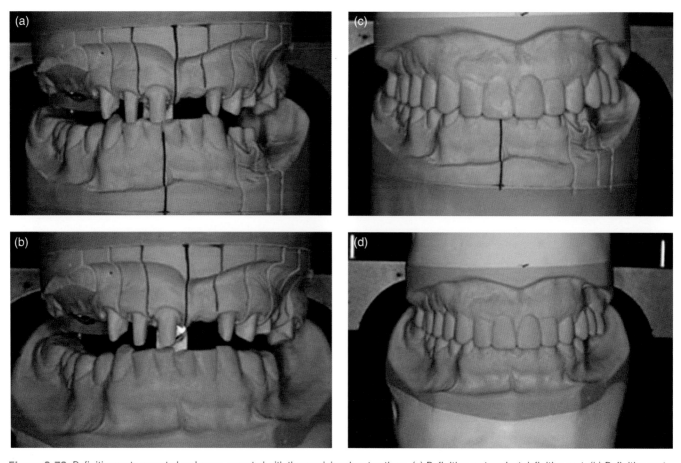

Figure 6.72 Definitive casts mounted and cross-mounted with the provisional restorations. (a) Definitive cast against definitive cast. (b) Definitive cast against cast of provisional restorations. (c) Cast of provisional restorations against definitive cast. (d) Cast of provisional restorations against cast of provisional restorations.

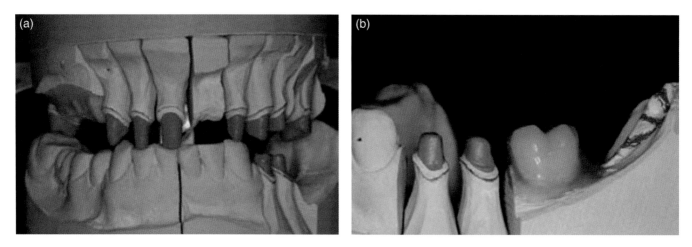

Figure 6.73 (a) Die relief placed on dies. (b) Acrylic resin artificial tooth placed in position of No. 19 to establish occlusal plane at a height equal to half the height of the retromolar pad (marked in red).

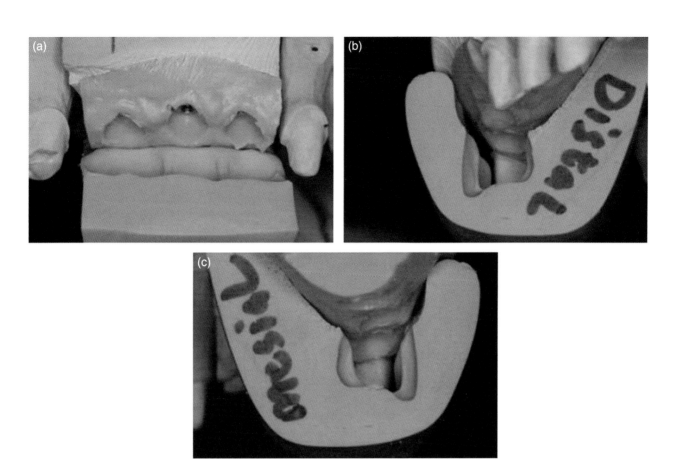

Figure 6.74 Putty index of the provisional restoration was made to provide a three-dimensional view of the available space for custom abutments for implants. (a) Facial view. (b and c) Proximal views.

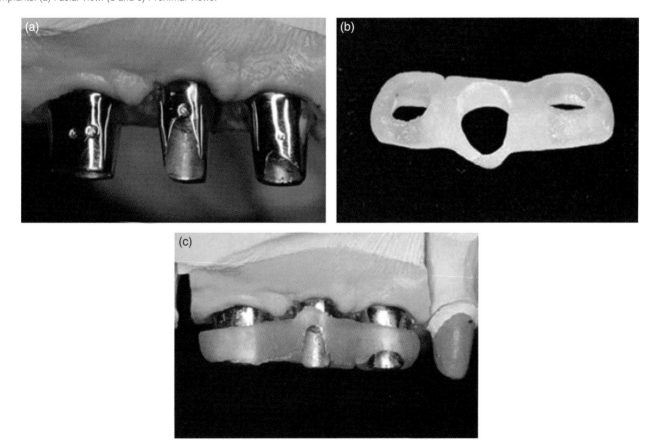

Figure 6.75 (a) Custom abutments were fabricated. (b and c) Verification jig was made.

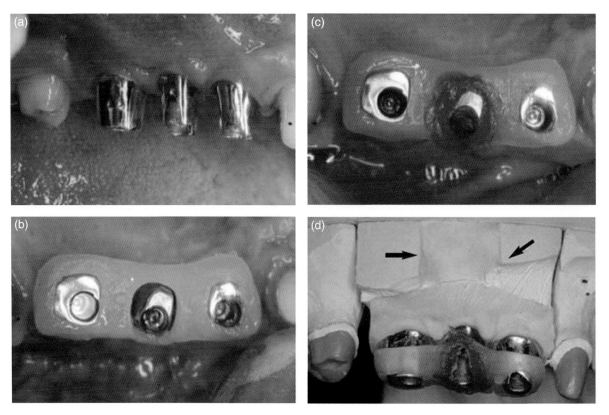

Figure 6.76 (a) Try-in of custom abutments. (b) Verification jig indicated that custom abutment for No. 4 was malpositioned. Jig was hollowed out in area of No. 4. (c) Autopolymerizing acrylic resin was used to register correct position of custom abutment. (d) Position was transferred to definitive cast, and cast was altered. Note pink stone where cast was altered (*arrows*).

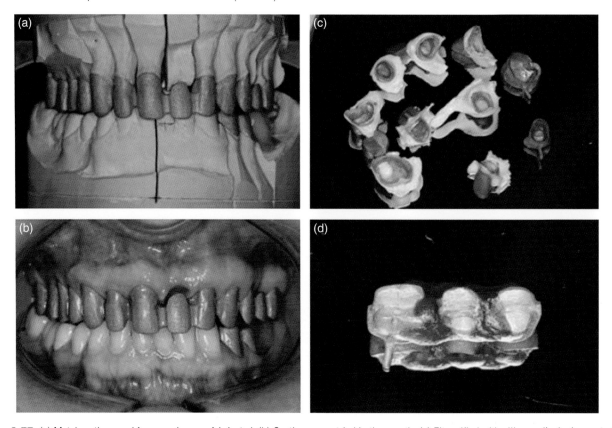

Figure 6.77 (a) Metal castings and frameworks were fabricated. (b) Castings were tried in the mouth. (c) Fit verified with silicone disclosing material (Fit Checker). (d) Metal framework for implant-supported splinted crowns, Nos. 3–5, was sectioned, and reconnected with autopolymerizing acrylic resin in preparation for soldering.

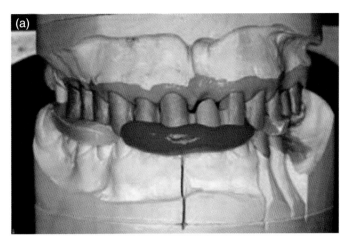

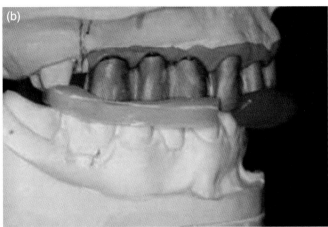 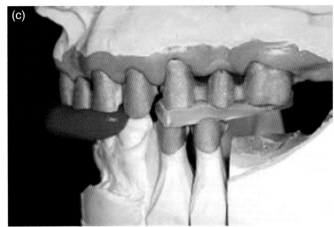

Figure 6.78 At the final try-in appointment, new jaw relation records were made at the established VDO, and a pick-up impression was made of the maxillary castings. The maxillary cast was mounted. (a) Frontal view. (b and c) Side views.

were then sent for final glazing. At the day of final delivery, gold screws for the custom abutments Nos. 3, 4, and 5 were torqued to 32 N·cm with a torque wrench (Torque Indicator; 3I, Palm Beach Gardens, FL, USA). The abutments were then torqued again to 32 N·cm after a 10-minute waiting period to compensate for embedment relaxation of the screws.

All restorations were cemented with Rely-X Luting resin-modified glass ionomer cement, with the exception of the implant-supported restorations Nos. 3–4–5, which were cemented with temporary cement (Temp Bond) after sealing the screw holes with a temporary sealer (Dura-Seal;

Reliance, Worth, IL, USA). Temporary cement was used for the implant-supported restorations to ensure retrievability (Figures 6.79 and 6.80).

Maintenance Phase

The maintenance phase included recall visits every three to four months.

Prognosis

The overall prognosis for the treatment provided (short and long term) is favorable.

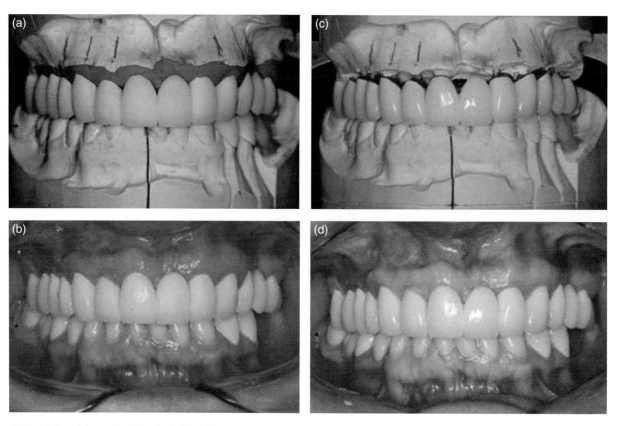

Figure 6.79 (a) Porcelain applied, Vita shade B1. (b) Restorations tried in the mouth and adjusted. (c) Porcelain glazed and metal finished and polished. (d) Final cementation.

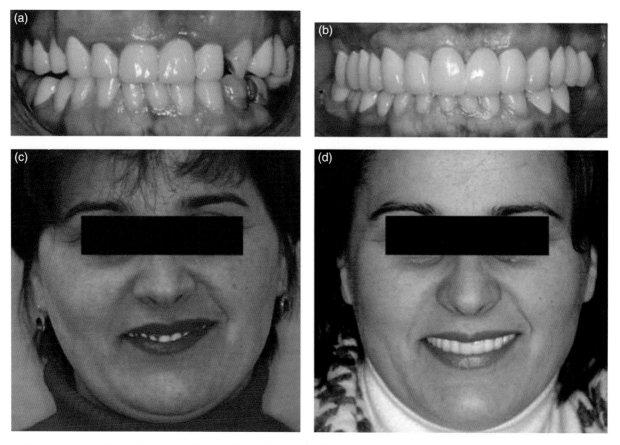

Figure 6.80 Intraoral views before (a) and after (b). Smile before (c) and after (d).

CONCLUSION

The overall quality of dental care depends on a concerted effort among the various dentists involved, a thorough and complete diagnosis that addresses all disease processes, and a realistic, carefully sequenced treatment plan that offers a favorable prognosis.

REFERENCES

AAP position paper (1997). Periodontal considerations in the management of cancer patients. Committee on Research, Science and Therapy of the American Academy of Periodontology. *J. Periodontol.* 68: 791–801.

Becker, W., Berg, L., and Becker, B. (1984). The long-term evaluation of periodontal treatment and maintenance in 95 patients. *Int. J. Periodont. Restor. Dent.* 2: 55–72.

Buser, D., Bragger, U., Lang, N.P. et al. (1990). Regeneration and enlargement of jaw bone using guided tissue regeneration. *Clin. Oral Implants Res.* 1: 22–32.

Buser, D., Dula, K., Hirt, H.P. et al. (1996). Lateral ridge augmentation using autografts and barrier membranes: a clinical study with 40 partially edentulous patients. *J. Oral Maxillofac. Surg.* 54: 420–432.

Chase, R. Jr. and Low, S.B. (1993). Survival characteristics of periodontally-involved teeth: a 40-year study. *J. Periodontol.* 64: 701–705.

Davies, R. (1993). Antibiotic prophylaxis in dental practice. *Br. Med. J.* 307: 1210–1211.

Dibart, S. and Karima, M. (2006). *Practical Periodontal Plastic Surgery*. Ames, IA: Wiley Blackwell.

Flocken, J.E. (1980). Electrosurgical management of soft tissues in restorative dentistry. *Dent. Clin. N. Am.* 24: 247–269.

Glickman, I. (1958). *Clinical Periodontology*, 2e, 694–696. Philadelphia: W.B. Saunders.

Listgarten, M.A. (1972a). Normal development, structure, physiology and repair of gingival epithelium. *Oral Sci. Rev.* 1: 3–67.

Listgarten, M.A. (1972b). Ultrastructure of the dento-gingival junction after gingivectomy. *J. Periodontal Res.* 7: 151–160.

Lucia, V.O. (1983). *Modern Gnathological Concepts – Updated*, 83–107. Chicago: Quintessence.

McGuire, M. (1991). Prognosis versus actual outcome: a long-term survey of 100 treated periodontal patients under maintenance care. *J. Periodontol.* 62: 51–58.

Mealey, B.L. and Oates, T.W. (2006). Diabetes mellitus and periodontal diseases. *J. Periodontol.* 77: 1289–1303.

Miller, S.C. (1950). *Textbook of Periodontia*, 3e, 125. Philadelphia: Blackstone.

Morgano, S.M. and Brackett, S.E. (1999). Foundation restorations in fixed prosthodontics: current knowledge and future needs. *J. Prosthet. Dent.* 82: 643–657.

Morgano, S.M., Garvin, P.M., Muzynski, B.L., and Malone, W.F. (1989). Diagnosis and treatment planning. In: *Tylman's Theory and Practice of Fixed Prosthodontics*, 8e (eds. W.F. Malone, D.L. Koth, E. Cavazos Jr. et al.), 1–23. St Louis: Ishiyaku EuroAmerica.

Rosenberg, E.S., Garger, D.A., and Evian, C.I. (1980). Tooth lengthening procedures. *Compend. Cont. Educ. Dent.* 1: 161–173.

Seibert, J. (1983). Reconstruction of deformed, partially edentulous ridges, using full thickness onlay grafts. Part I. Technique and wound healing. *Compend. Cont. Educ. Dent.* 4: 437–453.

Soileau, K.M. (2006). Oral post-surgical complications following the administration of bisphosphonates given for osteopenia related to malignancy. *J. Periodontol.* 77: 738–743.

Thomson, W.M., Lawrence, H.P., Broadbent, J.M., and Poulton, R. (2006). The impact of xerostomia on oral-health-related quality of life among younger adults. *Health Qual. Life Outcomes* 4: 86 (published online before print November 8, 2006).

Wooltorton, E. (2005). Health and drug alerts: patients receiving intravenous bisphosphonates should avoid invasive dental procedures. *Can. Med. Assoc. J.* 172: 1684.

Chapter 7 The Contribution of Periodontics to the Correction of Vertical Alveolar Ridge Deficiencies

Serge Dibart

ALVEOLAR DISTRACTION OSTEOGENESIS SURGERY

History

Alveolar distraction surgery is an application of Ilizarov's distraction osteogenesis method to the maxillofacial skeleton. Between 1954 and 1971, Gavriel Ilizarov, a Russian orthopedic surgeon, developed a novel surgical approach for reconstruction of skeletal deformities (Ilizarov 1971). This involved the use of a mechanical device (the distractor) and the formation of new bone between the bone segments that were gradually separated by incremental traction (Birch and Samchukov 2004). This traction generated tension that stimulated new bone formation parallel to the vector of distraction (Cope and Samchukov 2001; Samchukov et al. 1998). This technique had the added advantage of displacing and preserving the soft tissue with the mobilized bony segment. This is particularly useful in the process of alveolar distraction where the alveolar housing and the surrounding soft tissue are displaced together in a single, simultaneous process (Block et al. 1996; Chin and Toth 1996; McCarthy et al. 1995; Ortiz Monasterio et al. 1997).

Indications

- Combined deficiencies in hard and soft tissue not allowing for dental implant placement

- Vertical alveolar ridge deficiency impairing the placement of a dental implant or fixed partial denture (Figures 7.1 and 7.2)

- Axial correction of misaligned osseointegrated dental implants or ankylosed teeth

- Orthodontics: Therapy of local open bite

Limitations

- Must have a minimum of 6 mm of residual bone height

- Must have adequate bone width (otherwise block graft necessary before distraction)

- Thin residual bony arch, presenting the risk of fracture

- Patients on bisphosphonates

- Irradiated patients (>40–60 Gy)

- Malignancies

- Heavy tobacco use

Advantages

See Chiapasco et al. (2004).

- Eliminates the need to harvest bone

- Less operating time

- Distraction histogenesis

- Lower risk of morbidity of the surgical site

- Crestal part of the distracted segment has lower risk of resorption

- Greater vertical bone gain

Armamentarium

- Standard surgical kit, as described in *Practical Periodontal Plastic Surgery* plus:

- Alveolar Distraction Track Plus Kit (KLS Martin, Jacksonville, FL, USA) and oscillating and sagittal microsaws (KLS Martin, Jacksonville, FL, USA)

Technique for the Anterior Segment

After proper local anesthesia (infiltration with xylocaine 2% with 1 : 100 000 epinephrine and 1 : 50 000 epinephrine for hemostasis), an incision is made in the vestibule using a No. 15 blade. The incision is made high enough in the mucosa to allow for proper mobilization of the flap (Figure 7.3). The incision may be done in two steps: incision of the mucosal layer first, then incision of the connective tissue, muscles, and periosteum. Keep the blade oriented toward the alveolar bone. The incision has to be long enough to allow for easy blunt dissection with a periosteal elevator.

Practical Advanced Periodontal Surgery, Second Edition. Edited by Serge Dibart.
© 2020 John Wiley & Sons, Inc. Published 2020 by John Wiley & Sons, Inc.
Companion website: www.wiley.com/go/dibart/advanced

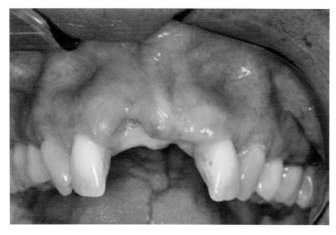

Figure 7.1 Patient presenting with a vertical height defect subsequent to the loss of teeth Nos. 8 and 9.

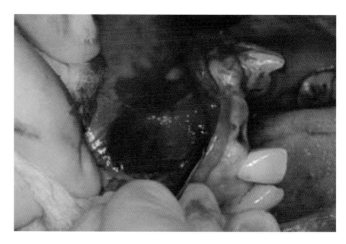

Figure 7.4 The full-thickness flap is reflected using a periosteal elevator.

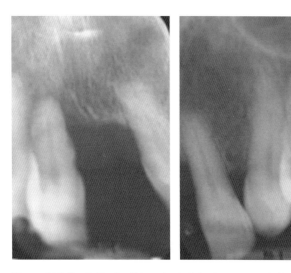

Figure 7.2 Tooth No. 8 will be extracted due to severe periodontal disease. Notice the lack of vertical height of the alveolar bone.

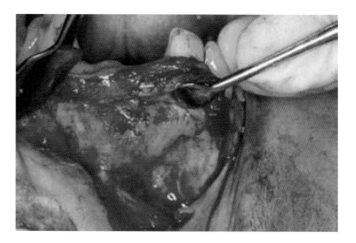

Figure 7.5 Reflection stops at the alveolar crest.

The role of the elevator is to now reflect the flap all the way up to the alveolar crest of the edentulous site but not beyond (Figures 7.4 and 7.5). It is critical to leave the palatal or lingual periosteum attached to the bone, because it will be the only source of vascularization of the bony fragment during the distraction process. Once the bony area is exposed, it is useful to draw a picture of the segment to be distracted on the bone using a sterile No. 2 pencil (Figure 7.6). The base of the bony segment should be wider at the crest than apically (Figure 7.7) to allow for unimpaired sliding movement during the traction process. Also at this point, it is important to remember that the distracted segment should be no shorter than 5 mm.

Once the segment is visualized, it is time to adapt the distractor to fit the clinical picture. This is the most time-consuming part of the operation, because one has to adapt (cut) and bend the upper and lower arms of the distractor to fit the underlying bone architecture, while preserving the proper direction of the vector (Figures 7.8–7.10). Distractors are available in 6-, 9-, 12-, and 15-mm

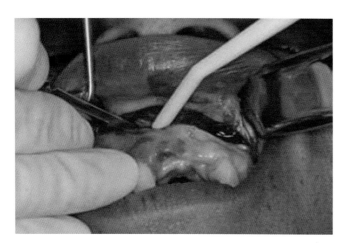

Figure 7.3 The incision is high up in the vestibule to allow for flap mobilization and access.

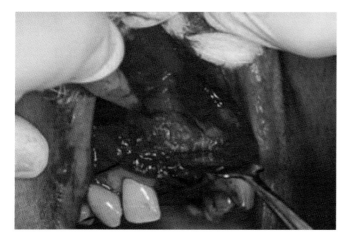

Figure 7.6 The segment to be distracted is delineated with a sterile No. 2 pencil.

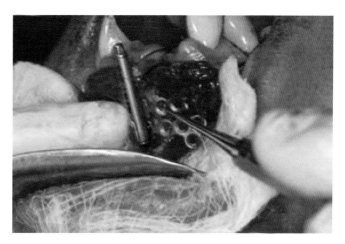

Figure 7.9 The distractor is placed, verifying the correct direction of the distraction vector.

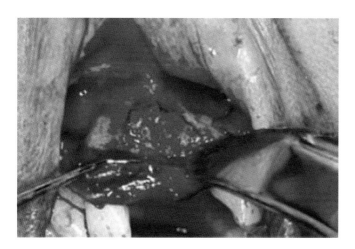

Figure 7.7 The segment to be cut is drawn on the bone. Notice the divergence of the cuts that will allow for free movement of the segment.

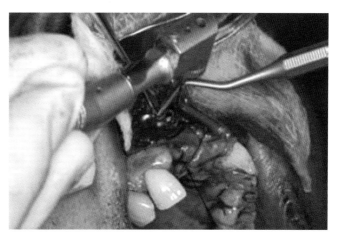

Figure 7.10 One hole in each arm of the distractor is predrilled; this will allow accurate repositioning of the device.

lengths. After predrilling one hole for each arm while holding the distractor in place, the sagittal saw (set at 20 000 RPM) is used to cut the bone (Figure 7.11). It is better not to do a through-and-through cut at the beginning but to get as close as possible to the palatal/lingual bony plate (Figure 7.12). Also, the orientation of the saw should always be kept slightly angled toward the alveolar crest; this will prevent invasion of anatomical structures (i.e. the nasal spine, the nasal cavity, or the genial tubercules).

The bony segment is gently detached from the maxilla or mandible using a very fine chisel and mallet while holding the segment palatally or lingually with the finger (Figure 7.13). At this point, the mobile segment is connected to the palatal or lingual gingiva only through the palatal/lingual periosteum. Once the segment is freed from the surrounding bone, the distractor is put back in place and secured through the use of screws that will engage in the predrilled holes previously mentioned (Figure 7.14). A minimum number of five screws is

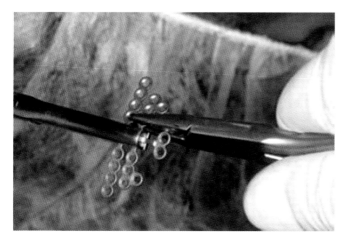

Figure 7.8 The distractor is modified to fit the clinical picture.

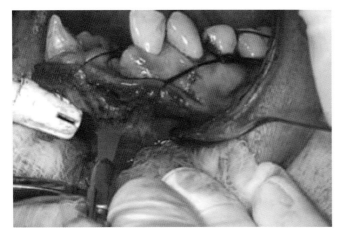

Figure 7.11 Using the oscillating microsaw (KLS Martin, Jacksonville, FL, USA), the osteotomy is started.

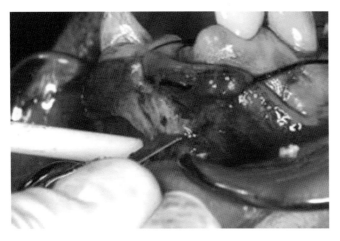

Figure 7.12 It is important to get as close as possible to the palatal/lingual cortical plate but not go through it with the sagittal microsaw, so as not to injure the palatal/lingual periosteum.

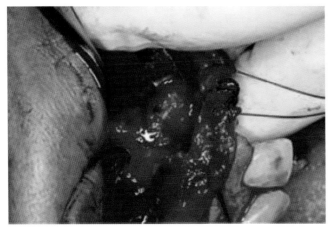

Figure 7.13 A fine osseous chisel (or modified spatula) is used very carefully with a mallet in order to detach the segment to be distracted. Notice the finger on the palate; it is used to counteract and control the force of the blow.

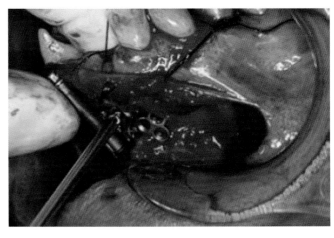

Figure 7.14 The distractor is repositioned very accurately due to the previously drilled holes and secured with the screws.

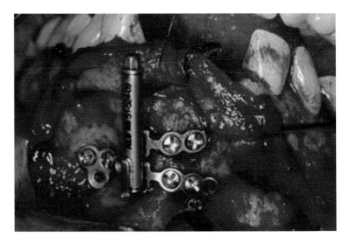

Figure 7.15 The distractor is securely in place.

recommended to secure the distractor (two screws for the upper segment and three screws for the lower segment).

These screws are self-drilling, but it is better to use the drill and predrill; this way, you will avoid running the risk of splitting the bony segment to be distracted. It is customary to use the 5-mm-length screws (Figure 7.15).

Once the distractor is securely in place, it is useful to activate it and see how the bony segment glides upward (Figure 7.16). This is critical because if there is an impediment to the smooth trajectory of the segment to be distracted, it should be corrected at this point. This is usually the case when the mesial and distal cuts are somewhat parallel to each other instead of being divergent. This can be corrected using a fine fissure bur. The distractor is put back in its inactive mode, and a small opening is made in the gingiva ("button hole") to allow for the passage of the distractor's arm (Figure 7.17). The suturing is done in two layers, using chromic gut sutures (Figures 7.18 and 7.19).

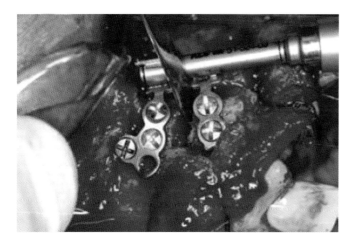

Figure 7.16 The distractor is activated to make sure that there will be no interferences during the distraction process.

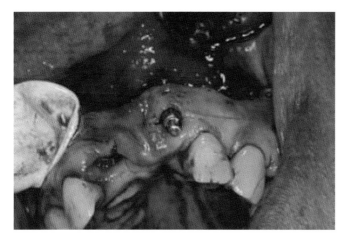

Figure 7.17 After bringing back the segment to its original position, a small incision is made close to the gingival crest to accommodate the head of the distractor post.

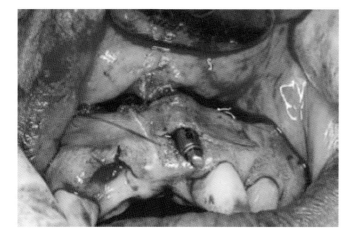

Figure 7.18 A two-layer suturing technique is used to close the wound. First, the deeper layers (muscles, etc.) are sutured with an internal horizontal or vertical mattress suture. You must use resorbable material such as chromic gut for this first suture.

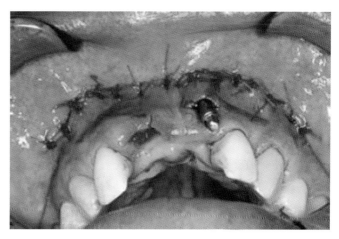

Figure 7.19 Now that the deeper layers are sutured, the second layer will approximate the edges of the wound without tension and the area will heal by primary intention. You can use resorbable or nonresorbable material for this suture (here, 4-0 chromic gut was used).

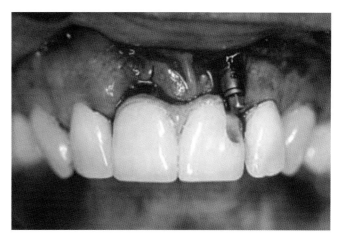

Figure 7.20 The temporary removable prosthesis is adjusted, so that it will not interfere with the distractor. It will be ground down gradually as the distraction progresses and the bone and tissues extend vertically.

The removable temporary partial denture is adjusted to fit the new clinical situation (Figures 7.20 and 7.21).

The patient is seen seven days after the surgery (latency period), and the distractor is then activated with one complete turn of the screw (0.3 mm) (starting of the distraction period). The patient is given the "distractor key" and asked to repeat the procedure twice a day (0.6 mm/day of distraction). The patient is monitored weekly until the desired vertical bone height is achieved (Figures 7.22 and 7.23). At this point, the consolidation period begins.

This is a three-month rest period that allows for bone remodeling and consolidation. After two months, the distractor is removed (Figures 7.24 through 7.26), the wound

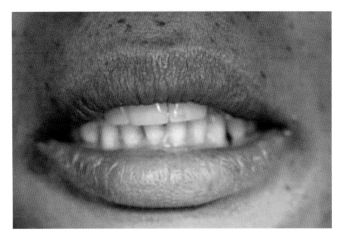

Figure 7.21 The patient with the adjusted prosthesis in place. The device is not noticeable.

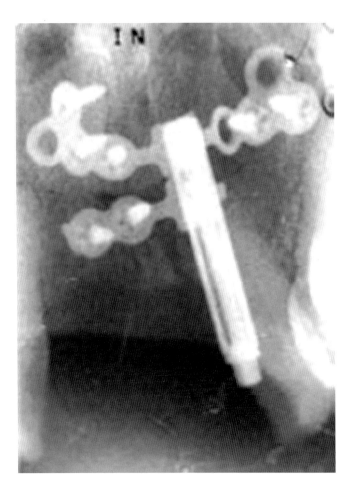

Figure 7.22 Periapical radiograph of the segment at the end of the alveolar distraction process.

is sutured, and the patient is sent home for another month (Figure 7.27). At the end of the three months (2 + 1) of consolidation, the patient is sent for a CT scan evaluation and the implants are placed. It is important to place the

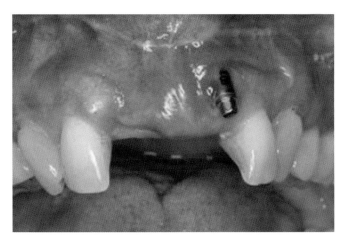

Figure 7.23 The bone has been distracted to the desired length. We ask the patient to stop activating the device. In two months, the distractor will be removed.

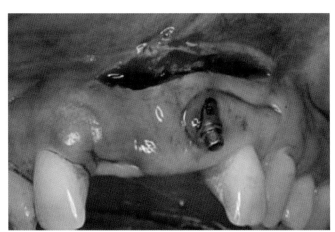

Figure 7.24 Two months after the end of the distraction period, the device is removed using a smaller incision.

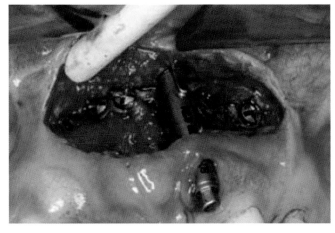

Figure 7.25 The distractor is exposed by blunt dissection with a periosteal elevator.

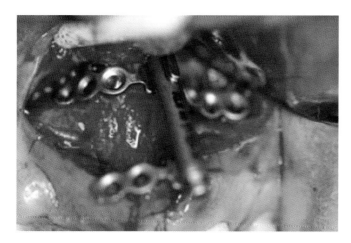

Figure 7.26 The screws are removed, as well as the device. Notice the amount of bone gained in the vertical dimension in less than one month.

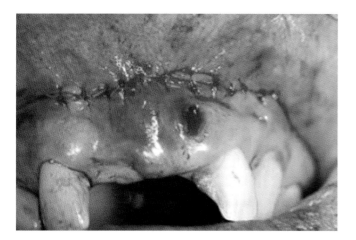

Figure 7.27 The surgical wound is closed with internal and external sutures, as before, and the area is left to heal undisturbed for one month before placing the implants.

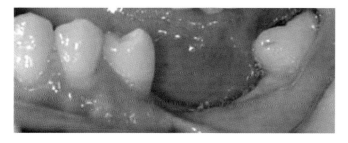

Figure 7.28 A 30-year-old patient presenting with a posterior vertical height defect. Tooth No. 17 cannot be used as an abutment for a fixed or removable partial denture.

implants shortly after the removal of the distractor; otherwise, you may run the risk of losing the newly formed bone.

Technique for the Posterior Segment

The posterior segment is much more challenging (Figure 7.28) than the anterior segments because of

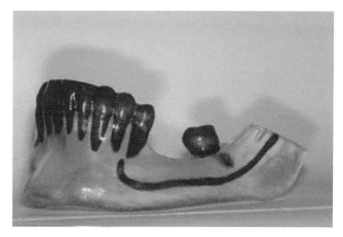

Figure 7.29 An exact replica of the patient's mandible. This model (ClearView Anatomical Model; Medical Modeling LLC, Golden, CO, USA) obtained from the patient's CT scan will allow the critical landmarks (mental foramen, mandibular canal, roots, etc.) to be located precisely. This in turn will make for guess-free and stress-free surgery.

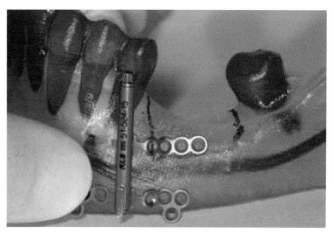

Figure 7.30 Radiographic images (CT scan of the patient's mandible) showing the mandibular nerve, mental foramen, etc. Notice the posterior vertical bony ledge due to the alveolar bone loss and its distance from the mandibular nerve.

anatomical limitations, access, and proximity of vital structures (mandibular nerve, maxillary sinus). It is very useful to visualize the anatomy of the mandible using a plastic model (Figure 7.29). This model (ClearView Anatomical Models; Medical Modeling LLC, Golden, CO) can be obtained after the CT scan is sent to the company (Figure 7.30). The incisions are planned on this extremely accurate model, and the distractor is bent and adapted beforehand (Figure 7.31). This will save considerable time, stress, and aggravation during the surgery.

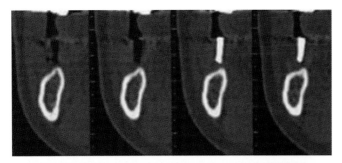

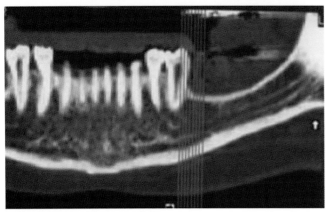

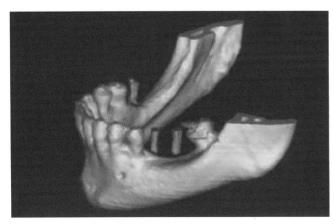

Figure 7.31 The segment to be distracted is drawn on the model and will be replicated in the mouth precisely during the surgery. The distractor arms are modified and bent prior to the surgery to fit the clinical situation. This will save a lot of time and aggravation during the surgery.

A Few Words of Caution

- Pay special attention to the direction of the vector in the lower anterior mandibular region (Figures 7.32 and 7.33).

- Make sure that the distractor does not interfere with the occlusion.

- Select patients who are reliable and compliant.

- Always "overdistract" by a couple of millimeters to ensure you will have enough bone.

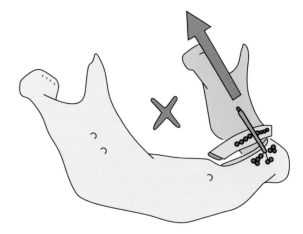

Figure 7.32 The *arrow* shows an incorrect vector of distraction. The bony segment will be too lingual and therefore could not be used for proper dental implant placement.

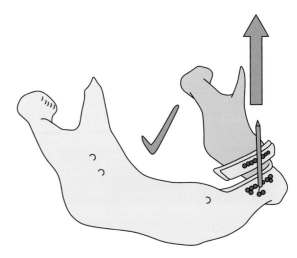

Figure 7.33 The *arrow* shows a correct vector of distraction. The bony segment will be distracted parallel with the long axis of the adjacent teeth. Dental implants can be placed in the proper alignment.

Preoperative Instructions

- Antibiotherapy (i.e. amoxicillin 500 mg three times a day starting the day of surgery and for seven days) is indicated.

- Mild oral sedation could be useful (i.e. diazepam 5 mg the night before and 5 mg one hour before the procedure).

- Analgesics are recommended (i.e. ibuprofen 600 mg one hour before the surgery).

Postoperative Instructions

- Corticosteroids for five days: dexamethasone 0.75 mg, five tablets the day of surgery, then four tablets the next day, then three tablets, and so on, to control the swelling

- Analgesics: acetaminophen with codeine (Tylenol #3) or ibuprofen 600 mg (Motrin 600) to control the pain

- Ice pack 20 minutes on/20 minutes off for the first 24 hours

- Chlorhexidine rinses twice a day for seven days

Possible Complications

- Possible necrosis of the bony segment if it is too small or completely detached from the periosteum

- Fibrous tissue formation at the end of the traction period: this is more likely to occur if the traction has been too vigorous (i.e. 1 mm/day or more)

- Infection

- Fracture of transport segment

- Fracture of anchorage segment

- Premature consolidation

- Undesirable transport vector

- Fracture of the distraction rod or of the transport disc (Mazzonetto et al. 2007)

REFERENCES

Birch, J.G. and Samchukov, M.L. (2004). Use of the Ilizarov method to correct lower limb deformities in children and adolescents. *J. Am. Acad. Orthop. Surg.* 12 (3): 144–154.

Block, M.S., Chang, A., and Crawford, C. (1996). Mandibular alveolar ridge augmentation in the dog using distraction osteogenesis. *J. Oral Maxillofac. Surg.* 54 (3): 309–314.

Chiapasco, M., Consolo, U., Bianchi, A., and Ronchi, P. (2004). Alveolar distraction osteogenesis for the correction of vertically deficient edentulous ridges: a multicenter prospective study on humans. *Int. J. Oral Maxillofac. Implants* 19 (3): 399–407.

Chin, M. and Toth, B.A. (1996). Distraction osteogenesis in maxillofacial surgery using internal devices: review of five cases. *J. Oral Maxillofac. Surg.* 54 (1): 45–53.

Cope, J.B. and Samchukov, M.L. (2001). Mineralization dynamics of regenerate bone during mandibular osteodistraction. *Int. J. Oral Maxillofac. Surg.* 30 (3): 234–242.

Dibart, S. and Karima, M. (2006). *Practical Periodontal Plastic Surgery*. Ames, IA: Wiley Blackwell.

Ilizarov, G.A. (1971). Basic principles of transosseous compression and distraction osteosynthesis. *Orthop. Travmatol. Protez.* 32 (11): 7–15.

Mazzonetto, R., Allais, M., Maurette, P.E., and Moreira, R.W. (2007). A retrospective study of the potential complications during alveolar distraction osteogenesis in 55 patients. *J. Oral Maxillofac. Surg.* 36: 6–10.

McCarthy, J.G., Staffenberg, D.A., Wood, R.J. et al. (1995). Introduction of an intra-oral bone lengthening device. *Plast. Reconstr. Surg.* 96 (4): 978–981.

Ortiz Monasterio, F., Molina, F., Andrade, L. et al. (1997). Simultaneous mandibular and maxillary distraction in hemifacial microsomia in adults: avoiding occlusal disasters. *Plast. Reconstr. Surg.* 100 (4): 852–861.

Samchukov, M.L., Cope, J.B., Harper, R.B., and Ross, J.D. (1998). Biomechanical considerations of mandibular lengthening and widening by gradual distraction using a computer model. *J. Oral Maxillofac. Surg.* 56 (1): 51–59.

Chapter 8 Papillary Construction After Dental Implant Therapy

Peyman Shahidi, Serge Dibart, and Yun Po Zhang

HISTORY

The presence of a "black triangle" due to the absence of interproximal papilla between two adjacent implants has become a steady concern among implant surgeons and restorative dentists. Three main surgical methods have been proposed in the past at second-stage surgery (uncovering) to correct the problem. Palacci (1995) suggested that a full-thickness flap be raised from the palatal side of the implant and a portion of it be rotated 90° to accommodate the interproximal space of the implant. Possible compromise of the blood supply of the rotated small flap, limited amount of pedunculated soft tissue for some larger interproximal areas, and lack of keratinized tissue in cases with a narrow band of attached gingiva on the facial seem to be some of the limitations of this technique. In 1999, Adriaenssens et al. introduced a novel flap design, the "palatal sliding strip flap," to help form papillae between implants and between natural teeth on the anterior area of the maxilla. The flap was designed and managed in a way that allowed the palatal mucosa to slide in a labial direction after dissection of two mesial and distal strips (to create papillae and at the same time augment the labial ridge).

Nemcovsky et al. (2000) introduced a U-shaped flap raised toward the buccal; the nature of this design was essentially the same as the one introduced earlier by Adriaenssens, with some minor differences. In 2004, Misch et al. modified Nemcovsky et al.'s technique further by raising the U-shaped flap toward the palatal rather than the buccal side. In 2004, Shahidi developed a surgical procedure with the goal of guiding the soft tissue that formerly covered the implant over to the sides of the implant and to gently squeeze this piece of tissue after insertion of the healing abutment. This was done to provide enough soft tissue in the interproximal spaces to allow for papilla generation.

In brief, there is not one single technique that is universally accepted to be the one that works 100% of the time. Tissue engineering, with the implantation of fibroblasts in the papillary area, may, in the future, help solve this problem by providing more predictability.

INDICATIONS

- At second-stage dental implant uncovering, between an implant and a tooth or between two or more implants, to minimize the formation of a "black triangle"

- Thick periodontal biotype

CONTRAINDICATIONS

- Thin periodontal biotype

- Lack of keratinized gingiva around the implant(s)

- Need to correct underlying bone

ARMAMENTARIUM

- A basic surgical set as described in *Practical Periodontal Plastic Surgery* (Dibart and Karima 2006)

- Implant kit

- Healing abutments

TECHNIQUE

In the single implant model, a small U-shaped flap is created to allow mobilization of the tissue in the mesial direction. Another U-shaped flap, mirror image of the first one and sharing the same buccolingual incision, allows mobilization of the tissues to the distal direction. Occlusally, these full- or partial-thickness U-shaped flaps form an H-shape design (Figure 8.1). The exact location of the implant is obtained using periapical/bitewing radiographs in

Practical Advanced Periodontal Surgery, Second Edition. Edited by Serge Dibart.
© 2020 John Wiley & Sons, Inc. Published 2020 by John Wiley & Sons, Inc.
Companion website: www.wiley.com/go/dibart/advanced

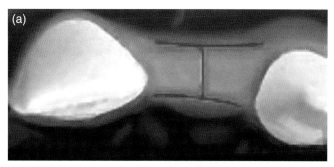

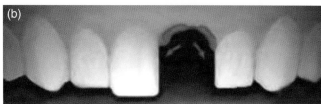

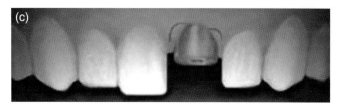

Figure 8.1 Diagram showing the uncovering incision and procedures for a single implant occlusally (a) and buccally (b) and with the healing abutment in place (c).

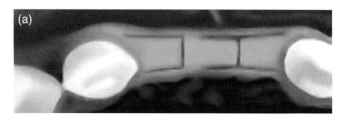

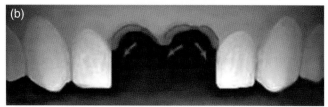

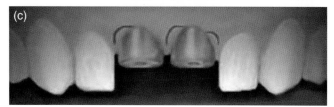

Figure 8.2 Diagram showing the uncovering incision and procedures for two implants side by side, occlusally (a) and buccally (b) with the healing abutments in place (c).

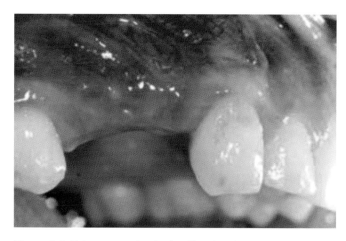

Figure 8.3 Before uncovering implant Nos. 4 and 5.

combination with alveolar ridge mapping with an explorer following local anesthesia.

In a multiple implant model (Figure 8.2), the covering tissue of the most mesial implant provides the proximal papilla (i.e. mesial) of that implant using the U-shape design; the second implant provides the contralateral papilla (i.e. distal) of the first implant.

After proper local anesthesia (Figure 8.3), the initial incisions, made using a No. 15 blade, are done as follows:

1. The first incision is done in a buccopalatal–lingual direction. The location ranges from the distal edge of the platform of the implant to the middle of the platform, depending upon the amount of tissue needed between implants or between implant and adjacent tooth.

2. The second step involves the placement of a mesio-distal incision on the buccal side for each implant, perpendicular to the first buccolingual incision. The incision is continued in a slight parabola buccally when there is adequate keratinized gingiva on the buccal to create a gingival margin around the implant. The incision is continued in a slight parabola palatally if there is insufficient keratinized gingiva on the buccal. Precautions must be taken to preserve buccal keratinized tissue. The incision passes the mesial or distal platform of the implant and ends halfway between the platform and the adjacent implant or tooth.

3. The third step involves the placement of a mesiodistal incision on the lingual/palatal parallel to the incision on the buccal. The incision for the anterior implants curves slightly off buccally in the middle, as the top of the papilla should be smaller than its base in the buccolingual direction. In posterior implants, the incision is also placed slightly palatally, because the width of the platform of a posterior implant is usually smaller than the

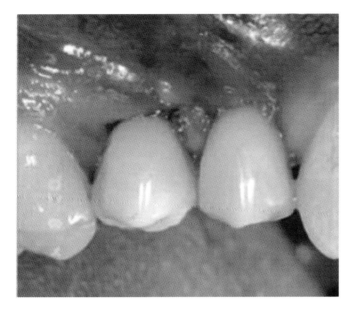

Figure 8.4 The abutment and provisional restorations for Nos. 4 and 5 in place. Notice how the gingiva has been folded and maintained via the temporary restorations.

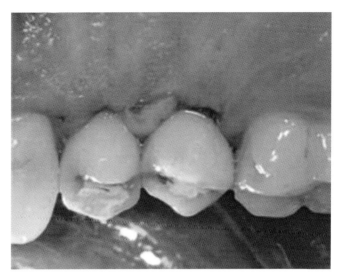

Figure 8.5 The palatal view. The U- and H-shaped flaps have been folded, creating papillae.

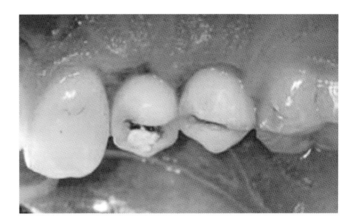

Figure 8.6 Two weeks postoperatively. The area has healed uneventfully.

width of its crown. This is essential in gaining an adequate buccolingual/palatal papilla or col. width to cover the interproximal space.

4. Flaps are elevated by using the tip of the blade and the tip of an Orban knife. First, the soft tissues are reflected from the underlying implant; then each mini-flap is undermined by the No. 15 blade and the Orban knife, and the full- or partial-thickness mini-flap is extended to about 1 mm from the adjacent implant or tooth.

Flaps are mobilized and pushed in the mesial and distal directions to open a "window" and place the healing abutment. The application of gauze in the area for a few minutes facilitates the molding of the tissues while pushing the tissues to the sides. After removing the cover screw, a healing abutment with proper height, width, and shape is inserted into the implant with or without a provisional restoration. This shapes the future papilla by pushing the tissues to the sides and holding them upright (Figures 8.4 and 8.5). The same technique is repeated for implant(s) distal to the first implant. No sutures are applied, because healing abutments hold the tissues in the proper position.

The patient then receives postoperative instructions and is scheduled for a follow-up visit within 7–10 days.

POSTOPERATIVE INSTRUCTIONS

The patient is advised to rinse with chlorhexidine gluconate (PerioGard oral rinse; Colgate Palmolive) twice daily for one week and take ibuprofen (Advil) 200 mg in case of discomfort. Postsurgical care after the first week of healing involves regular brushing with a soft bristle toothbrush (Colgate 360-degree toothbrush) and rinsing for another week with chlorhexidine gluconate.

SURGICAL INDEXING

This should be considered to increase predictability and esthetic outcome.

POSSIBLE COMPLICATIONS

- Complications are very unusual due to the minimally invasive nature of the procedure.

- Infection is always a possibility and should be treated with local antibiotherapy and antiseptic mouth rinses.

HEALING

The results are very stable 1.5 years postsurgery (Figures 8.6–8.9).

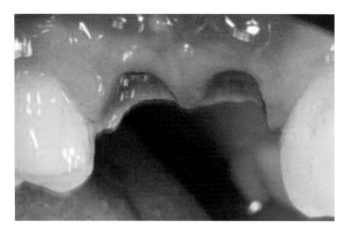

Figure 8.7 Five months postoperatively. Notice the formation of the papilla between implant Nos. 4 and 5.

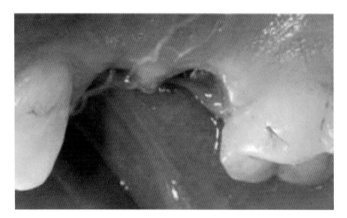

Figure 8.8 Five months postoperatively (palatal view). Notice the presence of a papilla between implant Nos. 4 and 5.

The efficacy of this new uncovering technique compared with the conventional one for papilla generation has been tested on 33 patients with 67 implants that were adjacent to either teeth or implants (Shahidi 2004). The mean difference between the two surgical methods revealed that this new technique provided 1.5 mm greater papilla height ($P < 0.001$) than the conventional one (mean difference for height of a papilla between an implant and a tooth was 1.71 mm

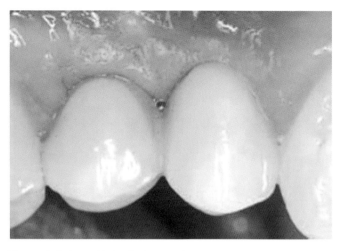

Figure 8.9 Area with the final restorations at 20 months postoperatively.

[$P < 0.001$], mean difference papilla height between implants was 0.78 mm [$P < 0.138$] at six months). The papilla generation between an implant and a tooth was more stable and predictable than papilla generation between two implants.

REFERENCES

Adriaenssens, P., Hermans, M., Ingber, A. et al. (1999). Palatal sliding strip flap: soft tissue management to restore maxillary anterior esthetics at stage 2 surgery: a clinical report. *Int. J. Oral Maxillofac. Implants* 14: 30–36.

Dibart, S. and Karima, M. (2006). *Practical Periodontal Plastic Surgery*. Ames, IA: Blackwell Publishing.

Misch, C.E., Al Shammori, K.E., and Wang, H.L. (2004). Creation of inter-implant papillae through split finger technique. *Implant Dent.* 13: 20–27.

Nemcovsky, C.E., Moses, O., and Artzi, Z. (2000). Interproximal papillae reconstruction in maxillary implants. *J. Periodontol.* 71: 308–314.

Palacci, P. (1995). *Optimal Implant Positioning and Soft Tissue Management for the Branemark System*, 35–39. Chicago: Quintessence.

Shahidi, P. (2004). Efficacy of a new papilla generation technique in implantology. MS thesis. Boston: Boston University.

Chapter 9 Dental Implant Placement Including the Use of Short Implants

Albert Price and Ming Fang Su

HISTORY

Branemark's exploration of the vascular supply to healing bone evolved into the concept referred to as *osseointegration*. The geometry of his prototype dental implant was that of a 3.0 mm titanium cylinder milled with an external thread depth of 0.375 or 0.5 mm and finished with an apical taper inward and a coronal flare outward to 4.1 mm final diameter. The restorative coronal platform presented a 0.7 mm high hexagonal shaped extension which had a screw chamber tapped through its center into the body of the cylinder for fixation of a variety of external devices (Figure 9.1).

According to Branemark's surgical protocol for edentulous areas, a full-thickness pedicle flap with a partial thickness margin was reflected and the bone crest surface exposed. The required buccal–lingual dimension was at least 6.0 mm leaving 1 mm of circumferential bone around the standard 4.0 mm implant after the osteotomy. The implant receptor site or osteotomy was initiated by creating a cylindrical hole through the compact bone of the crest and extending it vertically through intermediate trabeculated bone into the compact bone at the opposing base of bone in the mandible, floor of the nose, or floor of the sinus.

This initial cylindrical hole in the bone represented the body of the implant (3.0 mm in diameter) without threads (Figures 9.2 and 9.3) Threads were then tapped into the sides of the osteotomy when necessary. The coronal entry was subsequently countersunk in line with the cylinder drill axis to enlarge the coronal aspect to accommodate the 4.0 mm flared implant geometry. After installation of the implant a cover screw was placed over the external hex platform to seal the attachment chamber. The entire preparation was done with careful attention to measurement marks embedded in the drilling sequence so that in the finished installation the cover screw lay flush with the bone surface. The entry flap could then be sutured passively with the marginal incision providing primary connective tissue approximation and rapid healing.

Branemark's surgical technique required adherence to principles based on the results of his wound healing studies. Most of these early studies were done on edentulous subjects with severe vertical bone loss (primarily in basal bone):

1. A minimally traumatic bone preparation should be done with careful attention to minimizing heat production. This required constant irrigation with a sterile saline.

2. Primary surgical stability should be achieved with bicortical stabilization between the compact bone of opposing cortical plates.

3. Spacing of multiple implants was regulated to be 7.0–7.5 mm on center in the mandibular anterior which preserved sufficient vascular supply to the interproximal compact bone usually present in this area. Slightly closer approximation was allowed in the maxillary anterior due to the more cancellous nature of this bone.

4. A passive bone healing interval with no immediate direct load was prescribed to allow undisturbed bone and implant surface "osseointegration."

5. A minimum of 1 mm circumferential, vital bone was necessary for long term success (early bone chamber studies found at least 0.5 mm zone of osteocyte destruction with the most careful osteotomy protocol.

Many of the early Branemark and Branemark clone implants were placed in the mandible between the mental foramina and in the maxillary anterior/first bicuspid regions. Most of these early patients had complete loss of alveolar bone and minimal vestibule. The objective was to create a fixed alternative to an inadequate removable prosthesis. Implants have now become a standard of care and the treatment of choice for replacement of missing teeth. With the advancement in bone grafting techniques all areas of the mouth have been restored, and while the threaded cylinder and tapered cylinder implants are still the dominant forms, new surface treatments and attachment profiles have evolved.

Practical Advanced Periodontal Surgery, Second Edition. Edited by Serge Dibart.
© 2020 John Wiley & Sons, Inc. Published 2020 by John Wiley & Sons, Inc.
Companion website: www.wiley.com/go/dibart/advanced

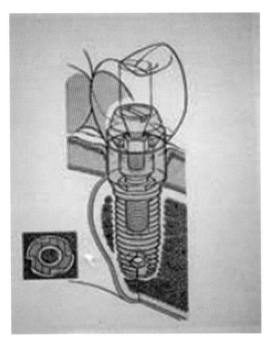

Figure 9.1 Image of a Branemark implant depicting design and surface structure. Source: Reprinted with permission from Branemark et al. (1985). *Tissue-Integrated Prostheses.* Quintessence, Chicago.

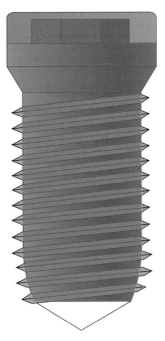

Figure 9.3 Implant fitted into the osteotomy site (cylindrical shape) Threads were pre-tapped or formed by self-tapping implant design upon insertion of implant.

(a)   (b)

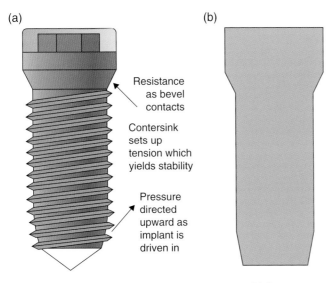

Resistance as bevel contacts

Contersink sets up tension which yields stability

Pressure directed upward as implant is driven in

Figure 9.2 (a) Branemark's prototype implant geometry. (b) Osteotomy outline created by cylinder and countersink burs representing the flared neck and body shape plus allowance for the cover screw without thread tapping. This protocol resulted in the cover screw flush with existing bone surface.

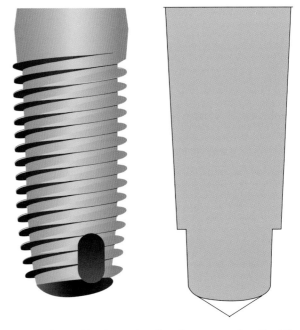

Figure 9.4 Tapered implant and outline of osteotomy site without thread tapping.

The current basic geometries include the cylinder with screw threads (Branemark's design), the tapered cylinder with threads (e.g. Zimmer [Figures 9.4 and 9.5]), and the plate form without threads, (e.g. Bicon [Figure 9.6] and Endopore). The microarchitecture of the bone influences the choice and effectiveness of these forms to gain the necessary stability at time of placement. (See bone microarchitecture in Figures 3.2, 3.4, 3.5, Chapter 3.)

Branemark stressed bicortical stabilization as essential to secure his implant system. The mechanical shape of his design created stability by the resistance of the countersink flare to the draw or pull of the threads into the bony preparation (Figure 9.2a and b); this requires heavy compact bone at each end of the osteotomy (the type of bone profile usually found in his test cases of severe

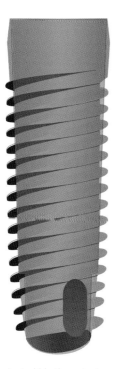

Figure 9.5 Tapered implant within the osteotomy site.

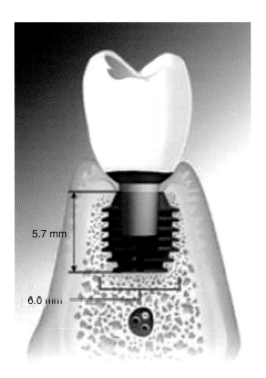

5.7 mm

6.0 mm

Figure 9.6 Bicon short implant (5.7×6 mm) placed in the mandible (especially useful in cases with insufficient bony height).

resorption). To ensure maximum use of bone and bicortical engagement (CT was not available then), the suggestion was made to place the finger firmly against the base of the mandible and to feel that the bur had penetrated the cortex. In the maxillary anterior, the surgeon was to place the finger in the nasal areas to feel the penetration of the floor of the nose (cortex). If the intermediate internal architecture had trabeculae of sufficient bulk, then the engagement of the more compact border areas was not needed. However, if the trabeculae were thin and widely spaced, such as in most areas of the upper posterior, then the screw pressures could break or strip the bone threads in the body and apical area of the implant or collapse the coronal bevel and result in a "spinner." It is possible to engage the cortical bone at the top of the mandibular canal, but this was not recommended. As the scope of placement widened to include more compromised posterior areas, single tooth sites, and even immediate placement in recent extraction sites, the need for alternate designs which increase surface contact area within a shorter bone profile evolved. (See Figure 9.6.)

The tapered screw form provides an alternative method of achieving surgical stability. Its wedge-shaped screw form achieves compression of the tapered osteotomy along its entire surface (see Figures 9.4 and 9.5). Originally referred to as the "root form implant" it was designed to fit tapered cross sectional sites with natural depressions like the incisal fossa (see oblique x-section#27 in Figure 9.7) and the depressions found over the upper first bicuspid. The tapered form is especially useful in areas of thin, lightly trabeculated bone.

INDICATIONS

Dental implants are used to:

1. Replace individual teeth
2. Support fixed and removable dental prostheses
3. Anchor maxillofacial prostheses
4. Act as anchorage for orthodontic appliances

SURGICAL TECHNIQUE

Anesthesia

Some practitioners prefer only infiltration so that the patient "feels" the proximity to vital structures and thus avoid potential damage to nerves. Block anesthesia, however, is the most efficient. Marcaine supplemented with lidocaine provides three to four hours of good working anesthesia with minimal local reinforcement. Oral sedation with diazepam 5.0 mg can be used to complement this for most nervous patients.

Pre-op visualization: Clinical observation of external bone form and well directed periapical radiographs coupled with sound anatomic knowledge is usually adequate in single tooth placement. In more advanced cases reformatted CT or CBCT images, with a distortion level of 1% or less, can be used with confidence (Figures 9.7–9.9).

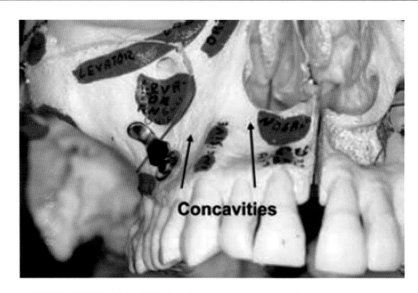

Concavities

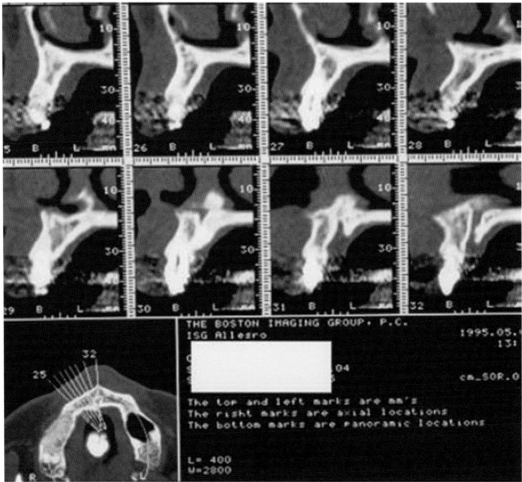

Figure 9.7 Dry skull and CT scan showing limiting anatomic features both internal (incisal canal on palatal of central incisors #31–32) and external (incisal fossa over lateral incisor #27) and varied trabeculation of the maxillary bone. (See also Figures 9.16 and 9.17.)

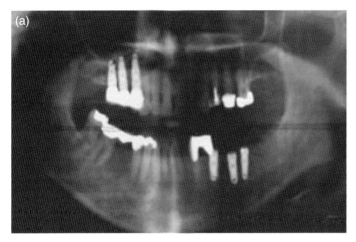
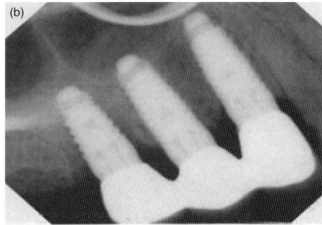

Figure 9.8 (a) Panoramic radiograph (distortion ±25%). (b) Periapical radiograph (distortion ±15%).

IMPLANT PLACEMENT

Entry Incision

The objective of the entry incision is to minimize marginal bone exposure at the site where the osteotomy is to be placed and to minimize vascular disruption to sensitive bone areas (Figure 9.10).

1. If one-stage implant or immediate load, a mid crestal incision with intrasulcular extensions buccal and lingual is used. This requires retraction of two flaps during osteotomy.

2. If classic delayed, two-stage implant, then

   a. In the maxillary arch, a horizontal incision is usually made just to the palatal of line angles and two vertical incisions sparing the proximal papillae are extended through the mucogingival junction (MGJ) on the buccal. The flap is reflected into the vestibule. Incisions vary with site objective and history of local trauma covered with a gauze pad and no retraction is needed (Figures 9.10 and 9.11).

   b. In the mandibular arch, an incision can be made just to the buccal of buccal line angles, or if the MGJ is close to this area, the incision is made below the MGJ and reverse split for about 2 mm to leave a small bed of periosteum behind. Vertical incisions sparing the papillae are extended over the crest and through the lingual MGJ. The flap is reflected to the lingual and usually placement of a protective gauze pad in the lingual vestibule maintains access.

3. If dealing with multiple implants in a severely resorbed lower arch with no vestibular depth, then an incision is made in the middle of available keratinized tissue, reflecting enough to expose the crest.

SITE PREPARATION

The only time one needs to reduce bone height at the site is a requirement for increased restorative space. It should be kept in mind that reducing the bone increases the crown–root ratio of the prosthesis, which increases stress–strain relationships at the abutment/implant and implant/bone interface.

(Vertical restorative space is the distance from the implant restorative platform to the opposing occlusal surfaces. This space varies for different restorative modes. Minimum vertical space needed for a crown direct to an implant with no abutment [screw retained] = 4.5 mm, vertical space required for abutment + cemented crown requires 6.5–7.0 mm, while a hybrid restoration with bar or bar overdenture requires 11–12 mm accommodation.)

The Osteotomy: Single Implant

The primary objective is to place the dental implant in the position which satisfies all the biologic and esthetic needs of the restoration. The ideal position is centered beneath the crown form both buccal–lingual and mesio-distal and vertically at least 3 mm below adjacent soft tissue level to allow for appropriate development of crown emergence profile. At the same time there must be at least 1.0 mm of bone circumferential to allow healing and long term osseointegration. It was estimated that at least 0.5 mm of bone is necrosed in the most careful surgery (Rhinelander 1974a, b).

Preparation

1. Using a small round bur approximating the size of the first cylinder bur (Figure 9.12), the mesial–distal, buccal–lingual location is marked with a small depression. This is remeasured and accepted or revised, and then the preparation is deepened for 2–3 mm to initiate penetration of

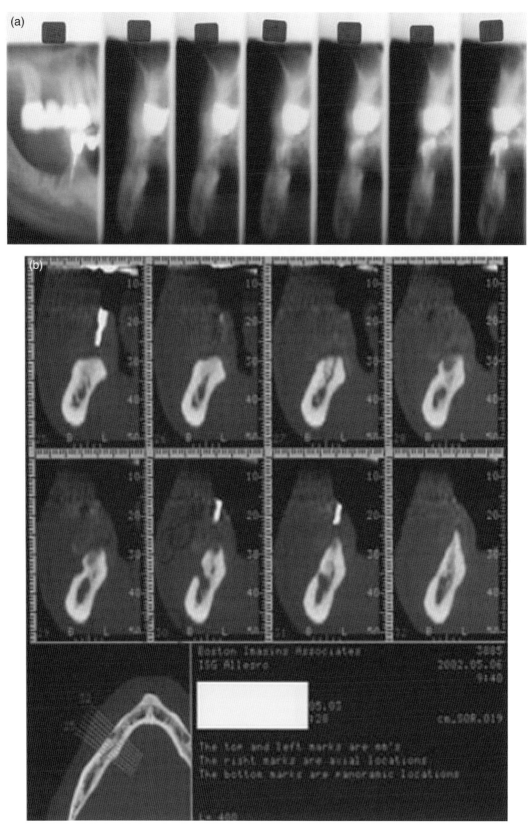

Figure 9.9 Two radiographic techniques – same patient area: (a) Conventional tomography technique. The "foggy" quality is due to slice thickness (5 mm) which distorts image. (b) Axial CT scan: distortion ±1% (reformat slice thickness ≤0.5 mm with 2 mm spacing).

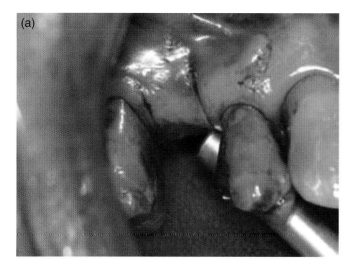

(a)

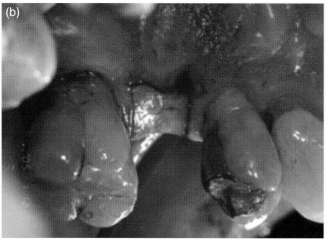

(b)

Figure 9.10 Incision design buccally (a) and palatally (b) before the placement of implant No. 4.

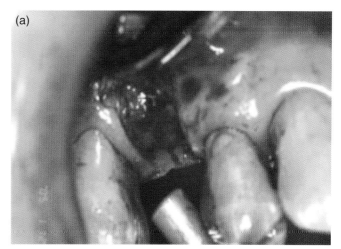

(a)

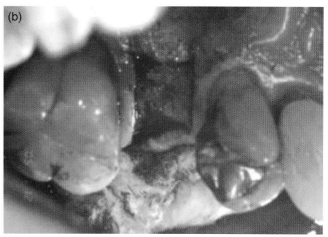

(b)

Figure 9.11 Full-thickness flap reflected to the buccal, exposing alveolar crest, buccal, and palatal.

the crestal cortex. In some sites, after penetrating 1–2 mm, the bur may suddenly drop. If this happens, a periodontal probe should be inserted and pushed until resistance is detected. The probe may drop 10 mm in areas of very little trabecular content. A revised strategy of under-preparation should be utilized to achieve surgical stability. In contrast excessively dense compact bone might require a smaller round bur first.

2. The starting cylinder bur is usually 2.0–2.5 mm in diameter (Figure 9.13) (in very dense bone, starting with a 1.5-mm bur is more efficient). The burs should have guide marks to mark vertical depth, and these should be checked against a common rule (periodontal probe) for actual depth and reference to CT scan measurements. Please note that many drill systems do not count the bevel at tip of bur, and the markings may not represent millimeters but instead a preferred depth for ideal placement of that particular implant system. A CT scan

or some method of judging distance to vital structures should be used in treatment planning visualization prior to surgery.

At this initial stage, it is prudent to drill only as deep as needed with the cylinder bur to check vertical angulation (7–8 mm) with a direction guide. If a change is to be made in position or direction, then it should be done before proceeding to larger drills. Sometimes it is necessary to use the round bur again to force this change in direction. The direction guide with string attached should be placed (Figures 9.14 and 9.15). The cylinder bur is aligned with this guide and then reoriented to the new direction. (In a given site the nature of internal microarchitecture can be quite different from buccal to lingual – see Figures 3.4 and 3.5 in Chapter 3. This difference in "structural density" can cause the bur to drift into unintended angulation or drift to buccal or lingual.) The guide is pulled, and the correction is made. Once the new direction is acceptable, the site is drilled to final depth. If the vertical dimension of bone allows, over-drill the depth of the site by about 1.0 mm in

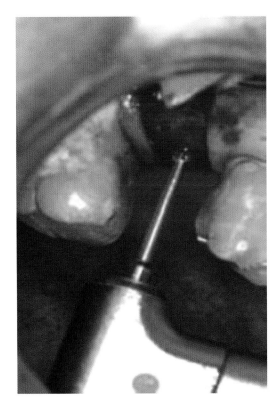

Figure 9.12 Using a pilot or round bur, future site of implant osteotomy is marked.

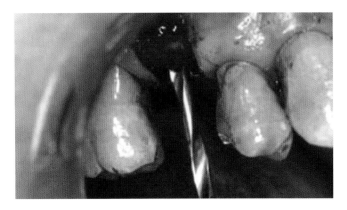

Figure 9.13 Initial cylinder drill is used to initiate the osteotomy.

the initial drill steps. This allows more flexibility as larger burs are used because they are not efficient end-cutters and can generate heat if pushed too hard trying to achieve increased depth at later stages. (Internally irrigated burs have not been found practical, because they constantly clog, and irrigation fails.)

Once the initial burs have created place and angulation, the site is gradually enlarged and deepened to the final size according to the steps recommended by the implant system guide. (Remember bur drift can occur at every step in the drilling sequence since internal microarchitecture varies. The surgeon must sense this and correct as needed.)

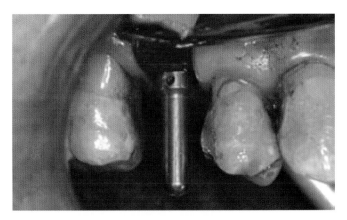

Figure 9.14 Directional guide used to check the proper alignment and 2 dimensional position of the implant.

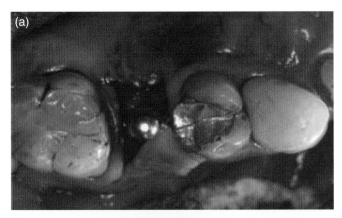

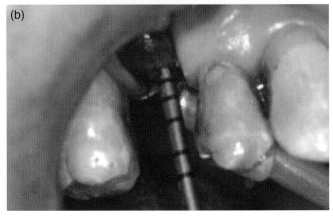

Figure 9.15 (a) Directional guide shows the proper alignment of the implant occlusally. (b) Using a periodontal probe, the proper depth of the osteotomy is being assessed.

WARNING: DRILL SPEED: Each drill system has been engineered to be run at certain speeds; failure to follow recommendations may overheat bone. Irrigation should be constant, and drilling is done in a pumping action to remove bone filings, especially in very compact bone. (In the lower anterior, it is sometimes necessary to change to a new bur after one osteotomy; remember that the smaller burs are being used in every case.)

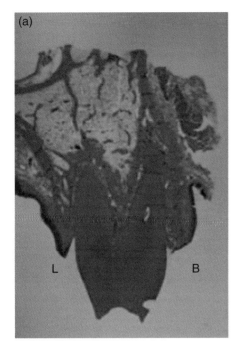
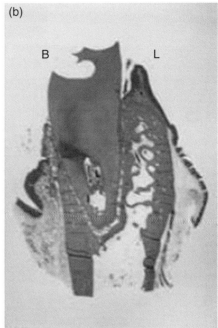

Figure 9.16 Internal architecture notches on buccal of crown. (a) Maxillary bicuspid. (b) Mandibular first bicuspid. Note different cortex and trabecular thickness. B, buccal area; L, lingual area.

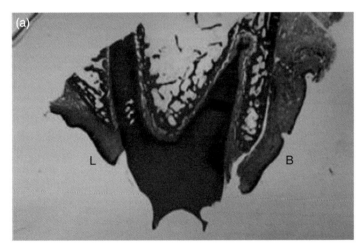
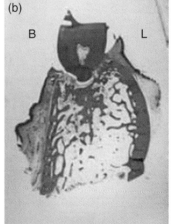

Figure 9.17 Internal architecture of furcation area of first molars. (Notches in tooth crown are too buccal.) (a) Maxillary first molar. (b) Mandibular first molar. Note differences in cortical plates and trabecular dimensions at the maxillary versus mandibular sites. B, buccal; L, lingual.

During the final drill stages, a judgment needs to be made about whether to tap threads. Reflecting on the internal arrangement of trabeculae seen in the pictures (Figures 9.16 and 9.17), it is possible to start "soft" and end "hard" as the last bur encounters heavy trabeculation or the inner aspect of bordering cortex or the residual compact socket framework from a recently extracted tooth.

If tapping threads is necessary, it should be done by hand or very low handpiece speed; the same speed used for placement of the implant (30–50 rpm). After tapping

threads, the osteotomy should be flushed free of debris and then restimulated to bleed by probing the apical area.

In some systems, a final coronal shaping is needed to countersink or expand the coronal for a slightly enlarged collar. If resistance or drill debris has been minimal during the preparation, then one can eliminate or reduce these last steps. If the implant site is not bleeding enough to fill the site after any of these steps, then have the patient open and close several times after stimulating with a probe. This "pumps" the maxillary artery and results in the desired fill of the osteotomy with blood.

THE FIXTURE (IMPLANT) INSTALLATION

The implant fixture may be placed by hand or with a machine-controlled drill speed and torque. A torque-metered speed of 30–50 rpm is preferred with torque set at a low value to start. The resistance sensed during the drilling sequence used to prepare the site should give one a sense of the torque needed. If one is in doubt, it is best to start the fixture placement with low torque of 15–20 N/cm. If the insertion stalls, then reverse the driver for a half turn and proceed with next highest torque. This reversal strategy clears the threads of bone chips and allows for momentum at the next torque/speed combination. If fixture is stalled at 40 N/cm at collar level – the last 3–4 mm is still exposed – then it should be reversed out and the osteotomy modified before proceeding. Note should be made of final insertion torque on record, and this is used to determine waiting period for integration and/or loading. Hand installation does not allow this objective measure of torque, but sometimes it is preferred in very "delicate" sites. Hand insertion after stalling at 40 N/cm or above with an unmetered ratchet wrench is discouraged because excess stress can fracture buccal plates and/or strip threading, over compress site or, worse, it can result in fracture of implant collar. (EVERY IMPLANT SYSTEM HAS A RECOMMENDED MAXIMUM INSERTION TORQUE – READ THE DIRECTIONS.) A surgical insertion torque of 20 N/cm would probably call for a six-month wait while insertion at 35–45 N/cm could be loaded immediately. Experience will guide in this judgment. After the fixture is adjusted to its final position, either a cover screw or healing abutment is placed. If trabeculation is light or thin and insertion torque is minimal, then a passive healing period is required and the final result should be at or slightly below crest with cover screw in place (Figures 9.18 and 9.19).

POSSIBLE PROBLEMS AND COMPLICATIONS

Common Drilling Problems

1. *Underdrill of site depth:* This can result in thread stripping as implant bottoms before engaging bevel; pertains to Branemark style hex top with countersunk neck or rapid taper like the Astra ST.

2. *Excess drill speed over the implant system's recommended speeds and/or lack of irrigation:* Burns bone, kills osteocytes, and results in early fixture loss.

3. *Failure to "read" bone external contours:* Perforation of buccal or lingual concavities (Figures 9.7 and 9.20). This can be very dangerous with postoperative swelling and closure of airway in case of lingual lower cuspid site; roughly the area where the sublingual gland is located; see multiple vascular supplies to this area (Figure 9.22), see Chapter 3. Inferior alveolar artery distribution.

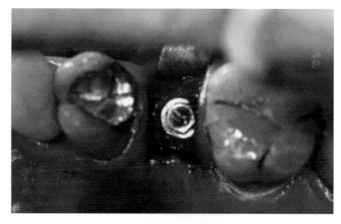

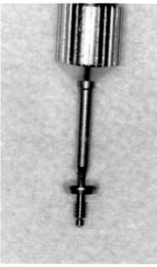

Figure 9.18 The cover screw is used to seal the coronal portion of the implant before flap closure.

4. *Tipping or angulation of drill* as depth increases from use of finger rest on tooth and rotating around the finger rest instead of vertical pumping movement.

5. *Overdrilling depth* or *irregular uneven osteotomy* can result in loss of implant into the sinus (Figure 9.21) or within the mandible when there is a "hollow" anatomy (previous pontic area of bridge often has absence of trabeculae), see Chapter 3, Figure 3.5b.

In addition to drilling problems, several local site variables may complicate placement. These include:

1. Surface slopes mesial–distal and/or buccal–lingual or both

2. Vestibular depth may be very shallow (1–2 mm)

3. Thin cortex at crest and thin trabeculae internally (maxillary posterior)

4. Dense 1- to 2-mm crest with subjacent very poor internal trabecular distribution (mandibular posterior;

(a)

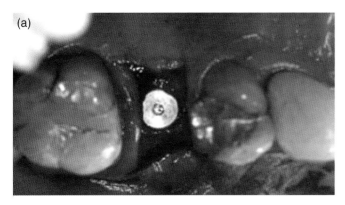

(b)

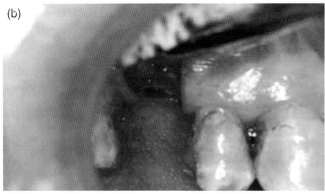

Figure 9.19 (a) Cover screw is seated. (b) Implant is at level or below alveolar crest.

especially after failed bridge where pontic has covered site)

5. Inadequate vertical height; maxillary first molar/sinus, lower posterior over canal

6. Buccal concavities: incisal fossa, cuspid fossa (Figures 9.7 and 9.20)

7. Lingual concavities: submandibular gland below lower molars, sublingual gland below lower cuspid/lateral areas (Figures 9.20 and 9.22)

Slopes: Major discrepancies in site restorative platform location (mesial–distal or buccal–lingual) should be corrected with grafting. Minor contour differences can be adjusted for by interplay between implant anatomy and site anatomy. For example, if a site has a 2-mm deficiency from mid crest to buccal line angles, then a Branemark style implant can be used by placing the implant at the level of the lingual crest. This intentionally leaves the buccal bevel exposed, but at one year, this bone would have been lost in the cupping resorption usually seen with this style implant. As long as the palatal bone and half the mesial and distal bone serve the purpose of creating surgical stability, the implant used in this example can be left at a reasonable height and the C/R ratio is not affected.

Minimal vestibular depth: This often happens in the lower anterior with severe resorption, classic Branemark case. If the crest was leveled and the implants are placed by the standard protocol, then the connections could fall below the floor and vestibular depth. By ignoring the buccal and lingual deficiencies and seating implants at mesial and distal bone level, the implants can be left above the floor and still retain maximum bone integration. It is even possible to leave the majority of the bevel above the crest, but this must be planned ahead and use of mid crestal incision is necessary.

Thin bone and minimal internal support: The site can be underprepared (stop one drill diameter short of final or use final bur for ½ vertical depth), laterally compressed with osteotomes, or site abandoned and allowed to reheal or even grafted internally and revisited at three to four months.

Inadequate vertical height: Site can be grafted with a block graft, or short implants with increased surface area can be used (Figure 9.23). Current protocols call for all-on four to angle implants to distal over sinus or mental foramen but this only gains 2–3 mm of extra distalization at best.

Buccal concavities: This can present the most difficulty. Sometimes threaded implants are placed and then grafted. The implant may be placed at an acute angle and restored with an angled abutment. This often results in a "knee" at gingival margin, which with time and recession can expose the restorative margin. Another alternative in multiple site cases may be to skip this site and bridge it with a pontic.

Lingual concavities: In the mandibular second molar, one can change the inclination with the direction closer to that of the Curve of Wilson; however, it is necessary to avoid encroaching on tongue space. Lower cuspid lingual concavity has multiple vascular supplies, so it is very dangerous to perforate this area; with the potential for submylohyoid swelling and closure of airspace (see Figure 9.22). A CT scan is advised if anatomy too hard to read clinically.

Multiple sites: Most of the issues with multiple sites are solved by good prosthetic guidance. In general, the implants need to be placed in the center of the respective crown shape.

The limits of placement proximity are different for implant-to-implant versus implant-to-tooth. The general rule is to have at least 2 mm of bone between implant surfaces. This proximity is problematic for two reasons: Tarnow et al. (2003) published data supporting the need for at least 3 mm to support interdental papillae. This would apply to Branemark style implants where the cupping

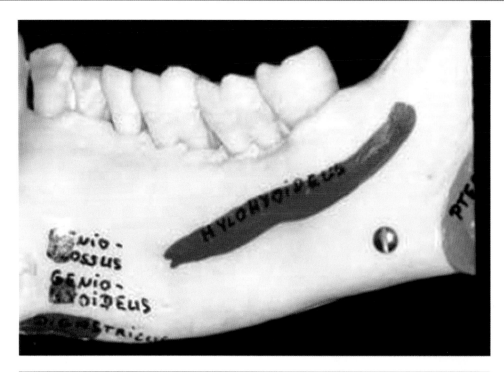

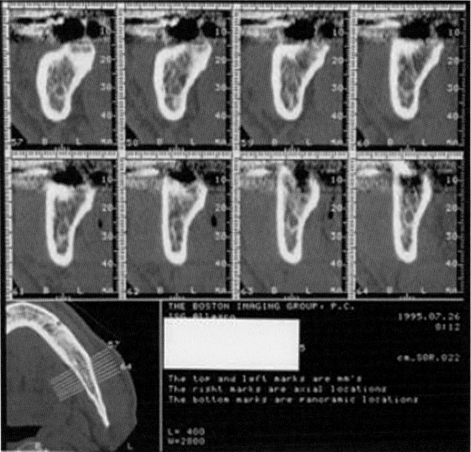

Figure 9.20 Mylohyoid insertion line (concavity below, submandibular gland) and canal proximity can limit angle and vertical depth of implant placement.

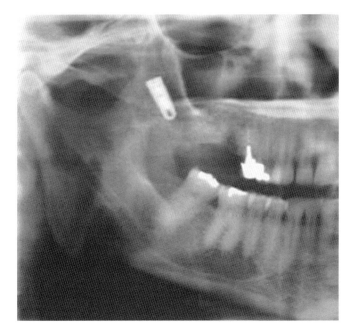

Figure 9.21 Implant displaced into maxillary sinus. Student failed to sense resistance to abutment torque.

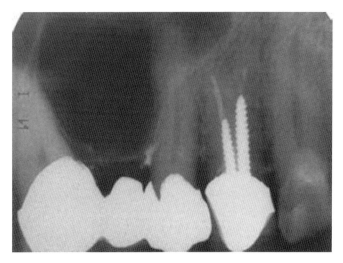

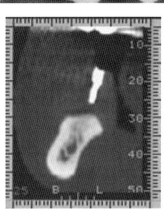

Figure 9.23 Anatomic limits. Sinus extension, resulting in less than 1 mm bone at the alveolar crest (*top*). Crestal resorption: there is less than 7 mm bone above the mandibular canal, impairing standard implant placement (*bottom*).

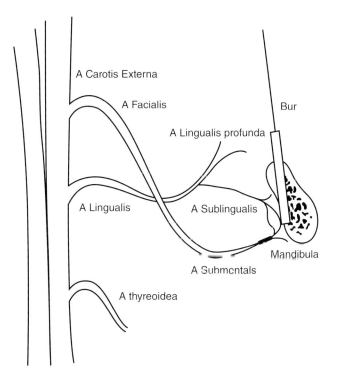

A Carotis Externa

A Facialis

A Lingualis profunda

Bur

A Lingualis

A Sublingualis

Mandibula

A Submentals

A thyreoidea

Figure 9.22 Diagram showing sublingual and submental arteries that can be injured during implant placement in the canine/premolar area due to the presence of a lingual concavity. Source: Reprinted with permission from *JOMI* 1993; 8[3]:329–333.

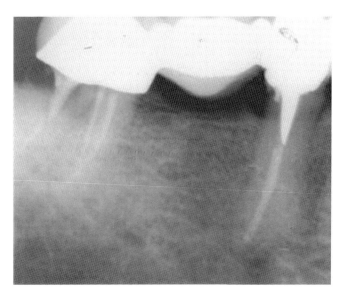

Figure 9.24 Periapical radiograph showing mandibular molar necessitating extraction and replacement with implants. Due to insufficient vertical bony height above the mandibular canal, short implants were selected to restore missing dentition.

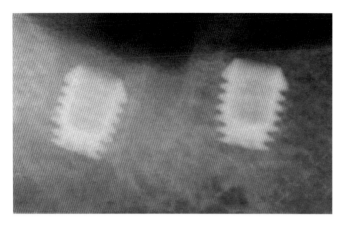

Figure 9.25 Short implants (Bicon, Boston, MA, USA) were placed to overcome vertical limitation.

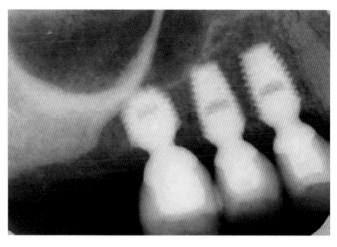

Figure 9.28 Short implants were used to overcome the anatomical limitations of sinus proximity (avoiding extensive sinus grafting).

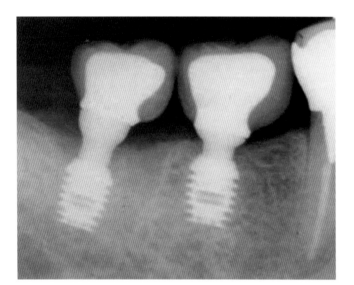

Figure 9.26 Periapical radiograph showing implants restored.

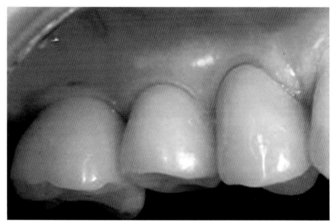

Figure 9.29 Clinical picture of final implant-supported restoration.

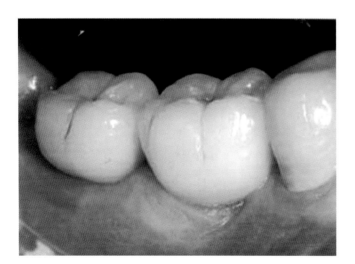

Figure 9.27 Clinical picture of restored short implants.

around adjacent implants would overlap and drop interproximal bone and then the soft tissue above leaving the "black triangle." Other implant geometries may not present this problem. In addition, if one is dealing with narrow buccal–lingual but heavy compact bone such as found in the lower anterior, then placing implants too close endangers the endosseous vascular supply between them and there is the risk of bone necrosis between and loss of both implants and bone. (Branemark isolated this by trial and error – suggesting 7.0 mm on center to allow 3 mm of bone between the standard 4.1 mm implant head.)

Implants can be placed closer to teeth because they have an increased vascular net in their periodontal ligamnet (PDL), which is connected through numerous spaces to the adjacent marrow.

It may be more prudent to skip an implant and bridge a site if mesial–distal proximity becomes a problem. For example, in the upper anterior, it might be better to skip the lateral site if inadequate spacing exists and/or to use the lateral and skip the central position if an overly large incisal foramen is present. (Note – the incisal foramen can sometimes be grafted with minimal post-op sequelae.) The general concept is to pay attention to the micro-architecture of bone.

Short implants: In the past, statistical analysis has shown decreased success rates with implants less than 10 mm. This is being challenged by newer forms and changed surface textures and treatments. Roughened surfaces, square threads, and plate form implants with greater surface area have been used successfully (Gentile et al. 2005). While success rates may not be 100%, it is still possible and judicious to use short implants in selected cases, especially when patients refuse extensive graft placement (Figures 9.24–9.29).

REFERENCES

Branemark, P.-I., Zarb, G.A., and Albrektsson, T. (eds.) (1985). *Tissue-integrated prostheses: osseointegration in clinical dentistry.* Chicago: Quintessence Publishing Co.

Bruggenkate, C.M., Krekeler, G., Kraaijenhagen, H.A. et al. (1993). Hemorrhage of the Floor of the Mouth Resulting from Lingual Perforation During Implant Placement: A Clinical Report. *Int. J. Oral Maxillofac. Implants* 8: 329–334.

Gentile, M., Chuang, S.K., and Dodson, T. (2005). Survival estimates and risk factors for failure with 6 × 5.7 mm implants. *Int. J. Oral Maxillofac. Implants* 20 (6): 930–937.

Rhinelander, F.W. (1974a). Tibial blood supply in relation to fracture healing. *Clin. Orthop.* 105: 34.

Rhinelander, F.W. (1974b). The normal circulation of bone and its response to surgical intervention. *J. Biomed. Mater. Res.* 8: 87.

Tarnow, D., Elian, N., Fletcher, P. et al. (2003). Vertical distance from the crest of bone to the height of the interproximal papilla between adjacent implants. *J. Periodontol.* 74: 1785–1788.

Chapter 10 Periodontal Medicine Including Biopsy Techniques

Vikki Noonan and Sadru Kabani

GINGIVAL NODULES

Nodular proliferations on the gingiva are frequently encountered and represent a number of distinct entities with different etiologies and treatment strategies. While most represent reactive or inflammatory processes, occasionally lesions arise that are developmental in nature, perhaps resulting from stimulation of residua of odontogenesis that persist in the oral mucosa following tooth development.

PARULIS

Inflammatory infiltrates at the apices of nonvital teeth occasionally channelize through medullary alveolar bone, penetrate the cortical bone and soft tissue, and drain into the oral cavity. These inflammatory infiltrates typically follow a path of least resistance. Given this trend, in most regions inflammatory apical lesions will drain into the oral cavity through a sinus tract on the buccal aspect of the alveolar bone due to decreased thickness of the buccal cortical plate compared with the lingual cortex. Exceptions to this rule are the mandibular second and third molars, the palatal roots of maxillary molars, and the maxillary lateral incisors, which typically perforate lingually. At the orifice of the sinus tract, a focal nodular proliferation of inflamed granulation tissue may arise, termed a "parulis" or "gum boil" (Figure 10.1).

The parulis represents a focus of communication between a pathologic cavity associated with an odontogenic infection and the oral cavity. Therefore, it is frequently possible to insert a gutta-percha point into the sinus tract and trace its path to the tooth that represents the source of the infection. If the sinus tract remains patent, chronic drainage will allow the offending tooth to be asymptomatic. If the sinus tract becomes obstructed, symptoms of odontogenic infection will typically arise. A parulis typically resolves following endodontic therapy or extraction of the offending tooth; however, residual microorganisms and inflammation that persist along a sinus tract following treatment may cause the parulis to persist. In such instances, excision may be required.

FIBROMA

A fibroma represents a nodular proliferation of dense fibrous connective tissue that arises secondary to trauma or focal irritation. Representing the most common reactive proliferation of the oral cavity, fibromas typically present as smooth-surfaced firm nodular lesions that are similar in color to the surrounding mucosa (Figure 10.2). If the lesion is frequently traumatized or subjected to constant irritation, surface ulceration or hyperkeratosis may result. One form of fibroma with distinctive clinicopathologic characteristics termed the *giant cell fibroma* appears to have no association with trauma and is often described clinically as having a papillary surface architecture. With a predilection for occurring on the gingiva (Magnusson and Rasmusson 1995), the giant cell fibroma is typically diagnosed in patients under age 30. The histopathologic appearance is distinctive due to the presence of multinucleated and stellate cells throughout the densely collagenized connective tissue stroma thought to be derived from the fibroblast lineage (Souza et al. 2004); however, the presence of these stellate and multinucleated fibroblasts in this lesion is of no known clinical significance.

PERIPHERAL OSSIFYING FIBROMA

Representing a reactive nodular proliferation of fibrous and mineralized tissue, the peripheral ossifying fibroma is a frequently encountered lesion arising exclusively on the gingiva, most often from the region of the maxillary interdental papilla (Figure 10.3). More common in females, the lesion typically presents in young patients anterior to the first molars (Cuisia and Brannon 2001) and may exhibit surface ulceration (Buchner and Hansen 1979). Although the pathogenesis is not completely understood, the peripheral ossifying fibroma is thought to represent a reactive process that frequently arises secondary to local irritation.

Practical Advanced Periodontal Surgery, Second Edition. Edited by Serge Dibart.
© 2020 John Wiley & Sons, Inc. Published 2020 by John Wiley & Sons, Inc.
Companion website: www.wiley.com/go/dibart/advanced

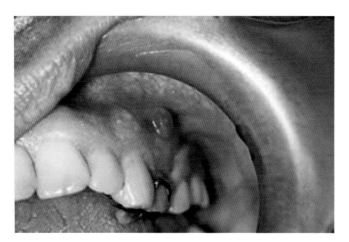

Figure 10.1 Nodular erythematous mass of granulation tissue near the mucobuccal fold and associated with an asymptomatic nonvital premolar. Source: Image courtesy of Dr. Helen Santis.

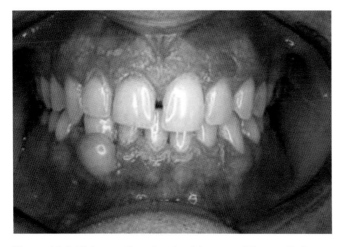

Figure 10.2 Pink, smooth-surfaced nodular mass of the mandibular attached gingiva. Source: Image courtesy of Dr. Helen Santis.

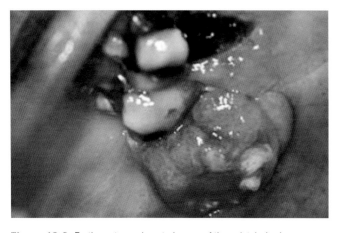

Figure 10.3 Erythematous ulcerated mass of the palatal gingiva.

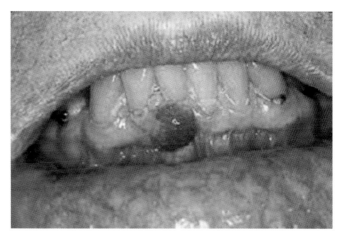

Figure 10.4 Erythematous nodular mass arising from the mandibular anterior gingiva.

PYOGENIC GRANULOMA

The pyogenic granuloma represents an acquired vascular lesion of the skin and mucous membranes that occurs in patients over a wide age range. Clinically presenting as a nodular lesion remarkable for rapid growth and frequently exhibiting surface ulceration, the pyogenic granuloma often bleeds on subtle provocation secondary to its vascular nature. Pyogenic granulomas of the oral cavity most commonly present on the gingiva in areas of focal chronic irritation (Figure 10.4).

These lesions have been reported to occur with greater frequency in pregnant women. This increased incidence is likely related to increased levels of estrogen and progesterone, which have been shown to enhance angiogenesis in traumatized tissues (Yuan et al. 2002).

PERIPHERAL GIANT CELL GRANULOMA

Arising exclusively on the gingiva, the peripheral giant cell granuloma presents as an exophytic sessile or pedunculated nodular lesion that is often dark red or purple. Although seen over a wide age range, the peripheral giant cell granuloma typically presents during the fifth to sixth decades of life, is more commonly encountered in females, and is seen with greater frequency in the mandible anterior to the first molars (Bodner et al. 1997; Buduneli et al. 2001) (Figure 10.5). Focal irritation is typically deemed the causative agent rather than a true neoplastic process. At least one study suggests diminished salivary flow rate and altered salivary composition may increase susceptibility to such lesions due to reduced ability to clear local irritants (Bodner et al. 1997). A pressure resorptive defect of the underlying bone may be appreciated in association with the peripheral giant cell granuloma having a "scooped-out" radiolucent appearance.

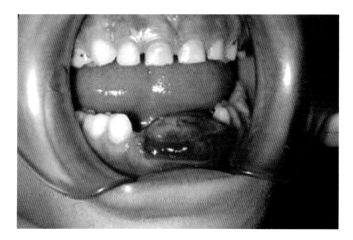

Figure 10.5 Ulcerated reddish-purple mass of the mandibular anterior gingiva.

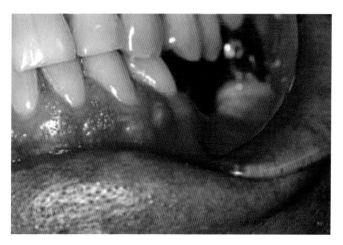

Figure 10.6 Fluid-filled lesion in the mandibular premolar region of the attached gingiva.

DIAGNOSIS AND TREATMENT OF REACTIVE GINGIVAL NODULES

Treatment of reactive gingival nodules, including the gingival fibroma, the peripheral ossifying fibroma, pyogenic granuloma, and peripheral giant cell granuloma, includes both a thorough excision of lesional tissue and removal of local irritants such as calculus or overextended restorations. Despite a diligent effort at complete excision, the recurrence rate for these lesions approaches 20% (Buduneli et al. 2001; Carrera Grano et al. 2001; Walters et al. 2001). To reduce the likelihood of recurrence, some suggest that reactive gingival lesions be excised to bone. In lesions recalcitrant to treatment, a wider excision including periosteum and curettage of the periodontal ligament may be indicated to prevent recurrence (Buduneli et al. 2001; Carrera Grano et al. 2001; Walters et al. 2001).

GINGIVAL CYST OF THE ADULT

The gingival cyst of the adult represents an infrequently encountered lesion of odontogenic origin. Thought to originate from rests of dental lamina, the gingival cyst of the adult presents as a fluid-filled swelling typically arising on the labial attached gingiva of the premolar-canine region of the mandible (Buchner and Hansen 1979; Nxumalo and Shear 1992) (Figure 10.6). Reported to primarily present during the fifth and sixth decades of life (Nxumalo and Shear 1992; Giunta 2002), the gingival cyst of the adult may occasionally cause a pressure resorptive defect of the subjacent alveolar bone that may cause the entity to be mistaken for a lateral periodontal cyst (Giunta 2002). Rare examples of multiple lesions have been described (Shade et al. 1987; Giunta 2002). Treatment consists of simple surgical excision with submission of lesional tissue for histopathologic examination.

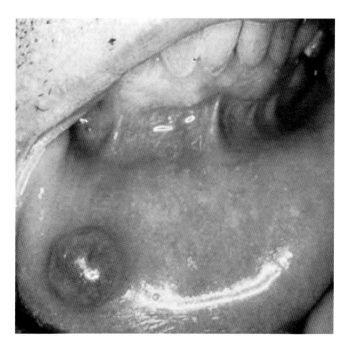

Figure 10.7 Bluish fluctuant swelling of the lower labial mucosa. Source. Image courtesy of Dr Helen Santis.

MUCOCELE

The mucocele is a frequently encountered lesion of the oral mucosa characterized by extravasated mucoid material that leads to a fluctuant nodular swelling of the mucosa, often remarkable for a bluish hue. Typically found on the lower labial mucosa lateral to the midline (Figure 10.7) but noted in the buccal mucosa, floor of the mouth (ranula), and the anterior ventral tongue, mucoceles frequently arise secondary to a focal traumatic injury that causes rupture of an excretory duct with subsequent spillage of mucin into the surrounding connective tissue. The feeder salivary gland typically retains its capacity to produce secretion;

however, the damaged duct prevents passage of saliva into the oral cavity. Patients typically complain of the lesion waxing and waning as the gland produces saliva and then empties. Occasionally, mucoceles are found on the posterior palate, posterior buccal mucosa, and retromolar trigone; most frequently, these lesions represent superficial mucoceles. These lesions typically present as small fluid-filled vesicles that rupture, leaving ulcerative lesions that occasionally recur. Tartar control toothpaste (Navazesh 1995) has been linked to the formation of these lesions, and they have also been described to occur more frequently at mealtime.

Additionally, superficial mucoceles have been reported in early stages of graft-versus-host disease (Garcia et al. 2002). A *mucous cyst* represents a true cystic lesion; the lining is derived from salivary ductal epithelium. These lesions are frequently located in the lips and buccal mucosa and are seen in association with ductal obstruction such as sialolithiasis that may increase intraluminal pressure; however, true developmental cystic lesions are seen.

DESQUAMATIVE GINGIVITIS

Desquamative gingivitis is a clinically descriptive term that is characterized by sloughing, erythematous areas of the attached gingiva. These desquamative gingival changes may be appreciated in the context of vesiculoerosive conditions, including pemphigus vulgaris, mucous membrane (cicatricial) pemphigoid, erosive lichen planus, linear IgA disease, graft-versus-host disease, paraneoplastic pemphigus, epidermolysis bullosa acquisita, systemic lupus erythematosus, chronic ulcerative stomatitis, contact hypersensitivity reactions, and foreign-body gingivitis (2003). (Portions reprinted with permission from the *Journal of the Massachusetts Dental Society* 2005 Fall; 54 (3): 38.)

LICHEN PLANUS

Lichen planus represents an immunologically mediated mucocutaneous disease that affects the oral cavity in as much as 2% of the population. Typically presenting in the fourth to fifth decades of life, lichen planus is characterized by a variety of clinical manifestations including the reticular, erosive, and atrophic forms of the disease. The most commonly affected site is the buccal mucosa, followed by the tongue, gingiva, labial mucosa, and lower labial vermilion (Eisen 2002). In just under 10% of patients lichen planus presents exclusively on the gingiva (Eisen 2002; Mignogna et al. 2005) (Figure 10.8). These cases typically present as the reticular or erosive forms of the disease involving wide areas of marginal and attached gingiva and most commonly affect women (Mignogna et al. 2005). A number of medications (especially antihypertensive agents), flavoring agents, oral hygiene products, and candies and chewing gum can elicit a mucosal

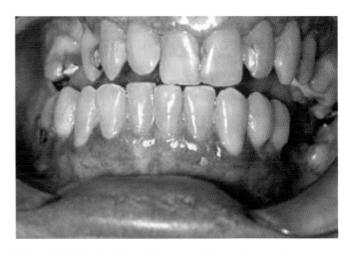

Figure 10.8 Erosive lichen planus presenting as desquamative gingivitis with erythema and discomfort. Source: Image courtesy of Dr. Helen Santis.

reaction clinically indistinguishable from lichen planus. Termed *lichenoid mucositis*, clinical features, when correlated with histopathologic findings, help to distinguish the entity from bona fide lichen planus (Thornhill et al. 2006). Diagnosis is based on a process of elimination of suspected stimuli. This is frequently based on trial and error and is time consuming. If there is a reason to suspect medication-induced mucositis, consultation with the patient's physician may be helpful to explore the possibility of substituting the medication. It is reasonable to treat this affliction with topical corticosteroids to control symptoms. *Chronic ulcerative stomatitis* represents an infrequently encountered condition that shares clinical features of erosive lichen planus superficially and may present as desquamative gingivitis. While the tongue and buccal mucosa are more commonly affected, gingival involvement is clinically indistinguishable from the erosive form of lichen planus (Solomon et al. 2003). This condition typically presents in women and is characterized by episodes of waxing and waning. Differences in the immunofluorescence profile aid in distinguishing chronic ulcerative stomatitis from lichen planus. The immunopathologic pattern for lichen planus is nonspecific but frequently consists of shaggy deposition of fibrinogen along the epithelial–connective tissue interface, whereas that of chronic ulcerative stomatitis consists of IgG autoantibodies directed against parabasal and basal stratified squamous epithelial cell nuclei. In some instances, a lichenoid appearance of the gingiva is seen secondary to the impregnation of dental materials into the gingiva during dental treatment. The term *foreign body gingivitis* is used to describe this entity. More common in females, foreign body gingivitis typically presents as an erythroplakic or erythroleukoplakic lesion of the gingiva (Figure 10.9) that does not respond to improved oral hygiene measures or minimal improvement with topical steroid therapy as a result of its anti-inflammatory effect (Gordon 2000).

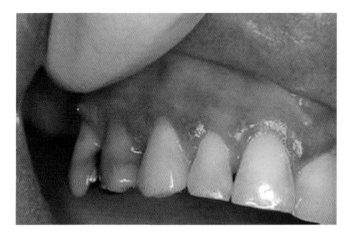

Figure 10.9 Focal areas of painful erythematous marginal gingiva.

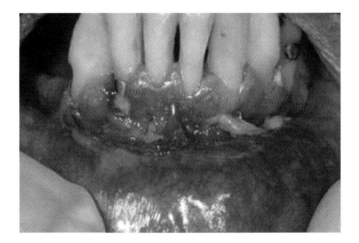

Figure 10.10 Erosive lesions affecting the anterior mandibular gingiva and mandibular mucobuccal fold.

PEMPHIGUS VULGARIS

Pemphigus vulgaris represents an autoimmune-mediated mucocutaneous disease characterized by autoantibody attack against components of desmosomes. Frequently representing the initial manifestation of the disease, oral lesions are found in most instances and typically present as blisters or erosive lesions of the oral and pharyngeal mucosa. Often the onset is insidious with lesions getting progressively worse over time. Desquamative gingivitis in the absence of other clinical features is a frequently encountered clinical presentation. Here, blisters and/or erosive lesions are seen often extending to the free gingival tissues (Mignogna et al. 2001) (Figure 10.10). Direct immunofluorescence findings from tissue submitted in Michel's media shows IgG or IgM antibodies and complement (typically C3) deposited in the intercellular areas of the epithelium. A condition linked to underlying lymphoproliferative disease termed *paraneoplastic pemphigus* may present with oral mucosal involvement yielding clinical characteristics indistinguishable from pemphigus vulgaris.

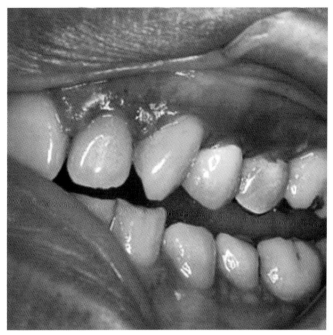

Figure 10.11 Desquamative gingival lesions representing the only affected site in this patient. Source: Image courtesy of Dr. Helen Santis.

In this condition, circulating autoantibodies produced in response to lymphoid neoplasia cross-react with antigens associated with epithelial desmoplakins and desmosomal proteins. Involvement of the oral mucosa is frequently seen and has been reported as the only manifestation of the disease (Bialy-Golan et al. 1996; Wakahara et al. 2005). Clinically, painful oral erosions and blister formation are appreciated on any mucosal surface including the labial vermilion. Skin eruptions are typically seen. Direct immunofluorescence findings for paraneoplastic pemphigus show deposition of IgG and complement intercellularly within the epithelium and in a linear fashion along the basement membrane. These findings together with a history of lymphoproliferative disease and unique circulating autoantibody profile help to distinguish paraneoplastic pemphigus from other vesiculobullous disorders.

MUCOUS MEMBRANE (CICATRICIAL) PEMPHIGOID

Mucous membrane (cicatricial) pemphigoid represents a group of immune-mediated mucocutaneous disorders in which autoantibodies are directed against basement membrane components. Although the disease typically affects patients in the fifth to sixth decades of life, rare examples of pemphigoid have presented in childhood; in some instances, lesions were limited exclusively to the gingiva (Laskaris et al. 1988; Sklavounou and Laskaris 1990; Cheng et al. 2001; Musa et al. 2002) (Figure 10.11). Characterized by subepithelial separation from the underlying connective tissue, cicatricial pemphigoid presents as areas of erosive or vesiculobullous change throughout the oral mucosa with subsequent scarring. Ocular involvement and conjunctival scarring caused by the disease can lead to blindness. A subgroup of patients more severely affected by the disease appear to have both IgG and IgA circulating anti-basement membrane zone antibodies and frequently require systemic management (Setterfield et al. 1998). One condition clinically indistinguishable from cicatricial pemphigoid termed *linear IgA disease* is characterized by deposition of IgA along the basement membrane. The immunostaining profile is distinct from that of cicatricial pemphigoid, which is characterized by linear deposition of IgG (and occasionally IgM and IgA) and C3 along the basement membrane and is used to distinguish the two disease processes.

DIAGNOSIS AND TREATMENT OF DESQUAMATIVE GINGIVAL LESIONS

Nonspecific inflammation frequently obscures critical features of underlying disease; therefore, it is recommended to avoid marginal gingiva when choosing a biopsy site for the diagnosis of mucosal fragility disorders. Prior to biopsy, verification of epithelial fragility should be sought by assessing the presence of the Nikolsky sign. Here, firm lateral pressure along the mucosal surface of clinically unremarkable tissue adjacent to involved mucosa will elicit bulla formation. Specimens representing the surface of a "de-roofed" vesicle may occasionally yield useful diagnostic information; therefore, any tissue obtained from clinical manipulation of the friable mucosa should be submitted for immunofluorescence analysis (Siegel and Anhalt 1993); however, a biopsy of perilesional tissue is recommended for diagnostic purposes. The specimen should be bisected with half submitted in formalin for routine hematoxylin and eosin staining, and the other half should be submitted in immunofluorescence medium such as Michel's for direct immunofluorescence. Immunofluorescence staining in conjunction with light microscopy is often required to make a definitive diagnosis of vesiculobullous disorders (Gallagher et al. 2005). Treatment of symptomatic lichen planus should begin after biopsy and histopathologic diagnosis. In mild cases, topical corticosteroids (0.05% fluocinonide gel [Lidex]) applied to the affected areas sparingly four times a day typically provides improvement in the symptoms and clinical appearance of the lesions within four weeks. For the most successful management, the patient is instructed to eat, brush, and then apply the gel with nothing per mouth for 30 minutes. It is important that the patient understands this is not a "cure" but rather an effort to maintain remission. More severe cases may require a brief course of systemic corticosteroid therapy in close consultation with the patient's physician. Once the patient is in remission, the patient can be maintained with topical steroids. With the use of topical or systemic corticosteroids, it is not uncommon for patients to develop superimposed candidiasis. A one-week course of fluconazole (Diflucan) 100-mg tablets (two tablets the first day and then one tablet each day following for two weeks) should provide relief in the absence of contraindications. In lesions consistent with foreign-body gingivitis, surgical excision of affected tissue is typically the requisite treatment approach (Gravitis et al. 2005). In some instances, it is possible to identify the source of the foreign material using energy-dispersive x-ray microanalysis (Daley and Wysocki 1990; Gordon and Daley 1997; Gordon 2000). Chronic ulcerative stomatitis is frequently recalcitrant to topical steroid therapy and may require management with hydroxychloroquine (Plaquenil) 200 mg/day; however, systemic side effects, including irreversible retinopathy, neuromyopathy, agranulocytosis, aplastic anemia, and toxic psychosis (Solomon et al. 2003), associated with this medication necessitates consultation with a patient's physician and close clinical follow-up. The management of pemphigus vulgaris and mucous membrane pemphigoid typically involves use of systemic corticosteroid therapy; however, a contemporary management approach involves treatment with rituximab and intravenous immune globulin (Ahmed et al. 2006). It is necessary to have patients evaluated by a physician knowledgeable about this contemporary approach to management.

PLASMA CELL GINGIVITIS

Plasma cell gingivitis represents a unique entity characterized by sharply demarcated erythema and enlargement of the free and attached gingiva (Figure 10.12). This condition generally represents a hypersensitivity reaction to flavoring agents in oral hygiene products, candies or chewing gum, medications, or a component of the diet (Macleod and Ellis 1989; Serio et al. 1991). Despite this fact, in many instances the offending antigen cannot be isolated.

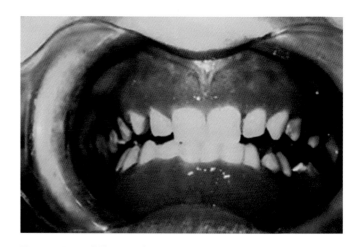

Figure 10.12 Diffuse, erythematous changes of the attached and free gingival tissues.

Biopsies of such lesions show a dense infiltrate of plasma cells within the connective tissue stroma subjacent to the epithelium. Because a neoplastic plasma cell proliferation cannot always be excluded on light microscopic examination alone, additional studies to determine the nature of the infiltrate may be indicated. In cases of idiopathic plasma cell gingivitis or cases representing a hypersensitivity reaction, the plasma cell infiltrate is polyclonal and does not show an atypical profile on immuno-electrophoresis. When other oral mucosal sites are involved, the condition is termed *plasma cell mucositis*. Here, diffuse, erythematous, and edematous changes may involve multiple areas of the oral mucosa (Kaur et al. 2001; Heinemann et al. 2006). Treatment of plasma cell gingivomucositis requires that the patient record all food intake and eliminate possible dietary culprits. Additionally, discontinuance of use of chewing gums, candies, and oral hygiene products remarkable for strong flavoring agents such as peppermint or cinnamon should be encouraged. Unfortunately, in some instances the underlying causative agent cannot be identified. Topical steroid agents (fluocinonide 0.05% gel [Lidex]) applied to the affected areas sparingly four times a day may provide some improvement. This regimen is most effective if the patient eats, brushes, and then applies the gel to the affected areas with nothing per mouth for 30 minutes following application. It is generally recommended that follow-up evaluation after four weeks of topical corticosteroid application be done, and the frequency of use adjusted until improvement is optimal.

ERYTHEMA MULTIFORME

Representing an acute hypersensitivity reaction involving the skin and the mucosa, erythema multiforme (EM) most typically presents in the third and fourth decades of life; however, a significant number of patients diagnosed with EM are children (Huff et al. 1983; Wine et al. 2006). Although the pathogenesis is poorly understood, the condition is likely an immune-mediated disorder. EM is induced by a variety of factors, of which the most common include bacterial and viral infectious agents and medications, most typically analgesics and antibiotics. Approximately 50% of cases arise subsequent to infection with herpes simplex virus. Two forms of EM are typically described: EM major and EM minor. EM minor presents with lesions involving the skin and oral mucosa. It is often recurrent, with the most frequent cause of recurrent EM being a herpes simplex virus infection (Huff et al. 1983; Sinha et al. 2006). EM major is also referred to as *Stevens Johnson syndrome* and is typically triggered by mycobacterium and medications (Huff et al. 1983). Here, in addition to cutaneous and lesions, ocular and/or genital mucosae are affected. Symblephara or bands of scar tissue within the conjunctiva can lead to blindness akin to ocular lesions of cicatricial pemphigoid. The most severe form of EM termed *toxic*

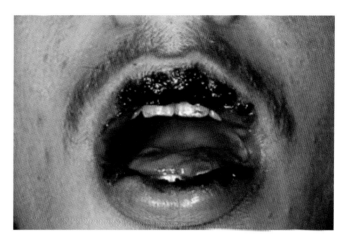

Figure 10.13 Ulceration and crusting lesions involving the labial vermilion.

epidermal necrolysis (Lyell's disease) involves sloughing and ulceration of large areas of the skin and mucosa. Mucosal lesions of EM are characterized by painful ulcerative lesions of acute onset (Figure 10.13), often involving the labial mucosa with crusting of the vermilion. Gingival involvement is rare but is occasionally reported. Classic skin eruptions are described as "target lesions" and are seen in approximately 25% of all patients presenting with EM (Ayangco and Rogers 2003). Here, concentric erythematous rings likened in appearance to a target or "bull's eye" are appreciated on the extremities initially and occasionally extending to involve other cutaneous sites. Unlike other vesiculobullous disorders, the attached mucosae including that of the gingiva and hard palate are typically unaffected by the process. In most instances, EM resolves spontaneously over the course of a two- to four-week period. Treatment is typically supportive and directed at managing symptoms. In severe cases one may consider systemic corticosteroid therapy. Here, prednisone tablets (10 mg) may be prescribed with the instruction to take six tablets in the morning until the lesions recede and then decrease by one tablet on each successive day (Arm et al. 2001). Dexamethasone (Decadron) elixir 0.5 mg/5 ml can also be used. Here, one can recommend the patient rinse with one tablespoonful (15 ml) for three days four times per day and swallow. Then, for three days, rinse with one teaspoonful (5 ml) four times a day and swallow. Then, for three days, rinse with one teaspoonful (5 ml) four times a day and swallow every other time. Last, the patient should rinse with one teaspoonful (5 ml) four times per day and expectorate (Arm et al. 2001). If recurrent EM is thought to be precipitated by herpes simplex virus, antiviral medications are typically prescribed such as systemic acyclovir (Zovirax) 400 mg capsules administering one tablet three times daily or valacyclovir (Valtrex) 500-mg capsules administering one tablet per day.

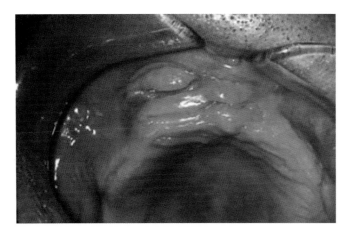

Figure 10.14 Redundant hyperplastic folds of tissue in the anterior maxillary associated with a maxillary denture.

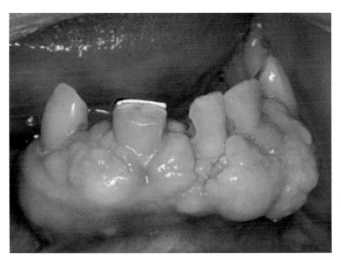

Figure 10.15 Marked gingival hyperplasia in a patient using calcium channel blocker agents.

GINGIVAL ENLARGEMENT

Gingival enlargement may be focal or diffuse in nature. Focal gingival enlargement is seen in association with a number of entities ranging from benign reactive proliferations to malignant epithelial neoplasia. Generalized gingival enlargement is likewise seen in association with a variety of conditions. Systemic medications, neoplastic infiltration, infection, and hereditary conditions may all present with generalized gingival enlargement. The diagnosis and treatment of such lesions are discussed later.

EPULIS FISSURATUM

Epulis fissuratum is characterized by folds of hyperplastic fibrovascular connective tissue that develop in association with an ill-fitting denture. These redundant folds of tissue frequently extend into the vestibule with invaginations to accommodate the denture flange (Figure 10.14). Treatment consists of surgical excision to ensure improved soft tissue contour for impression making and fabrication of a new prosthesis.

MEDICATION-INDUCED GINGIVAL OVERGROWTH

Numerous medications have been implicated as the causative agent for diffuse gingival enlargement. The medications most commonly associated with gingival overgrowth include calcium channel blockers (Figure 10.15), cyclosporine, and anticonvulsant medications. Although incompletely understood, it seems such medications target a common pathway of collagen degradation; interference with this pathway induces fibrosis and extracellular matrix overgrowth in the gingival tissues (McCulloch 2004; Kataoka et al. 2005). Introduction of the causative medication in childhood seems to increase the likelihood of occurrence. The most typical clinical course for the process begins as diffuse gingival enlargement of the facial surfaces of the gingiva most prominently along the interdental papillae several weeks following the initiation of a medication. Over time, the tissue overgrowth extends to the lingual surfaces of the gingiva and can completely cover the dentition. Typically, hyperplastic changes are not appreciated in edentulous areas unless the tissues approximate poorly fitting prostheses or surround dental implants. Oral hygiene dictates the clinical appearance of the hyperplastic gingival tissues. In patients with adequate oral hygiene, the hyperplastic tissues maintain a pink color and stippled appearance. In patients with marginal oral hygiene, the tissues may become friable and bleed on subtle provocation.

Treatment for medication-induced gingival hyperplasia includes substitution of the inciting medication with a different agent that is less likely to cause gingival hyperplasia when possible and encouraging meticulous oral hygiene. Additionally, supplementation with folic acid may reduce the incidence of medication-induced gingival overgrowth; however, the results of such efforts have been mixed (Drew et al. 1987; Backman et al. 1989; Brown et al. 1991; Prasad et al. 2004). Azithromycin has been shown to significantly reduce gingival overgrowth in patients taking cyclosporine (Tokgoz et al. 2004). In some instances, however, surgical intervention is indicated. Although a variety of surgical techniques may be used, such as gingivectomy or flap surgery, laser excision with submission of lesional tissue for histopathologic examination has been shown to represent a favorable method of management (Mavrogiannis et al. 2006).

HYPERPLASTIC GINGIVITIS

Diffuse erythematous enlargement of the gingival tissues is frequently seen secondary to poor oral hygiene (Figure 10.16). Diabetes mellitus (Mealey 2006) and

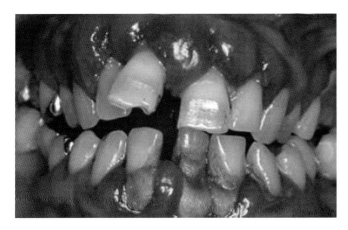

Figure 10.16 Diffuse enlargement and erythema of the marginal and papillary gingiva.

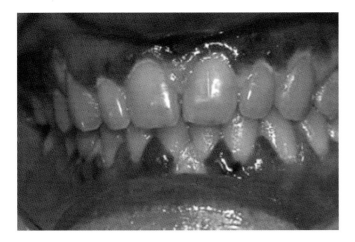

Figure 10.17 Diffuse gingival enlargement and hemorrhage in this patient subsequently diagnosed with monocytic leukemia.

smoking have also been implicated in the development of hyperplastic gingivitis. Treatment requires professional scaling and curettage and improved oral hygiene measures. Chemopreventive measures such as 0.12% chlorhexidine rinse may be used if debridement and improved oral hygiene measures alone do not provide resolution. Surgical recontouring of the gingival tissues using a scalpel or laser may be indicated for patients who are recalcitrant to conservative treatment.

LEUKEMIA

Leukemia represents a hematopoietic stem cell malignancy that produces a number of clinical signs and symptoms intimately associated with a proliferation of atypical leukocytes and subsequent reduced numbers of normal circulating leukocytes and erythrocytes. The most typical oral lesions associated with leukemia include ulcerative lesions, spontaneous gingival bleeding, and gingival hyperplasia (Weckx et al. 1990) (Figure 10.17). In many instances, oral lesions represent the first sign of the

disease. The systemic signs and symptoms of leukemia are numerous and include malaise, fever, fatigue, and lymphadenopathy. Gingiva ranks among the most common sites of extramedullary disease (Wiernik et al. 1996) and is most typically involved in patients with acute myeloid leukemia, particularly the subtypes of acute monocytic and myelomonocytic leukemia. Diffuse gingival enlargement characterized by a boggy consistency with spontaneous bleeding or bleeding on subtle provocation should be viewed with a high index of suspicion. A scalpel biopsy with submission of lesional tissue for histopathologic and immunohistochemical analysis is indicated.

GINGIVAL FIBROMATOSIS

Gingival fibromatosis represents a disorder characterized by progressive enlargement of gingival tissues secondary to increased numbers of collagen fiber bundles. While gingival fibromatosis may be idiopathic, it is often hereditary, with most cases showing autosomal dominant inheritance. While most cases represent isolated examples of the disorder, gingival fibromatosis is also seen in association with a number of hereditary syndromes. In addition to functional concerns such as difficulty eating, speaking, and maintaining oral hygiene, gingival fibromatosis causes esthetic concerns for the patient. Gingival fibromatosis is characterized by painless diffuse gingival enlargement of normal color and firm, fibrous consistency with minimal bleeding (Coletta and Graner 2006). Typically arising at the time of primary or permanent tooth eruption, gingival fibromatosis frequently causes malpositioning of teeth, retention of primary dentition, delayed eruption of the permanent dentition, and other functional and esthetic concerns.

Treatment traditionally involves gingivectomy using serial gingival resections together with strict oral hygiene measures. One recent report suggests a more aggressive surgical protocol of gingivectomy, odontectomy, and alveolar ridge ostectomy of an entire arch at a time eliminates recurrence (Odessey et al. 2006); however, the management strategy employed depends on the individual case and wishes of the patient.

LIGNEOUS GINGIVITIS AND CONJUNCTIVITIS

Ligneous gingivitis represents a rare disorder characterized by deposition of amyloid-like material within the gingival connective tissue subjacent to the oral mucosa. Ligneous conjunctivitis is frequently seen in association with gingival lesions and represents an autosomal recessive form of chronic membranous conjunctivitis (Bateman et al. 1986). Many cases of ligneous conjunctivitis are related to plasminogen deficiency and present in patients of Turkish origin (Gokbuget et al. 1997; Gunhan et al. 1999). It is hypothesized that plasminogen deficiency caused inability of fibrinolytic activity to clear fibrin deposits, allowing accumulation of this material. Clinical presentation can include gingival enlargement with multiple areas of ulceration involving both arches (Scully et al. 2001), a change that mimics gingival enlargement associated with leukemia. At least one case of ligneous gingivitis affecting the alveolar mucosa in the absence of conjunctivitis in a patient without plasminogen deficiency has been reported (Naudi et al. 2006). The best management strategy for these lesions at the present is uncertain. In individuals with plasminogen deficiency, intravenous purified plasminogen concentrate has been used (Schott et al. 1998); however, this therapy is not widely available.

WEGENER'S GRANULOMATOSIS

Wegener's granulomatosis represents a necrotizing granulomatous vasculitis most commonly involving the respiratory tract and kidneys. Oral lesions have been described and are characterized by gingival hyperplasia remarkable for a rough, granular appearance often likened to that of a strawberry, which bleed with subtle provocation (Manchanda et al. 2003). Isolated gingival lesions may represent the initial manifestation of the disease in approximately 7% of patients (Patten and Tomecki 1993) and begin initially in the interdental papilla spreading to the adjacent gingival tissues. In one case report, the disease initially presented as a poorly healing extraction socket in a young patient (Kemp et al. 2005). Other oral lesions may also be present, including mucosal ulcerations, nodular lesions of the labial mucosa, and palatal osteonecrosis. Biopsy with confirmation using antinuclear cytoplasmic antibody (ANCA) testing is critical. It is important to include Wegener's granulomatosis in a differential diagnosis of gingival hyperplasia, particularly in a patient with a history of sinusitis, given the poor prognosis associated with the condition if left untreated.

PIGMENTED LESIONS

Pigmented lesions are encountered with some frequency in the oral cavity. In some instances, these lesions represent generalized or diffuse changes; in other instances, the pigmented change is focal in nature.

PHYSIOLOGIC PIGMENTATION

Most commonly noted on attached gingiva in darker-skinned patients, physiologic pigmentation presents as a diffuse brown-black pigmentation secondary to increased melanocyte activity. Here, pigmentation develops during the first two decades of life. Physiologic pigmentation is typically bilaterally symmetrical in distribution and most prominent along the labial attached gingiva in the region of the maxillary and mandibular incisors. The distribution is likened to a ribbon-like band that spares the marginal gingiva (Eisen 2000) (Figure 10.18). Pigmentation may also

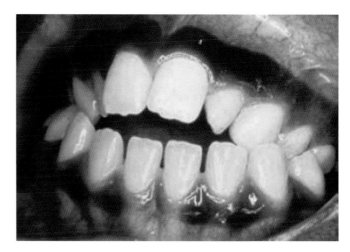

Figure 10.18 Band-like pigmentation of the attached gingiva. Source: Image courtesy of Dr. Helen Santis.

be appreciated within the buccal mucosa, lips, tongue (particularly of the fungiform papillae), and hard palate and is notable for a macular appearance with indistinct borders (Kauzman et al. 2004). Although physiologic pigmentation is not a medical concern, recent publications suggest social pressures influence some patients to request gingival depigmentation for esthetic purposes (Tal et al. 2003). The most significant factor for clinicians is to recognize the entity as a normal manifestation as opposed to a pathologic process.

MEDICATION-INDUCED PIGMENTATION

Drug-induced discoloration of the oral mucosa is caused by an increasing number of medications. The discoloration can occur after direct contact with the medication or following its systemic absorption. In some instances, medication stimulates melanocytes to increase melanin production; in other instances, medication causes formation of metabolites that are thought to be the cause of increased pigmentation. Medications typically associated with pigmentation of the oral mucosa include minocycline (Figure 10.19), antimalarial medications, estrogens, tranquilizers, phenolphthalein found in laxatives, chemotherapy medications, and medications used to manage patients with HIV infection (Abdollahi and Radfar 2003). In some instances, discoloration caused by medication resolves in the weeks following discontinuation of the medication; however, in some instances, the change is permanent. Many accounts of exposure to metals such as gold, lead, mercury, and silver have been historically documented in the literature with a classic presentation of linear pigmentation following the gingival margins described. Other presentations of drug-induced pigmentation vary but include diffuse pigmentation of the palate and rare descriptions of pigmentation changes of the soft tissues of the lips, tongue, eyes, and perioral skin.

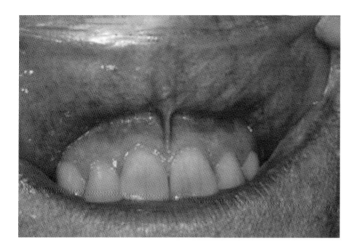

Figure 10.19 Pigmentation of the gingiva associated with use of minocycline.

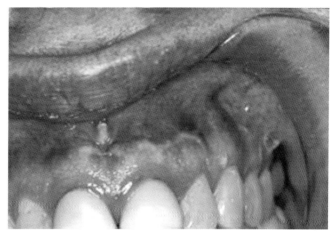

Figure 10.21 Multifocal areas of mucosal pigmentation at the apices of teeth treated with apical retrofill procedures. Source: Image courtesy of Dr. Helen Santis.

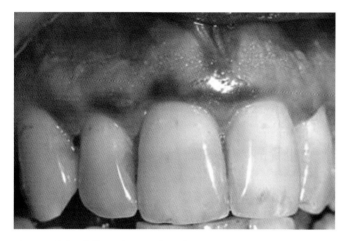

Figure 10.20 Diffuse pigmentation of the anterior attached gingiva in a heavy smoker. Source: Image courtesy of Dr. Brad Neville.

Antimalarial agents are typically linked to discoloration of the palate; minocycline use is frequently associated with palatal and occasionally skin lesions (Treister et al. 2004); phenolphthalein is associated with well-circumscribed macular pigmented lesions of the skin and mucosa; and estrogens are associated with diffuse melanosis and most typically seen in female patients. In some instances, a biopsy may be indicated to confirm the diagnosis and rule out the presence of underlying melanocytic pathology.

SMOKER'S MELANOSIS

Smoker's melanosis represents diffuse benign pigmentation of the oral mucosa, particularly noted on the anterior facial attached gingiva (Hedin 1977; Axell and Hedin 1982) (Figure 10.20). Typically, the distribution of pigmented changes begins in the interdental papilla region and may extend to form continuous ribbons involving the anterior attached gingiva with the apical extension of the lesions not exceeding the mucogingival junction (Hedin 1977). Unlike

physiologic pigmentation, smoker's melanosis does not spare the marginal gingiva, is of recent onset, and increases in intensity and number of lesions with an increase in the number of cigarettes used daily. In patients who consume alcohol in addition to smoking, areas of oral depigmentation surrounded by hyperpigmentation are frequently noted (Natali et al. 1991). In a study of dark-skinned patients, while most non-tobacco users exhibited some level of physiologic oral melanin pigmentation, tobacco smokers had significantly more oral surfaces pigmented than did the non-tobacco users (Ramer and Burakoff 1997). Reports have been described of reduction in smoking leading to the disappearance of smoking-induced melanosis (Hedin et al. 1993). Given that these lesions present in patients in adulthood and often darken progressively over time, biopsy is often indicated to rule out melanoma. (Portions reprinted with permission from the *Journal of the Massachusetts Dental Society* 2007 Spring; in press.)

AMALGAM TATTOO

An amalgam tattoo typically presents as a gray-blue macular lesion of the oral mucosa that occurs following implantation of dental amalgam into the oral soft tissues (Figure 10.21). Common clinical scenarios associated with this phenomenon include introduction of amalgam into the oral soft tissues by high-speed hand pieces, contamination of extraction sites with amalgam debris, and linear impregnation of interdental tissues with amalgam-laden dental floss following restorative procedures (Mirowski and Waibel 2002). Small radiopaque particles may be evident on radiographic examination to corroborate the clinical impression; however, the metallic particles are often too small to be appreciated. Over time, an amalgam tattoo may appear to enlarge as the amalgam-carrying macrophages migrate away from the initial site of implantation. In some

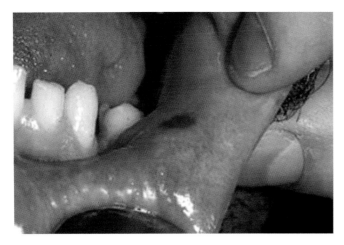

Figure 10.22 Well-demarcated brown macular lesion of the lower labial mucosa.

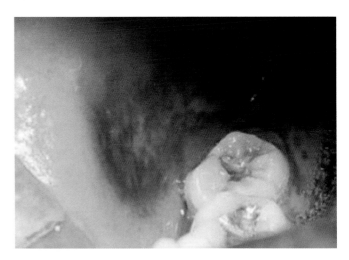

Figure 10.23 Smooth pigmented lesion of recent onset of the posterior buccal mucosa.

individuals, an inflammatory response to the amalgam may be accompanied by clinical discomfort that would predicate the need for biopsy. When a suspected amalgam tattoo presents in an unusual location, a biopsy may be indicated to exclude other pigmented lesions such as melanoacanthoma and melanoma. (Portions reprinted with permission from the *Journal of the Massachusetts Dental Society* 2005 Spring; 54 (1):55.)

MELANOTIC MACULE

The oral melanotic macule is a frequently encountered pigmented lesion of the oral mucosa. Typically found on the lower labial vermilion, buccal mucosa, gingiva, and palate, the oral melanotic macule is characterized as a solitary, well-demarcated, uniformly pigmented, macular brown lesion (Figure 10.22). Although exposure to ultraviolet radiation can clearly be excluded as a causative agent in intraoral lesions, the relationship between lesions of the lower labial vermilion and sun exposure is unclear. While the oral melanotic macule is generally not regarded as a lesion with potential to undergo malignant transformation, rare examples of malignant transformation have been reported in the literature (Kahn et al. 2005). Given the predilection for melanoma to present on the gingiva and palate, lesions presenting in these locations should be viewed with a high index of suspicion. Additionally, features such as asymmetry and color variegation are worrisome. Because malignancy cannot always be excluded on clinical presentation alone, an excisional biopsy may be indicated with submission of lesional tissue for histopathologic evaluation.

ORAL MELANOACANTHOMA (MELANOACANTHOSIS)

Oral melanoacanthoma represents an acquired melanocytic pigmentation that arises suddenly and most likely represents a reactive phenomenon. Presenting most

frequently in black females, the lesion is characterized by a brown-black appearance exhibiting a smooth to somewhat raised surface contour (Figure 10.23). Typically found on the buccal mucosa, oral melanoacanthoma has been reported to arise on the lip, palate, and gingiva (Flaitz 2000). As the lesion arises suddenly with marked growth potential, melanoacanthoma cannot be differentiated from other melanocytic lesions without biopsy. Distinctive histopathologic features, particularly the presence of dendritic melanocytes within the epithelial spinous cell layer, differentiate melanoacanthoma from other melanocytic lesions. Once definitive diagnosis is made, further treatment is unnecessary. Although rare, cases of spontaneous resolution of oral melanoacanthoma have been reported (Wright 1988; Fatahzadeh and Sirois 2002).

ORAL MELANOCYTIC NEVUS

Oral melanocytic nevi typically present as well-circumscribed papules that range in color from brown to black and may be devoid of pigmentation (Figure 10.24). The most common locations for melanocytic nevi in the oral cavity include the buccal mucosa, gingiva, lips, and palate (Buchner and Hansen 1987a, b, c). One form of melanocytic nevus termed the *blue nevus* typically presents on the palate (Buchner and Hansen 1987a, b, c). Oral melanocytic nevi are somewhat more common in women and occur over a wide age range, with most lesions noted in the third to fourth decades of life (Buchner et al. 2004). Although the malignant transformation potential of oral mucosal melanoma is not proved, given that oral melanocytic nevi frequently present on the palate, similar to oral mucosal melanoma, and are relatively uncommon lesions, excision with submission of lesional tissue for histopathologic evaluation is recommended.

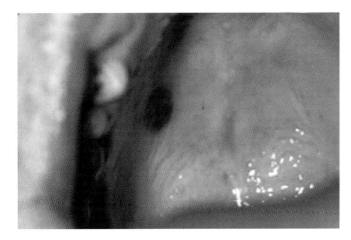

Figure 10.24 Slightly raised pigmented lesion of the posterior hard palate.

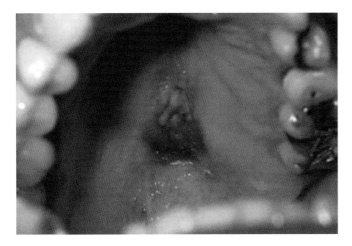

Figure 10.25 Irregular pigmented lesion of the posterior palate.

ORAL MELANOMA

Typically occurring on the palate, maxillary gingiva, and maxillary alveolar mucosa (Barker et al. 1997), oral melanoma represents an uncommon malignancy of the oral cavity. The five-year survival rate for oral melanoma persists unchanged since initially being reported in the literature and ranges from 1U to 20% (Eisen and Voorhees 1991). Oral melanoma presents as pigmented plaques remarkable for irregular asymmetric borders exhibiting brown-black coloration (Figure 10.25). Some melanomas are notable for lack of melanocytic pigmentation (Eisen and Voorhees 1991). Clinical evidence of ulceration, bone erosion, or frank invasion of bone is not uncommon. When intraoral melanoma represents metastatic rather than a primary oral lesion, such lesions typically present on the buccal mucosa, tongue, and at the site of a nonhealing extraction socket (Patton et al. 1994). Given that the prognosis of oral melanoma depends on the stage of the disease at the time of diagnosis and that the depth of most oral lesions at the time of diagnosis is advanced, early

detection is critical. Pigmented lesions with irregular borders presenting on the palate, maxillary gingiva, or alveolar mucosa should be viewed with suspicion. Treatment typically involves radical surgical excision together with neck dissection and adjuvant chemotherapy (Umeda and Shimada 1994).

SANGUINARIA-INDUCED LEUKOPLAKIA

Exposure of the oral cavity to chemical substances, medications, or dentifrice can lead to specific mucosal changes. Chronic use of mouth rinses containing sanguinaria extract (also known as bloodroot extract) has been shown to produce leukoplakic lesions with an implied potential for malignant transformation (Damm et al. 1999). The use of Viadent brand mouth rinse (Colgate Oral Pharmaceuticals, Canton, MA) containing sanguinaria extract, a product of the bloodroot plant, has been shown to produce leukoplakic lesions of the maxillary vestibule, a site that is uncommon for white lesions (Figure 10.26). It is generally recognized that these lesions frequently persist and even recur following discontinuation of the product. Because biopsy may show areas of mild to moderate epithelial dysplasia, these patients need to be kept under close surveillance (Eversole et al. 2000). Given the apparent association between sanguinaria-containing dentifrice and dysplastic leukoplakia, it is recommended that individuals presenting with leukoplakic lesions and history of exposure to Viadent submit for biopsy and discontinue use of the product (Damm et al. 1999). (Portions reprinted with permission pending from *Otolaryngol. Clin. N. Am.* (38) 2005 21–35.)

PROLIFERATIVE VERRUCOUS LEUKOPLAKIA

One particularly persistent and importunate form of leukoplakia can be difficult to distinguish from verrucous carcinoma. Proliferative verrucous leukoplakia (PVL) is

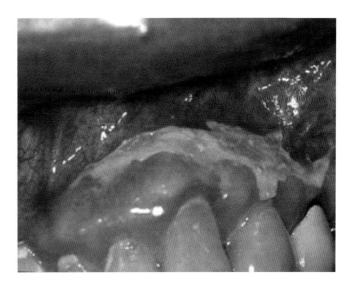

Figure 10.26 White plaque of the maxillary mucobuccal fold.

characterized as an extensive exophytic papillary proliferation that often involves multiple sites and is recalcitrant to treatment. Initial PVL lesions present in a solitary fashion characterized by thin hyperkeratosis and are well delineated from the surrounding mucosa. As the lesion evolves, it may develop a perceptually thickened quality with superficial undulations consistent with verrucous hyperplasia. The lesions become multifocal and recur following excision. Over time, the lesions progress to verrucous carcinoma or squamous cell carcinoma (Hansen et al. 1985).

Unique in its predilection for women nearly 4:1 over men, PVL is generally diagnosed in the seventh decade of life. Studies report from 70 to nearly 100% of PVL lesions progress to squamous cell carcinoma (Silverman and Gorsky 1997; Batsakis et al. 1999), with the gingiva and tongue being the sites showing the highest incidence of transformation (Silverman and Gorsky 1997). Months to years may transpire from the time of initial recognition of the process to its ultimate transformation to invasive carcinoma. No apparent link between use of tobacco products has been firmly established with regard to PVL (Silverman and Gorsky 1997; Fettig et al. 2000), and the link between human papilloma virus and PVL is controversial (Palefsky et al. 1995; Bagan et al. 2007). Given that PVL most likely represents a disease that is multifactorial in nature, it is difficult to anticipate specifically who is at high risk for developing the condition. (Portions reprinted with permission pending from *Otolaryngol. Clin. N. Am.* (38) 2005 21–35.)

MALIGNANT NEOPLASIA

Malignant neoplasia involving the oral cavity may represent primary disease or metastasis, particularly from the breast, lung, kidney, prostate, gastrointestinal tract, and thyroid gland.

SQUAMOUS CELL CARCINOMA

Oral squamous cell carcinoma represents the most common intraoral malignancy and is remarkable for a variety of clinical presentations ranging from erythroplakia to leukoplakia, or it may present as a combination of the two. Incipient lesions are typically painless; however, as the lesion progresses, areas of ulceration and induration may be seen, and the lesion may become more nodular. Fixation to underlying tissues and local-regional lymph node metastasis indicate further progression to an intermediate stage of malignancy. Late-stage lesions may present with bony involvement, tooth mobility, pain, and paresthesia (Zakrzewska 1999).

All forms of tobacco use are associated with an increased risk of developing oral squamous cell carcinoma. When combined, tobacco and alcohol work in synergy to potentiate the increased risk of developing invasive tumor (Zakrzewska 1999; Scully and Porter 2000). Additionally, exposure to ultraviolet radiation (lip) or betel quid (a mixture of slaked lime, areca nut, and tobacco wrapped in betel leaf and chewed – a social habit quite prevalent in the Indian subcontinent) may predispose susceptive individuals to submucous fibrosis, a condition that has an approximately 17% chance of malignant transformation and immunosuppression; these are well-recognized etiologic factors that when paired with a genetically susceptible individual may yield transformation to oral squamous cell carcinoma (Scully and Porter 2000).

The most common sites for oral squamous cell carcinoma are the posterior lateral and ventral tongue, floor of the mouth, and soft palate, although gingival lesions are also reported (Seoane et al. 2006) (Figure 10.27). In some instances, the similarities between gingival squamous cell carcinoma and periodontal disease may lead to a delay in diagnosis. The prognosis for oral squamous cell carcinoma is largely based on the stage of presentation (Sanderson and Ironside 2002) and the lesion's location. The presence of positive nodal involvement reduces long-term survival by as much as 50% (Sanderson and Ironside 2002).

Clinical presentations that warrant immediate action to rule out squamous cell carcinoma include nonhealing ulceration or unexplained swelling of approximately three weeks' duration and all red and/or white lesions. A biopsy is mandatory with definitive diagnosis via histolopathologic examination. Additionally, it is recommended that tooth mobility unrelated to periodontal disease receive thorough investigation (Sanderson and Ironside 2002).

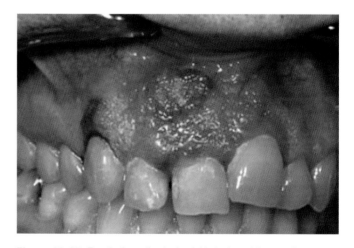

Figure 10.27 Exophytic erythroleukoplakic lesion of the anterior maxillary gingiva.

Early biopsy is recommended for any nonhealing or slowly resolving lesion even if the patient is young and/or denies exposure to tobacco products. Although extremely rare, occasional accounts of squamous cell carcinoma arising in pediatric patients have been made (Bill et al. 2001). Additionally, recent reports have shown an increased incidence of squamous cell carcinoma in female patients and in those patients younger than 40 years (Martin-Granizo et al. 1997). Ultimately, despite advances in treatment, prognosis depends heavily on tumor staging at the time of presentation. Thorough clinical examination and a high index of suspicion for mucosal alterations at high-risk sites provide the best chance for a positive outcome. (Portions reprinted with permission pending from *Otolaryngol. Clin. N. Am.* (38) 2005 21–35.)

VERRUCOUS CARCINOMA

Verrucous carcinoma represents a low-grade variant of squamous cell carcinoma with a characteristic papillary exophytic growth pattern (Figure 10.28). A superficial insidious neoplasm principally due to its indolent growth course, verrucous carcinoma can be extensive and multifocal at the time of clinical presentation. Within the oral cavity, the most common sites of occurrence are the buccal mucosa and gingiva, sites typically not considered "high risk" with regard to traditional squamous cell carcinoma (Koch et al. 2001).

Although verrucous carcinoma is not confined exclusively in presentation to the upper aerodigestive tract, a significant link between oral verrucous carcinoma and tobacco products has been made (Ferlito and Recher 1980; Medina et al. 1984; Spiro 1998). Surgical excision is

advocated as the standard of care for treatment, and many years of follow-up are required to capture additional foci, as dictated by the multicentric nature of the process and apparent increased likelihood that recurrent lesions may prove to be more poorly differentiated than their predecessor (Ferlito and Recher 1980; Medina et al. 1984; Spiro 1998). Further, studies have reported a near 20% incidence of squamous cell carcinoma arising in lesions of verrucous carcinoma. Clinical distinction cannot be made between traditional verrucous carcinoma lesions and those containing foci of invasive squamous cell carcinoma (Medina et al. 1984). This finding dictates thorough surgical excision extending deep into connective tissue to allow adequate assessment of the epithelial–connective tissue interface histologically and that multiple levels through the specimen be subjected to histologic evaluation. Given the propensity for verrucous carcinoma lesions to grow in a slow fashion, adequate surgical excision coupled with rigorous clinical follow-up provides the most optimistic prognosis (McCoy and Waldron 1981). (Portions reprinted with permission pending from *Otolaryngol. Clin. N. Am.* (38) 2005 21–35.)

METASTATIC DISEASE

Although metastatic disease is uncommon in the oral cavity, representing less than 1% of oral neoplasia (van der Waal et al. 2003), in at least one third of patients, metastasis to the jawbones or oral soft tissues represents the first clinical sign of the disease (Hirshberg and Buchner 1995; van der Waal et al. 2003; D'Silva et al. 2006). Of lesions inclined to metastasize to the oral soft tissues, metastatic disease from the lung is the most commonly encountered (Hirshberg and Buchner 1995). When lesions metastasize to the gingiva, lesions typically

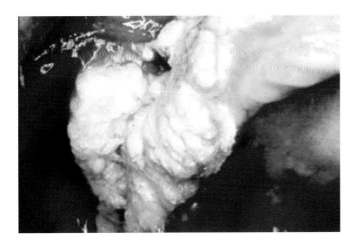

Figure 10.28 Extensive exophytic white papillary lesion involving the edentulous maxillary alveolar ridge and vestibule.

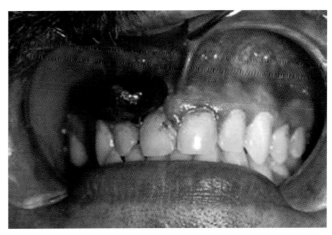

Figure 10.29 Metastatic melanoma to the anterior maxillary gingiva.

present as polypoid masses that may be mistaken for a benign reactive gingival nodule (Ramon Ramirez et al. 2003) (Figure 10.29), and the most common primary tumors to metastasize to the gingiva are those originating in the lung, kidney, breast, bone, and liver (Elkhoury et al. 2004). Obviously, it is of utmost importance to distinguish metastatic disease from benign lesions that can share similar clinical features. Biopsy with submission of lesional tissue for histopathologic analysis is important to ensure the best prognosis.

INFECTIONS

The oral cavity is susceptible to infections with fungal, bacterial, and viral organisms. Infections with herpes simplex virus and oral manifestations of HIV infection are discussed later.

HERPES

Primary herpetic infection typically presents as gingivo-stomatitis with the recurrence manifesting as cutaneous/mucocutaneous disease. Symptoms of primary herpetic stomatitis arise after an incubation period of up to three weeks following infection. The prodromal symptoms are not pathognomonic and include malaise, fever, headache, nausea, anorexia, and irritability. Acute onset of pain in the oral cavity is seen with the development of numerous small vesicular lesions that quickly coalesce and ulcerate. These lesions may involve any area of the oral cavity, including the gingiva, buccal mucosa, tongue, palatal mucosa, vermilion, perioral skin, and oropharynx. A severe complication of primary herpetic gingivostomatitis is ocular involvement. After initial infection, oral herpes simplex virus remains latent in the trigeminal ganglion. Upon activation, the virus utilizes the axons of sensory neurons as a means to reach overlying tissues. Symptomatic recurrences are common and can be preceded by a prodrome of "tingling" or discomfort in the affected region, sometimes initially mistaken for a toothache. The typical clinical presentation for recurrent intraoral herpetic infection is of multiple "punched-out" painful areas of ulceration that may coalesce and often follow the distribution of the greater palatine nerve. Recurrences are frequently attributed to manipulation of oral tissues during routine dental procedures. The distinction between recurrent herpetic lesions and recurrent apthous stomatitis (canker sores) is that herpetic ulcerations typically involve keratinized tissues (Figure 10.30) and recurrent apthous ulcerations are seen on moveable mucosa. Systemic antiviral therapy is generally accepted as being effective for management of primary herpetic stomatitis using acyclovir (Zovirax) 200-mg capsules administering one capsule five times a

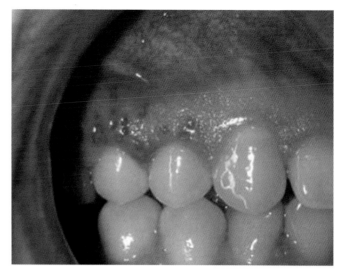

Figure 10.30 Multiple painful punctate areas of ulceration involving the maxillary attached gingiva.

day for five to seven days; however, the effectiveness of other antiviral medications such as famciclovir or valaciclovir has not been fully evaluated (Arduino and Porter 2006). Further, the optimal timing of initiating therapy and optimum dose are not fully defined. Reduction of clinical signs and patient symptoms has been reported for recurrent herpetic stomatitis using acyclovir (Zovirax) cream (5%) one application topically every three to four hours for five days and penciclovir (Denavir) cream (1%) every two hours for five days, but studies are still needed to determine which is more effective (Arduino and Porter 2006). A recent report advocates the utility of oral famciclovir (Famvir) in the management of herpes labialis (Spruance et al. 2006). Here, 1,500 mg is taken within one hour of the onset of prodromal symptoms. This protocol was reported to reduce duration of symptoms by approximately two days. In immunocompromised patients, topical therapeutics offer little benefit. Acyclovir remains the medication of choice (Arduino and Porter 2006). As self-inoculation is possible, it is recommended patients be advised to avoid touching the lesions and then touching the eyes, genitalia, or other body areas to prevent infection at new sites. (Portions reprinted with permission from the *Journal of the Massachusetts Dental Society* 2005 Winter; 53 (4):55.)

HIV-ASSOCIATED GINGIVITIS

Initially termed "HIV-related gingivitis," linear gingival erythema presents as a red band involving the free gingival margin. This change is typically most prominent in the region of the anterior dentition but extends to involve the posterior quadrants with some frequency (Reznik 2005). Mild bleeding on subtle provocation has been reported, and efforts at improved oral hygiene do not lead to resolution. Some reports suggest this pattern of gingivitis represents a form of candidiasis (Velegraki et al. 1999). Lesions typically resolve following professional plaque removal and rinses with a 0.12% suspension of chlorhexidine gluconate twice per day for two weeks. Additional HIV-related conditions involving the gingiva include *necrotizing ulcerative gingivitis* (NUG) involving necrosis of one or more intordental papillae and *necrotizing ulcerative periodontitis* with features of NUG in addition to rapidly progressing loss of periodontal attachment. Treatment for these conditions includes gentle debridement with povidone-iodine irrigation. The standard management approach includes rinsing with a suspension of 0.12% chlorhexidine. Follow-up with additional debridement at 24 hours and again every 7–10 days is required. In the acute phase with systemic symptoms of fever and malaise, antibiotic therapy is indicated (amoxicillin 2 g a day for seven days or metronidazole).

ORAL SOFT TISSUE BIOPSY TECHNIQUES

It is usually prudent to recommend a biopsy on lesions that have persisted for over two weeks after the removal of a potential irritant. Lesions that are related to infection, inflammation, or local trauma may resolve during this time.

Biopsies can be incisional or excisional depending on the nature of the lesion and the comfort level and skills of the practitioner. If the lesion is large or malignancy is suspected, an incisional biopsy is indicated in order to not compromise the definitive treatment of the potentially malignant lesion. If the lesion is benign, located away from vital structures and of small diameter (less than 1 cm), an excisional biopsy could be recommended. In both cases, it is important to include some of the surrounding healthy tissue in the biopsy specimen. The incision should be made parallel to the normal course of nerves, arteries, and veins to minimize injury (Ellis 2003). Also, when opting for an incisional biopsy you should keep in mind that "deeper is better" and it is much better to take a deep, narrow biopsy rather than a broad, shallow one in order to not miss the cellular changes at the base of the lesion (Ellis 2003). Because of the size and morphology of the lesion requiring an incisional approach, it is sometimes necessary to obtain more than one biopsy sample of the same lesion (different locations).

The following methods are used to collect tissue samples from the oral cavity (Campisi et al. 2003; Ellis 2003).

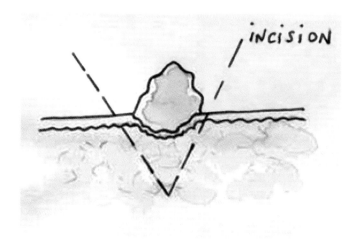

Figure 10.31 Excisional biopsy. Notice the angulation of the blade, which will create a wedge, as well as the amount of healthy tissue removed.

- Needle biopsy
- Tissue punch biopsy
- Scalpel biopsy
- Laser biopsy

This chapter will be limited to describing techniques using scalpel biopsy.

ARMAMENTARIUM

Surgical set that is recommended is given in *Practical Periodontal Plastic Surgery* (Dibart and Karima 2006).

INCISIONAL SCALPEL BIOPSY

After proper local anesthesia is achieved by infiltrating the area 1 cm peripheral to the lesion with xylocaine 2% with 1 : 100 000 epinephrine, the surgeon focuses on the area where the incision will take place. With a No. 15 blade, a small wedge that is approximately 3 mm deep, 5 mm long, and 3 mm wide is excised. The specimen needs to include a portion of the margin as well as some healthy tissue. The specimen is then very delicately transferred to a biopsy container with 10% formalin. It is very important not to crush the tissues during excision or transfer into the fixative solution as that may interfere with the proper oral pathology diagnosis. The surgical site can be closed with a single suture; the patient is given some mild analgesics (acetaminophen 500 mg) and advised to rinse with an antiseptic mouthwash (chlorhexidine 0.12%) for one week.

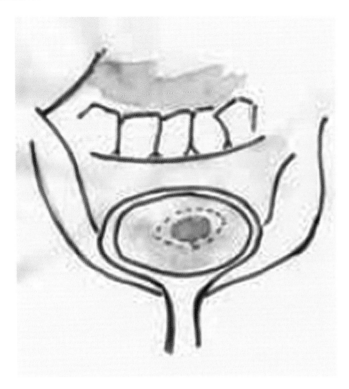

Figure 10.32 Elliptical incision to remove a growth located on the lower lip. The lip is stabilized here with a Chalazion clamp.

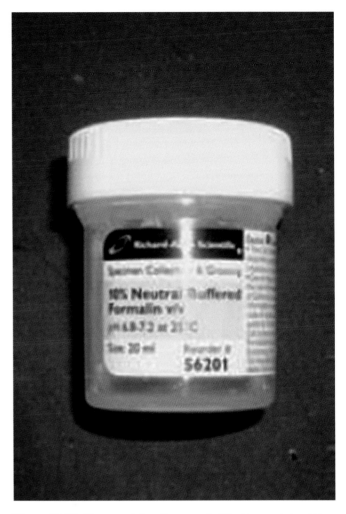

Figure 10.33 Biopsy container, the amount of liquid present should be sufficient to completely cover the biopsy specimen.

EXCISIONAL SCALPEL BIOPSY

After proper local anesthesia is achieved by infiltrating the area 1 cm peripheral to the lesion with xylocaine 2% with 1 : 100 000 epinephrine, an elliptical incision is made around the lesion with the blade angled toward the lesion (Figure 10.31). Tissue stabilization and hemostasis can be achieved manually (assistant's fingers pinching the soft tissue on both sides of the biopsy) or mechanically by using a clamp (i.e. Chalazion clamp for a biopsy of the lip) (Figure 10.32). Again, it is important to remember to remove some healthy tissue with the specimen. The rule of thumb for easy closure is to have an ellipse that is three times longer than wide. Also, depending on the location of the biopsy site and the size of the wound, there may be a need to undermine the mucosa (with scissors) in order to obtain tension-free closure. Primary closure of an elliptic wound is easily achieved provided that the margins of the wound are gently undermined.

Elliptical incisions on the attached gingiva or palate are not sutured but are left to heal by secondary intention. The excised specimen is then very delicately transferred to a biopsy container with 10% formalin for fixation (Figure 10.33). Again, it is very critical not to crush the tissues during excision or transfer into the fixative solution as that may interfere with the proper oral pathology diagnosis.

The patient is given some mild analgesics (acetaminophen 500 mg) and advised to rinse with an antiseptic mouthwash (chlorhexidine 0.12%) for one week.

BIOPSY DATA SHEET

Once the specimen has been placed in formalin and the patient discharged, the biopsy data sheet must be completed in its entirety. Patient's information including age and gender as well as the lesion's size, location of the biopsy, and a clinical diagnosis are typically required (Figure 10.34). This sheet must accompany the biopsy container and must be sent to the oral pathology laboratory without delay.

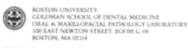

Figure 10.34 Biopsy data sheet used at Boston University School of Dental Medicine, Oral and Maxillofacial Pathology Laboratory.

REFERENCES

Abdollahi, M. and Radfar, M. (2003). A review of drug-induced oral reactions. *J. Contemp. Dent. Pract.* 4 (1): 10–31.

Ahmed, A.R., Spigelman, Z., Cavacini, L.A., and Posner, M.R. (2006). Treatment of pemphigus vulgaris with rituximab and intravenous immune globulin. *N. Engl. J. Med.* 355 (17): 1772–1779.

Arduino, P.G. and Porter, S.R. (2006). Oral and perioral herpes simplex virus type 1 (HSV-1) infection: review of its management. *Oral Dis.* 12 (3): 254–270.

Arm, R.N., Bowers, C., Epstein, J. et al. (2001). *Clinician's Guide to Treatment of Common Oral Conditions*, 5e (eds. M.A. Siegel, S. Silverman Jr. and T.P. Sollecito). New York: BC Decker.

Axell, T. and Hedin, C.A. (1982). Epidemiologic study of excessive oral melanin pigmentation with special reference to the influence of tobacco habits. *Scand. J. Dent. Res.* 90 (6): 434–442.

Ayangco, L. and Rogers, R.S. 3rd. (2003). Oral manifestations of erythema multiforme. *Dermatol. Clin.* 21 (1): 195–205.

Backman, N., Holm, A.K., Hanstrom, L. et al. (1989). Folate treatment of diphenylhydantoin-induced gingival hyperplasia. *Scand. J. Dent. Res.* 97 (3): 222–232.

Bagan, J.V., Jimenez, Y., Murillo, J. et al. (2007). Lack of association between proliferative verrucous leukoplakia and human papillomavirus infection. *J. Oral Maxillofac. Surg.* 65 (1): 46–49.

Barker, B.F., Carpenter, W.M., Daniels, T.E. et al. (1997). Oral mucosal melanomas: the WESTOP Banff workshop proceedings. Western Society of Teachers of Oral Pathology. *Oral Surg. Oral Med. Oral Pathol. Oral Radiol. Endod.* 83 (6): 672–679.

Bateman, J.B., Pettit, T.H., Isenberg, S.J., and Simons, K.B. (1986). Ligneous conjunctivitis: an autosomal recessive disorder. *J. Pediatr. Ophthalmol. Strabismus* 23 (3): 137–140.

Batsakis, J.G., Suarez, P., and el-Naggar, A.K. (1999). Proliferative verrucous leukoplakia and its related lesions. *Oral Oncol.* 35 (4): 354–359.

Bialy-Golan, A., Brenner, S., and Anhalt, G.J. (1996). Paraneoplastic pemphigus: oral involvement as the sole manifestation. *Acta Dermatol. Venereol.* 76 (3): 253–254.

Bill, T.J., Reddy, V.R., Ries, K.L. et al. (2001). Adolescent gingival squamous cell carcinoma: report of a case and review of the literature. *Oral Surg. Oral Med. Oral Pathol. Oral Radiol. Endod.* 91 (6): 682–685.

Bodner, L., Peist, M., Gatot, A., and Fliss, D.M. (1997). Growth potential of peripheral giant cell granuloma. *Oral Surg. Oral Med. Oral Pathol. Oral Radiol. Endod.* 83 (5): 548–551.

Brown, R.S., Di Stanislao, P.T., Beaver, W.T., and Bottomley, W.K. (1991). The administration of folic acid to institutionalized epileptic adults with phenytoin-induced gingival hyperplasia. A double-blind, randomized, placebo-controlled, parallel study. *Oral Surg. Oral Med. Oral Pathol.* 71 (5): 565–568.

Buchner, A. and Hansen, L.S. (1979). The histomorphologic spectrum of the gingival cyst in the adult. *Oral Surg. Oral Med. Oral Pathol.* 48 (6): 532–539.

Buchner, A. and Hansen, L.S. (1987a). The histomorphologic spectrum of peripheral ossifying fibroma. *Oral Surg. Oral Med. Oral Pathol.* 63 (4): 452–461.

Buchner, A. and Hansen, L.S. (1987b). Pigmented nevi of the oral mucosa: a clinicopathologic study of 36 new cases and review of 155 cases from the literature. Part I: a clinicopathologic study of 36 new cases. *Oral Surg. Oral Med. Oral Pathol.* 63 (5): 566–572.

Buchner, A. and Hansen, L.S. (1987c). Pigmented nevi of the oral mucosa: a clinicopathologic study of 36 new cases and review of 155 cases from the literature. Part II: analysis of 191 cases. *Oral Surg. Oral Med. Oral Pathol.* 63 (6): 676–682.

Buchner, A., Merrell, P.W., and Carpenter, W.M. (2004). Relative frequency of solitary melanocytic lesions of the oral mucosa. *J. Oral Pathol. Med.* 33 (9): 550–557.

Buduneli, E., Buduneli, N., and Unal, T. (2001). Long-term follow-up of peripheral ossifying fibroma: report of three cases. *Periodontal Clin. Investig.* 23 (1): 11–14.

Campisi, G., Di Fede, O., and Di Liberto, C. (2003). Incisional biopsy in oral medicine: punch vs traditional procedure. *Minerva Stomatol.* 52 (11–12): 481–488.

Carrera Grano, I., Berini Aytes, L., and Escoda, C.G. (2001). Peripheral ossifying fibroma. Report of a case and review of the literature. *Med. Oral* 6 (2): 135–141.

Cheng, Y.S., Rees, T.D., Wright, J.M., and Plemons, J.M. (2001). Childhood oral pemphigoid: a case report and review of the literature. *J. Oral Pathol. Med.* 30 (6): 372–377.

Coletta, R.D. and Graner, E. (2006). Hereditary gingival fibromatosis: a systematic review. *J. Periodontol.* 77 (5): 753–764.

Cuisia, Z.E. and Brannon, R.B. (2001). Peripheral ossifying fibroma – a clinical evaluation of 134 pediatric cases. *Pediatr. Dent.* 23 (3): 245–248.

D'Silva, N.J., Summerlin, D.J., Cordell, K.G. et al. (2006). Metastatic tumors in the jaws: a retrospective study of 114 cases. *J. Am. Dent. Assoc.* 137 (12): 1667–1672.

Daley, T.D. and Wysocki, G.P. (1990). Foreign body gingivitis: an iatrogenic disease? *Oral Surg. Oral Med. Oral Pathol.* 69 (6): 708–712.

Damm, D.D., Curran, A., White, D.K., and Drummond, J.F. (1999). Leukoplakia of the maxillary vestibule – an association with Viadent? *Oral Surg. Oral Med. Oral Pathol. Oral Radiol. Endod.* 87 (1): 61–66.

Dibart, S. and Karima, M. (2006). *Practical Periodontal Plastic Surgery*. Ames, IA: Blackwell Publishing.

Drew, H.J., Vogel, R.I., Molofsky, W. et al. (1987). Effect of folate on phenytoin hyperplasia. *J. Clin. Periodontol.* 14 (6): 350–356.

Eisen, D. (2000). Disorders of pigmentation in the oral cavity. *Clin. Dermatol.* 18 (5): 579–587.

Eisen, D. (2002). The clinical features, malignant potential, and systemic associations of oral lichen planus: a study of 723 patients. *J. Am. Acad. Dermatol.* 46 (2): 207–214.

Eisen, D. and Voorhees, J.J. (1991). Oral melanoma and other pigmented lesions of the oral cavity. *J. Am. Acad. Dermatol.* 24 (4): 527–537.

Elkhoury, J., Cacchillo, D.A., Tatakis, D.N. et al. (2004). Undifferentiated malignant neoplasm involving the interdental gingiva: a case report. *J. Periodontol.* 75 (9): 1295–1299.

Ellis, E. (2003). Principles of differential diagnosis and biopsy. In: *Contemporary Oral and Maxillofacial Surgery*, 4e (eds. L.J. Peterson, E. Ellis III, J.R. Hupp and M.R. Tucker), 458–478. Philadelphia: Elsevier.

Eversole, L.R., Eversole, G.M., and Kopcik, J. (2000). Sanguinaria-associated oral leukoplakia: comparison with other benign and dysplastic leukoplakic lesions. *Oral Surg. Oral Med. Oral Pathol. Oral Radiol. Endod.* 89 (4): 455–464.

Fatahzadeh, M. and Sirois, D.A. (2002). Multiple intraoral melanoacanthomas: a case report with unusual findings. *Oral Surg. Oral Med. Oral Pathol. Oral Radiol. Endod.* 94 (1): 54–56.

Ferlito, A. and Recher, G. (1980). Ackerman's tumor (verrucous carcinoma) of the larynx: a clinicopathologic study of 77 cases. *Cancer* 46 (7): 1617–1630.

Fettig, A., Pogrel, M.A., Silverman, S. Jr. et al. (2000). Proliferative verrucous leukoplakia of the gingiva. *Oral Surg. Oral Med. Oral Pathol. Oral Radiol. Endod.* 90 (6): 723–730.

Flaitz, C.M. (2000). Oral melanoacanthoma of the attached gingiva. *Am. J. Dent.* 13 (3): 162.

Gallagher, G., Kabani, S., and Noonan, V. (2005). Desquamative gingivitis. *J. Mass. Dent. Soc.* 54 (3): 38.

Garcia, F.V.M.J., Pascual-Lopez, M., Elices, M. et al. (2002). Superficial mucoceles and lichenoid graft versus host disease: report of three cases. *Acta Derm. Venereol.* 82 (6): 453–455.

Giunta, J.L. (2002). Gingival cysts in the adult. *J. Periodontol.* 73 (7): 827–831.

Gokbuget, A.Y., Mutlu, S., Scully, C. et al. (1997). Amyloidaceous ulcerated gingival hyperplasia: a newly described entity related to ligneous conjunctivitis. *J. Oral Pathol. Med.* 26 (2): 100–104.

Gordon, S. (2000). Foreign body gingivitis associated with a new crown: EDX analysis and review of the literature. *Oper. Dent.* 25 (4): 344–348.

Gordon, S.C. and Daley, T.D. (1997). Foreign body gingivitis: identification of the foreign material by energy-dispersive x-ray microanalysis. *Oral Surg. Oral Med. Oral Pathol. Oral Radiol. Endod.* 83 (5): 571–576.

Gravitis, K., Daley, T.D., and Lochhead, M.A. (2005). Management of patients with foreign body gingivitis: report of 2 cases with histologic findings. *J. Can. Dent. Assoc.* 71 (2): 105–109.

Gunhan, O., Gunhan, M., Berker, E. et al. (1999). Destructive membranous periodontal disease (Ligneous periodontitis). *J. Periodontol.* 70 (8): 919–925.

Hansen, L.S., Olson, J.A., and Silverman, S. Jr. (1985). Proliferative verrucous leukoplakia. A long-term study of thirty patients. *Oral Surg. Oral Med. Oral Pathol.* 60 (3): 285–298.

Hedin, C.A. (1977). Smoker's melanosis. *Arch. Dermatol.* 113: 1533–1538.

Hedin, C.A., Pindborg, J.J., and Axell, T. (1993). Disappearance of smoker's melanosis after reducing smoking. *J. Oral Pathol. Med.* 22 (5): 228–230.

Heinemann, C., Fischer, T., Barta, U. et al. (2006). Plasma cell mucositis with oral and genital involvement – successful treatment with topical cyclosporin. *J. Eur. Acad. Dermatol. Venereol.* 20 (6): 739–740.

Hirshberg, A. and Buchner, A. (1995). Metastatic tumours to the oral region. An overview. *Eur. J. Cancer B Oral Oncol.* 31B (6): 355–360.

Huff, J.C., Weston, W.L., and Tonnesen, M.G. (1983). Erythema multiforme: a critical review of characteristics, diagnostic criteria, and causes. *J. Am. Acad. Dermatol.* 8: 763–775.

Kataoka, M., Kido, J., Shinohara, Y., and Nagata, T. (2005). Drug-induced gingival overgrowth – a review. *Biol. Pharm. Bull.* 28 (10): 1817–1821.

Kaur, C., Thami, G.P., Sarkar, R., and Kanwar, A.J. (2001). Plasma cell mucositis. *J. Eur. Acad. Dermatol. Venereol.* 15 (6): 566–567.

Kauzman, A., Pavone, M., Blanas, N., and Bradley, G. (2004). Pigmented lesions of the oral cavity: review, differential diagnosis, and case presentations. *J. Can. Dent. Assoc.* 70 (10): 682–683.

Kemp, S., Gallagher, G., and Kabani, S. (2005). Case report: oral involvement as an early manifestation of Wegener's granulomatosis. *Oral Surg. Oral Med. Oral Pathol.* 100 (2): 187.

Koch, B.B., Trask, D.K., Hoffman, H.T. et al. (2001). National survey of head and neck verrucous carcinoma: patterns of presentation, care, and outcome. *Cancer* 92 (1): 110–120.

Laskaris, G., Triantafyllou, A., and Economopoulou, P. (1988). Gingival manifestations of childhood cicatricial pemphigoid. *Oral Surg. Oral Med. Oral Pathol.* 66 (3): 349–352.

Macleod, R.I. and Ellis, J.E. (1989). Plasma cell gingivitis related to the use of herbal toothpaste. *Br. Dent. J.* 166 (10): 375–376.

Magnusson, B.C. and Rasmusson, L.G. (1995). The giant cell fibroma. A review of 103 cases with immunohistochemical findings. *Acta Odontol. Scand.* 53 (5): 293–296.

Manchanda, Y., Tejasvi, T., Handa, R., and Ramam, M. (2003). Strawberry gingiva: a distinctive sign in Wegener's granulomatosis. *J. Am. Acad. Dermatol.* 49 (2): 335–337.

Martin-Granizo, R., Rodriguez-Campo, F., Naval, L., and Diaz Gonzalez, F.J. (1997). Squamous cell carcinoma of the oral cavity in patients younger than 40 years. *Otolaryngol. Head Neck Surg.* 117 (3 Pt 1): 268–275.

Mavrogiannis, M., Ellis, J.S., Seymour, R.A., and Thomason, J.M. (2006). The efficacy of three different surgical techniques in the management of drug-induced gingival overgrowth. *J. Clin. Periodontol.* 33 (9): 677–682.

McCoy, J.M. and Waldron, C.A. (1981). Verrucous carcinoma of the oral cavity. A review of forty-nine cases. *Oral Surg. Oral Med. Oral Pathol.* 52 (6): 623–629.

McCulloch, C.A. (2004). Drug-induced fibrosis: Interference with the intracellular collagen degradation pathway. *Curr. Opin. Drug Discov. Devel.* 7 (5): 720–724.

Mealey, B.L. (2006). Periodontal disease and diabetes: a two-way street. *J. Am. Dent. Assoc.* 137 (Suppl 2): 26S–31S.

Medina, J.E., Dichtel, W., and Luna, M.A. (1984). Verrucous-squamous carcinomas of the oral cavity. A clinicopathologic study of 104 cases. *Arch. Otolaryngol.* 110 (7): 437–440.

Mignogna, M.D., Lo Muzio, L., and Bucci, E. (2001). Clinical features of gingival pemphigus vulgaris. *J. Clin. Periodontol.* 28 (5): 489–493.

Mignogna, M.D., Lo Russo, L., and Fedele, S. (2005). Gingival involvement of oral lichen planus in a series of 700 patients. *J. Clin. Periodontol.* 32 (10): 1029–1033.

Mirowski, G.W. and Waibel, J.S. (2002). Pigmented lesions of the oral cavity. *Dermatol. Therapy* 15 (3): 218–228.

Musa, N.J., Kumar, V., Humphreys, L. et al. (2002). Oral pemphigoid masquerading as necrotizing ulcerative gingivitis in a child. *J. Periodontol.* 73 (6): 657–663.

Natali, C., Curtis, J.L., Suarez, L., and Millman, E.J (1991). Oral mucosa pigment changes in heavy drinkers and smokers. *J. Natl. Med. Assoc.* 83 (5): 434–438.

Naudi, K.B., Hunter, K.D., MacDonald, D.G., and Felix, D.H. (2006). Ligneous alveolar gingivitis in the absence of plasminogen deficiency. *J. Oral Pathol. Med.* 35 (10): 636–638.

Navazesh, M. (1995). Tartar-control toothpaste as a possible contributory factor in the onset of superficial mucocele: a case report. *Spec. Care Dentist.* 15 (2): 74–78.

Noonan, V., Kabani, S., and Gallagher, G. (2005). Recurrent intraoral herpes infection. *J. Mass. Dent. Soc.* 53 (4): 55.

Nxumalo, T.N. and Shear, M. (1992). Gingival cyst in adults. *J. Oral Pathol. Med.* 21 (7): 309–313.

Odessey, E.A., Cohn, A.B., Casper, F., and Schechter, L.S. (2006). Hereditary gingival fibromatosis: aggressive 2-stage surgical resection in lieu of traditional therapy. *Ann. Plast. Surg.* 57 (5): 557–560.

Palefsky, J.M., Silverman, S. Jr., Abdel-Salaam, M. et al. (1995). Association between proliferative verrucous leukoplakia and infection with human papillomavirus type 16. *J. Oral Pathol. Med.* 24 (5): 193–197.

Patten, S.F. and Tomecki, K.J. (1993). Wegener's granulomatosis: cutaneous and oral mucosal disease. *J. Am. Acad. Dermatol.* 28 (5 Pt 1): 710–718.

Patton, L.L., Brahim, J.S., and Baker, A.R. (1994). Metastatic malignant melanoma of the oral cavity. A retrospective study. *Oral Surg. Oral Med. Oral Pathol.* 78 (1): 51–56.

Prasad, V.N., Chawla, H.S., Goyal, A. et al. (2004). Folic acid and phenytoin induced gingival overgrowth – is there a preventive effect? *J. Indian Soc. Pedod. Prev. Dent.* 22 (2): 82–91.

Ramer, M. and Burakoff, R.P. (1997). Smoker's melanosis. Report of a case. *N. Y. State Dent. J.* 63 (8): 20–21.

Ramon Ramirez, J., Seoane, J., Montero, J. et al. (2003). Isolated gingival metastasis from hepatocellular carcinoma mimicking a pyogenic granuloma. *J. Clin. Periodontol.* 30 (10): 926–929.

Reznik, D.A. (2005). Oral manifestations of HIV disease. *Top. HIV Med.* 13 (5): 143–148.

Sanderson, R.J. and Ironside, J.A. (2002). Squamous cell carcinomas of the head and neck. *BMJ* 325 (7368): 822–827.

Schott, D., Dempfle, C.E., Beck, P. et al. (1998). Therapy with a purified plasminogen concentrate in an infant with ligneous conjunctivitis and homozygous plasminogen deficiency. *N. Engl. J. Med.* 339 (23): 1679–1686.

Scully, C., Gokbuget, A.Y., Allen, C. et al. (2001). Oral lesions indicative of plasminogen deficiency (hypoplasminogenemia). *Oral Surg. Oral Med. Oral Pathol. Oral Radiol. Endod.* 91 (3): 334–337.

Scully, C. and Porter, S. (2000). ABC of oral health. Oral cancer. *BMJ* 321 (7253): 97–100.

Seoane, J., Varela-Centelles, P.I., Walsh, T.F. et al. (2006). Gingival squamous cell carcinoma: diagnostic delay or rapid invasion? *J. Periodontol.* 77 (7): 1229–1233.

Serio, F.G., Siegel, M.A., and Slade, B.E. (1991). Plasma cell gingivitis of unusual origin. A case report. *J. Periodontol.* 62 (6): 390–393.

Setterfield, J., Shirlaw, P.J., Kerr-Muir, M. et al. (1998). Mucous membrane pemphigoid: a dual circulating antibody response with IgG and IgA signifies a more severe and persistent disease. *Br. J. Dermatol.* 138 (4): 602–610.

Shade, N.L., Carpenter, W.M., and Delzer, D.D. (1987). Gingival cyst of the adult. Case report of a bilateral presentation. *J. Periodontol.* 58 (11): 796–799.

Siegel, M.A. and Anhalt, G.J. (1993). Direct immunofluorescence of detached gingival epithelium for diagnosis of cicatricial pemphigoid. Report of five cases. *Oral Surg. Oral Med. Oral Pathol.* 75 (3): 296–302.

Silverman, S. Jr. and Gorsky, M. (1997). Proliferative verrucous leukoplakia: a follow-up study of 54 cases. *Oral Surg. Oral Med. Oral Pathol. Oral Radiol. Endod.* 84 (2): 154–157.

Sinha, A., Chander, J., and Natarajan, S. (2006). Erythema multiforme presenting as chronic oral ulceration due to unrecognised herpes simplex virus infection. *Clin. Exp. Dermatol.* 31 (5): 737–738.

Sklavounou, A. and Laskaris, G. (1990). Childhood cicatricial pemphigoid with exclusive gingival involvement. *Int. J. Oral Maxillofac. Surg.* 19 (4): 197–199.

Solomon, L.W., Aguirre, A., Neiders, M. et al. (2003). Chronic ulcerative stomatitis: clinical, histopathologic, and immunopathologic findings. *Oral Surg. Oral Med. Oral Pathol. Oral Radiol. Endod.* 96 (6): 718–726.

Souza, L.B., Andrade, E.S., Miguel, M.C. et al. (2004). Origin of stellate giant cells in oral fibrous lesions determined by immunohistochemical expression of vimentin, HHF-35, CD68 and factor XIIIa. *Pathology* 36 (4): 316–320.

Spiro, R.H. (1998). Verrucous carcinoma, then and now. *Am. J. Surg.* 176 (5): 393–397.

Spruance, S.L., Bodsworth, N., Resnick, H. et al. (2006). Single-dose, patient-initiated famciclovir: a randomized, double-blind, placebo-controlled trial for episodic treatment of herpes labialis. *J. Am. Acad. Dermatol.* 55 (1): 47–53.

Tal, H., Oegiesser, D., and Tal, M. (2003). Gingival depigmentation by erbium: YAG laser: clinical observations and patient responses. *J. Periodontol.* 74 (11): 1660–1667.

Thornhill, M.H., Sankar, V., Xu, X.J. et al. (2006). The role of histopathological characteristics in distinguishing amalgam-associated oral lichenoid reactions and/oral lichen planus. *J. Oral Pathol. Med.* 35 (4): 233–240.

Tokgoz, B., Sari, H.I., Yildiz, O. et al. (2004). Effects of azithromycin on cyclosporine-induced gingival hyperplasia in renal transplant patients. *Transplant. Proc.* 36 (9): 2699–2702.

Treister, N.S., Magalnick, D., and Woo, S.B. (2004). Oral mucosal pigmentation secondary to minocycline therapy: report of two cases and a review of the literature. *Oral Surg. Oral Med. Oral Pathol. Oral Radiol. Endod.* 97 (6): 718–725.

Umeda, M. and Shimada, K. (1994). Primary malignant melanoma of the oral cavity – its histological classification and treatment. *Br. J. Oral Maxillofac. Surg.* 32 (1): 39–47.

van der Waal, R.I., Buter, J., and van der Waal, I. (2003). Oral metastases: report of 24 cases. *Br. J. Oral Maxillofac. Surg.* 41 (1): 3–6.

Velegraki, A., Nicolatou, O., Theodoridou, M. et al. (1999). Paediatric AIDS – related linear gingival erythema: a form of erythematous candidiasis? *J. Oral Pathol. Med.* 28 (4): 178–182.

Wakahara, M., Kiyohara, T., Kumakiri, M. et al. (2005). Paraneoplastic pemphigus with widespread mucosal involvement. *Acta Derm. Venereol.* 85 (6): 530–532.

Walters, J.D., Will, J.K., Hatfield, R.D. et al. (2001). Excision and repair of the peripheral ossifying fibroma: a report of 3 cases. *J. Periodontol.* 72 (7): 939–944.

Weckx, L.L., Hidal, L.B., and Marcucci, G. (1990). Oral manifestations of leukemia. *Ear Nose Throat J.* 69 (5): 341–342, 345–346.

Wiernik, P.H., De Bellis, R., Muxi, P., and Dutcher, J.P. (1996). Extramedullary acute promyelocytic leukemia. *Cancer* 78 (12): 2510–2514.

Wine, E., Ballin, A., and Dalal, I. (2006). Infantile erythema multiforme following hepatitis B vaccine. *Acta Paediatr.* 95 (7): 890–891.

Wright, J.M. (1988). Intraoral melanoacanthoma: a reactive melanocytic hyperplasia. Case report. *J. Periodontol.* 59 (1): 53–55.

Yuan, K., Wing, L.Y., and Lin, M.T. (2002). Pathogenetic roles of angiogenic factors in pyogenic granulomas in pregnancy are modulated by female sex hormones. *J. Periodontol.* 73 (7): 701–708.

Zakrzewska, J.M. (1999). Fortnightly review: oral cancer. *BMJ* 318 (7190): 1051–1054.

Chapter 11 Sinus Augmentation Using Tissue-Engineered Bone

Ulrike Schulze-Späte, Luigi Montesani, and Lorenzo Montesani

HISTORY

Implant placement in the edentulous maxilla often represents a clinical challenge due to insufficient bone height after crestal bone resorption and maxillary sinus pneumatization. Surgical approaches that were developed over the past years aim to restore bone height in the posterior maxilla to create a sufficient implant bed. Boyne and James were the first ones to describe a procedure which utilizes existing space in the maxillary sinus by lifting up the Schneiderian membrane from its bony surface and filling this newly created space with augmentation material (Boyne and James 1980). Several modifications of the originally described surgical procedure were developed, however, the basic principle of increasing maxillary bone height by placing graft material in the maxillary sinus after detaching the Schneiderian membrane remained the same (Davarpanah et al. 2001; Fugazzotto and De Paoli 2002; Summers 1994). Grafting materials used to augment bone height in the posterior maxilla can be categorized into four groups: autogenous bone, allografts (from humans), xenografts (from a nonhuman species), and alloplasts (synthetic materials). Autogenous bone is the only grafting material with an osteogenic potential and it has been shown that its use in sinus augmentation can achieve predictable results. Furthermore, autogenous bone requires shorter healing times (4 months vs. 8–10 months) since it contains living cells and growth factors. Unfortunately, its availability is limited due to anatomical confines and donor site morbidity (Block and Kent 1997; Cammack 2nd et al. 2005; Froum 1998; Garg 1999; Pikos 1996; Wheeler 1997). Several current approaches aim to overcome those boundaries; one novel approach uses concepts previously established in the field of tissue engineering. In contrast to conventional one dimensional *in vitro* cell culture, tissue-engineering techniques aim to mimic an *in vivo* environment by using scaffolds, which arrange cells in a three-dimensional fashion (Risbud 2001). Living tissues which otherwise would be limited in their potential to grow can be contained and even expanded *in vitro* before being re-introduced *in vivo*.

Periosteum, a membrane that closely enfolds bone, consists of connective tissue and contains chondroprogenitor and osteoprogenitor cell populations (Hutmacher and Sittinger 2003). It has been shown that these progenitor cells can be isolated and stimulated *in vitro* to form cartilage and bone using tissue-engineering techniques (Arnold et al. 2002; Breitbach et al. 1998). In 2003, Schmelzeisen et al. described a clinical procedure, which substitutes autogenous bone graft material with tissue-engineered bone in a sinus augmentation procedure. Periosteal tissue was harvested from the oral cavity and its progenitor cells were isolated and expanded in a three dimensional bioabsorbable polymer fleece matrix *in vitro*. The matured transplants were inserted in the maxillary sinus in between the elevated Schneiderian membrane and the bony floor of the sinus. A number of follow-up publications and a prospective clinical study demonstrated successful remodeling of the graft material, therefore, establishing sinus augmentation with tissue-engineered bone as a possible option for overcoming current limitations of autogenous bone grafting in the posterior maxilla (Schimming and Schmelzeisen 2004; Schmelzeisen et al. 2003).

Implant placement can occur at the same surgical appointment (immediate placement) or following a healing period (delayed placement) depending on the remaining bone height. It is generally acknowledged that for an immediate placement at least 4–5 mm of remaining ridge height is necessary to achieve sufficient immobilization of implants during maturation of the sinus graft (Jensen et al. 1998).

INDICATIONS

- Insufficient bone height in the posterior maxilla for dental implant placement.

- Need for a large amount of autogenous bone grafting material

- Patient's refusal to have a bone graft from a source that is not his/her own.

Practical Advanced Periodontal Surgery, Second Edition. Edited by Serge Dibart.
© 2020 John Wiley & Sons, Inc. Published 2020 by John Wiley & Sons, Inc.
Companion website: www.wiley.com/go/dibart/advanced

CONTRAINDICATIONS

- The presence of uncontrolled diabetes, immune diseases, or other contraindicating systemic conditions.
- Thrombocytopenia or allergically induced thrombocytopenia (type II).
- Radiation therapy to the head and neck area in the 12 month period prior to proposed surgical treatment.
- Chemotherapy in the 12 month period prior to proposed surgical treatment.
- An active sinus infection or a history of persistent sinus infections.
- Hypersensitivity to bovine albumin, penicillin, gentamicin, amphotericin B.
- An excessive smoking habit.
- Alcohol and drug abuse.
- Physical and psychological handicaps.
- Pregnancy and lactating patients.

ARMAMENTARIUM

1. For the harvesting procedure, a basic surgical kit such as the one described in *Practical Periodontal Plastic Surgery* and an osseous coagulum collector (Citagenix Inc., Quebec, Canada) can be used.
2. For the sinus augmentation procedure, a basic surgical kit and the following can be used:
   - Angulated elevation instruments for separation of the Schneiderian membrane from the inner bony surface of the maxillary sinus (Hu-Friedy, Chicago, IL, USA)
   - CollaTape (Zimmer Dental, Carlsbad, CA, USA)
   - Bio-Oss (Geistlich Pharma North America Inc., Princeton, NY, USA)
   - Resorbable membrane: Bioguide (Geistlich Pharma North America Inc., Princeton, NY, USA); RCM (Bicon, Boston, MA, USA)

SINUS AUGMENTATION USING TISSUE-ENGINEERED BONE DISCS

Technique

Sinus augmentation using tissue-engineered bone requires two surgical procedures, harvesting and transplant implantation surgery.

Harvesting Procedure

Periosteal tissue can be obtained from several locations in the oral cavity. However, access to the lateral cortex of the mandibular body in the apical region of the first molar area is

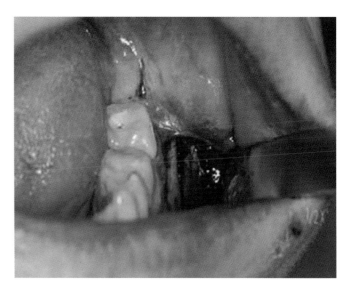

Figure 11.1 Collection of a periosteal biopsy. Periosteal tissue was harvested from the goniac angle of the mandible.

relatively easy and not too invasive. After administering local anesthesia, an intrasulcular or intravestibular incision parallel to the mucogingival junction is made using a #15 blade. The incision on the buccal side of the first mandibular molar should extend at least one and a half teeth toward the anterior and posterior in order to obtain sufficient access. A partial thickness flap is elevated to expose the underlying periosteum. After outlining the area with a #15 blade, the periosteal biopsy (approximately $1\,cm^2$) can be collected using a back action chisel or osseous coagulum collector (see Figure 11.1). Alternatively, an alveolar bone biopsy (8x10x2mm) can be taken from the same side or the tuberosity area after exposing the bone using a distal wedge incision. The collected tissue biopsy needs to be stored in appropriate sterile tissue containers and transferred to an *in vitro* cell/tissue facility for further culturing and tissue expansion. In addition, a blood sample (approximately 126ml of blood will be sufficient for 10 tissue-engineered discs) needs to be taken from the patient. This blood sample will be used to produce serum, which is essential for future culturing of the isolated periosteal cells (Schimming and Schmelzeisen 2004). The donor side can be sutured with either resorbable (5-0 chromic gut) or nonresorbable (5-0 silk) suture material.

Postoperative Management

Pain medications should be prescribed as needed. In addition, chlorhexidine rinses twice a day for 21 days starting 1 day after the surgery should be included in the postoperative regimen.

Treatment and Expansion of Periosteal Biopsies

The periosteal tissue biopsy can be cultured using a tissue engineering protocol described by Schmelzeisen et al.

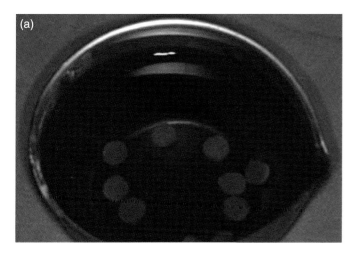
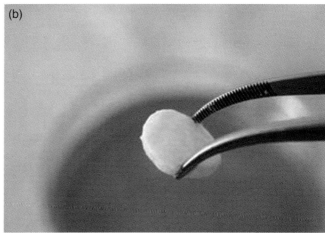

Figure 11.2 Tissue-engineered bone discs. (a) Discs were kept in transportation medium until implantation. (b) Scaffolds need to be carefully handled so as not to destroy the incorporated cells.

(Schmelzeisen 2003). In addition, commercial companies such as Bio Tissue Technology, Freiburg, Germany offer to overtake laborious cell culturing and provide the clinician with the finished tissue-engineered bone discs.

The periosteum needs to be enzymatically digested to isolate progenitor cells. Collagenase CLSII (*Clostridium histo lyticum*) at a concentration of 333 U/ml (Biochrom, Cambridge, UK) in 1 : 1 DMEM/Ham's F-12 (Dulbecco's modified Eagle's medium, Invitrogen, Carlsbad, CA, USA) can be used and the resulting cell suspension needs to be washed with phosphate buffered saline (PBS, Invitrogen, Carlsbad, CA, USA). Cells are counted using a hemocytometer and stained with trypan blue dye to determine the overall cell viability. Afterwards, they are resuspended in 1 : 1 DMEM/Ham's F-12 supplemented with 10% autologous serum and seeded into cell culture flasks. The flasks are cultured in a cell culture incubator adjusted to 37 °C, 3.5% CO_2 and 95% humidity. The medium needs to be replaced every two days until cells reach a 70% confluency. At this point, cells are trypsinized (0.02% trypsin and 0.02% EDTA in PBS) for five minutes and seeded at a density of 5000/mm². This step needs to be repeated four times to increase cell number. Following trypsinization, cells are now ready to be incorporated into the transplant discs (Perka et al. 2000). Several scaffold materials such as synthetic and natural polymers, composites, and ceramics have been tested in recent years (Sittinger et al. 2004). They need to be biocompatible and resorbable to facilitate integration of the future graft into an *in vivo* environment. To incorporate cells into the scaffold, cells are suspended in 1 : 1 DMEM/Ham's and mixed with human fibrinogen (TissueColl, Baxter Immuno, Austria) in a 3 : 1 ratio. The resulting cell solution is soaked into polymer fleeces (e.g. Ethicon, Cornelia, GA, USA) and subsequently polymerized by adding bovine thrombin (TissueColl, Baxter Immuno,

Austria) in a 1 : 10 PBS dilution. The transplant discs are cultured for an additional week in DMEM/Ham's supplemented with 5% autologous serum, dexamethasone 10-7 Mol, β-glycerophosphate 10 mM and ascorbic acid (50 mg/l). At this point (approximately seven weeks after the harvesting procedure), the transplants are ready for implantation. Each final disc contains around 1.5×10^6 cells and is circa 2×10 mm in size (see Figure 11.2a and b).

TRANSPLANT IMPLANTATION SURGERY (SINUS AUGMENTATION PROCEDURE USING TISSUE-ENGINEERED BONE DISCS)

Prior to the sinus augmentation procedure, a computed tomography (CT) scan or panoramic radiograph should be taken from the selected area (Figure 11.4a). The procedure can be performed under local anesthesia. A mid-crestal incision is made with mesial and distal releasing incisions extending well into the buccal fold. The mucoperiosteal flap is reflected in a full thickness manner and care needs to be taken to completely release the tissue for a tension-free access to the lateral wall of the maxillary sinus. There are three classical approaches to enter the maxillary sinus. In the Caldwell Luc approach the window is anterior to the zygomatic buttress, in a low position the window is situated next to the alveolar crest and in a mid-maxillary position the lateral window is situated between the alveolar crest and zygomatic buttress (Lazzara 1996; Summers 1994; Zitzmann and Scharer 1998). In the above introduced application, a lateral window approach is recommended. However, in any case, the osteotomy window should be placed according to the anatomical structure of the maxillary sinus and its inferior horizontal border should be 3–4 mm above the sinus floor. The oval window is outlined under continuous sterile saline irrigation with a highspeed handpiece and either a carbide or a diamond bur (see Figure 11.3a). As an alternative, piezoelectric surgery could be used, reducing the risks of underlying membrane perforation (Vercellotti et al. 2001). The bone covering the window can either be thinned uniformly all around or in a trap door manner, which uses the superior border as a hinge (see Figure 11.3b). In both techniques, the bony window is carefully pushed inward and at the same time the Schneiderian membrane gets detached from its underlying bony surface using angulated elevation instruments. Attention should be paid to preserving the integrity of the sinus membrane by keeping elevation instruments in constant contact with the internal bony sinus wall during the membrane elevation process. After elevation, membrane integrity can be checked with the valsalva maneuver (Charkawi et al. 2005). Occurring tears can be repaired. For small tears (less than 5 mm) a fast resorbing collagen membrane such as Collatape (Zimmer Dental, Carlsbad, CA, USA) can be used to cover the tear. Repair of larger perforations requires a more rigid and longer lasting membrane (Biomend, Zimmer Dental, Carlsbad, CA, USA) (Zimbler et al. 1998). In cases of major membrane destruction, it is recommended to abort the grafting procedure and wait six to nine months for membrane regeneration (Berengo et al. 2004). It is important to detach the membrane sufficiently from its walls since it has been shown that in an adequately elevated membrane tears can heal without complications. In contrast, laceration could stay open in membranes which are too stretched (Jensen et al. 1998). In addition, insufficient membrane elevation might subsequently result in a graft, which is not adequate in its dimensions to support future implants. Especially the medial and anterior walls are common regions to display insufficient grafting. Therefore, grafting the anterior wall first is a habit many surgeons have developed to prevent this problem. Furthermore, it is advised to hold up the membrane with a periosteal elevator while packing the bone graft against the medial wall to prevent packing against a Schneiderian membrane that has "come down" as a result of the patient's breathing.

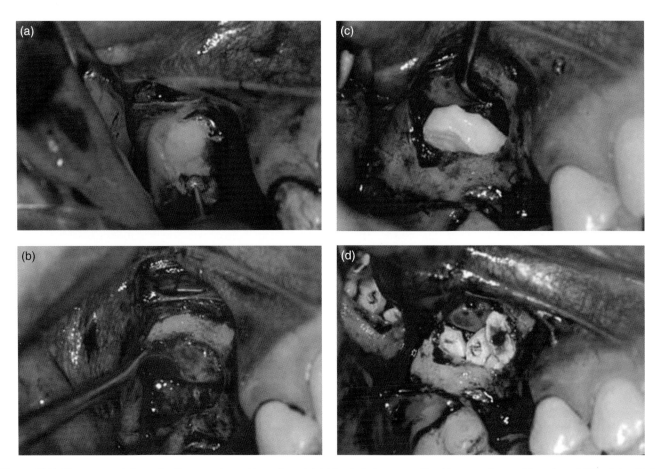

Figure 11.3 Sinus augmentation using tissue-engineered bone discs. (a) A lateral window was outlined to access the maxillary sinus. (b) The Schneiderian membrane was elevated from its bony surface to create space for the augmentation material. (c and d) Tissue-engineered bone discs were implanted into the maxillary sinus. (e) The discs were covered with Bio-Oss (Osteohealth) augmentation material (optional). (f) The grafted area was covered with a resorbable membrane (Bioguide, Osteohealth). (g) The flap was sutured in its original position with single interrupted sutures (Gortex, Gore Medical).

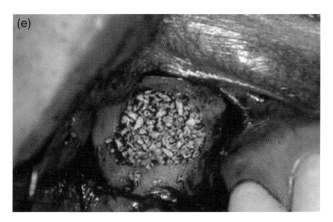

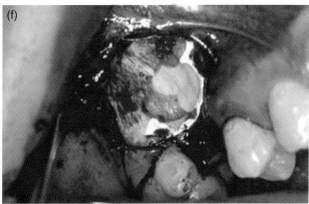

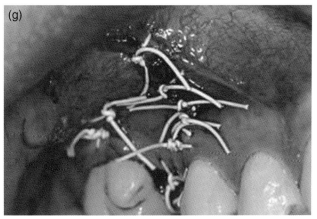

Figure 11.3 (*continued*)

It also should be kept in mind that the ostium which represents the connection in between the middle meatus of the nose and the maxillary sinus is approximately 25 mm above the floor of the sinus. A blockade due to extensive sinus grafting can result in a chronic infection of the maxillary sinus (Doud Galli et al. 2001).

Assuming that the membrane is elevated sufficiently, the tissue-engineered discs which can be kept in the transportation medium during the procedure are then inserted into the sinus and gently packed until the space in between sinus membrane and bony walls of the sinus is filled (see Figure 11.3c and d). In addition, bone augmentation material such as Bio-Oss (Osteohealth, Shirley, NY, USA) can be used as a protective layer on the outside of the graft (see Figure 11.3e). The window should be covered with a membrane that overlaps its outlines and therefore protects the grafted side. Either a nonresorbable membrane with securing tacks or a resorbable one can be used for this purpose (see Figure 11.3f). Afterwards, the mucoperiosteal flap is positioned back to cover the surgical site. It might be necessary to release the periosteum of the flap with a

#15 blade in order to facilitate a tension free closure. The flap can now be sutured with either resorbable (such as Vicryl, Ethicon, Carnelia, GA, USA) or nonresorbable (such as Gortex suture, Gore Medical, Flagstaff, Arizona) suture material in single interrupted sutures (see Figure 11.3g). Whenever necessary, these sutures can be replaced by a continuous suture and further secured with horizontal mattress sutures.

Postoperative Management

- Antibiotic therapy should be started the day before the procedure: 500 mg amoxicillin three times daily for seven days (300 mg clindamycin four times daily should be prescribed for penicillin sensitive patients)

- Analgesics: Acetaminophen + codeine (Tylenol #3) or ibuprofen (Motrin 600 mg) three times a day or as necessary.

- Anti-inflammatories: Dexamethasone can be prescribed for five days in the following manner (day of surgery: 3.75 mg; day 2: 3 mg; day 3: 2.25 mg: day 4: 1.5 mg; day 5: 0.75 mg). This will control the swelling and alleviate the discomfort.

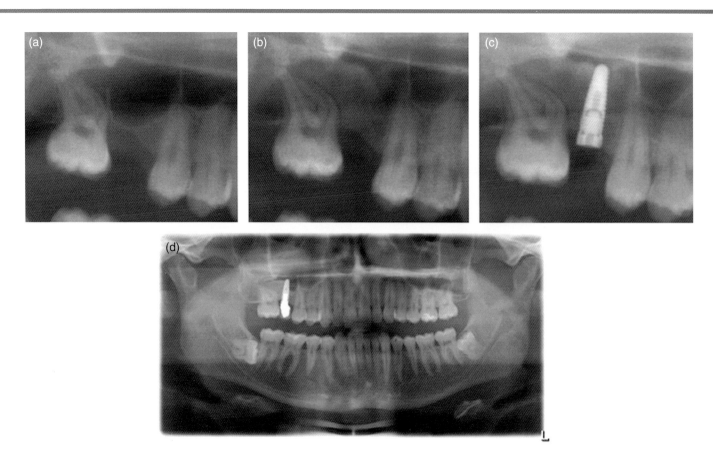

Figure 11.4 Radiographic evaluation of the grafted site. (a) A periapical radiograph was taken and revealed inadequate bone height prior to implant placement. (b) Radiograph depicting the augmented site prior to implant placement. (c) Implant was placed successfully in the grafted site achieving primary stability. (d) 10 year follow up. Graft material is still in place.

- Afrin spray: Patients should be given this spray to use in order not to blow their noses for two weeks, as that will impair proper healing of the graft.

- Antiseptic rinses: Chlorhexidine digluconate rinses twice a day for 21 days starting 1 day after the surgery are recommended.

- Patients can wear their complete dentures after the procedure; however, the buccal flange needs to be reduced and later on relined with a soft reliner. Partial dentures should only be worn if they have an acrylic base which allows appropriate relief and facilitates soft relining. However, it is recommended to advise that the denture is worn for esthetic reasons and not for function until the day of suture removal.

Healing

Studies revealed sufficient new bone formation four month after implantation of the tissue-engineered bone discs (Schmelzeisen et al. 2003). Therefore, dental implants can be placed four month after the grafting procedure (see Figure 11.4b and c). A core biopsy can be taken during the surgery and subjected to histological

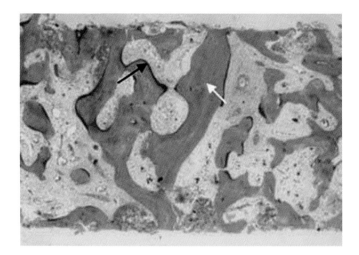

Figure 11.5 Histological staining of core biopsy taken from the future implant side. Goldner's staining shows mineralized bone (green; see white arrow) and newly formed osteoid (red; see black arrow).

staining to determine current mineralization status of the augmented bone (see Figure 11.5). Afterwards, implants can be restored according to standard protocols (see Figure 11.6).

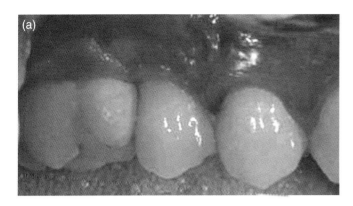

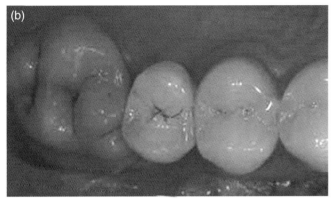

Figure 11.6 Clinical view of the restored implant. (a and b) Implant was restored with a single porcelain fused metal (PFM) crown.

SINUS LIFT USING AUTOGENOUS MESENCHYMAL CELLS PROCESSED CHAIRSIDE

This technique mixing a xenograft with autogenous mesenchymal cells taken from the posterior iliac crest allows for quick maturation of the bone and implant placement at four months (Duttenhoefer et al. 2014).

Harvesting Procedure

After loco-regional anesthesia, 60 ml of a bone marrow aspirate is taken from the posterior iliac crest of the patient (Figure 11.7). This material is then put through a centrifuge for 14 minutes according to the manufacturer's instruction (Harvest, Terumo BCT, Colorado USA) to separate the plasma from the mononuclear cells, granulocytes, thrombocytes, and erythrocytes (Figure 11.8). The plasma layer is discarded, and the cellular layers are mixed with the xenograft (Bio-Oss) (Figure 11.9). Following this the graft mixture is ready to be loaded in a syringe (Figure 11.10) and to be inserted into the sinus (Figure 11.11). The implants are placed simultaneously and after four months final impressions can be taken in most cases (Figure 11.12).

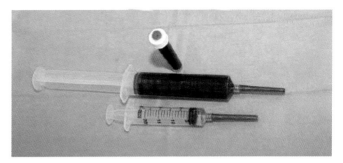

Figure 11.7 Material taken from the bone marrow through aspiration.

Possible Complications

Complications occurring after sinus augmentation with tissue-engineered bone should not be different from complications associated with other grafting materials assuming that the discs were prepared and transported under sterile conditions.

Swelling, Bruising, and Bleeding

Patients might experience swelling and bruising in the surgical areas after the procedure. Therefore, it is recommended to use cold pads for the initial 24 hours. Afterwards, the application of warm pads in combination with anti-inflammatory medications will help to reduce swelling and discomfort. It is not unusual for patients to report an exacerbated feeling of pain five days after the procedure since at this time point the corticosteroid regimen has ended. Therefore, patients should be informed beforehand and advised to continue taking non-steroidal anti-inflammatory drugs for a week.

In case of nasal bleeding due to laceration of the Schneiderian membrane, patients should be reassured (as this will happen after they have left your office), and pressure with a cotton ball should be applied to stop the nasal bleeding.

Infraorbital Nerve Paresthesia

Paresthesia of the area innervated by the infraorbital nerve can be caused by blunt retraction over the neurovascular bundle. It is usually transient and disappears within a few weeks. However, in some cases long-lasting paresthesia up to several months is possible.

Infection of the Grafted Site and Membrane Exposure

Infection spreading from an infected graft can lead to pansinusitis, spread to the orbit, dura, brain, and requires intervention. An early sign is the occurrence of an intraoral swelling one week post-surgery; however, signs of infection can be detected as early as three days. In case of an

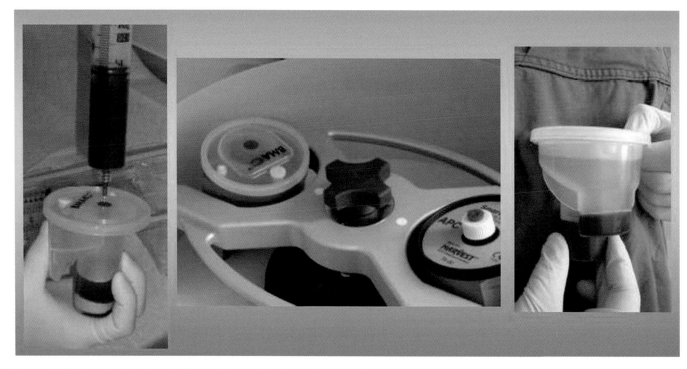

Figure 11.8 The material is placed in the centrifuge and the plasma is separated.

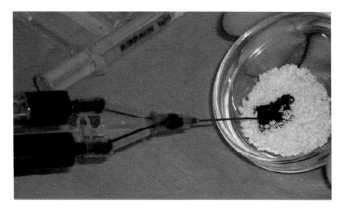

Figure 11.9 The stem cell-rich material is mixed with the xenograft (Bio-Oss).

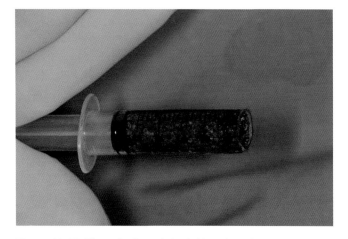

Figure 11.10 The graft mixture is loaded into the syringe.

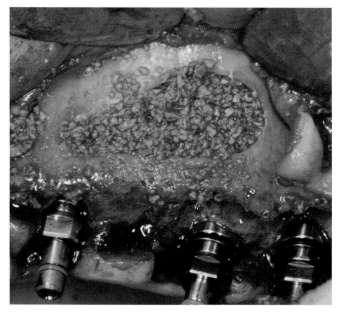

Figure 11.11 The bone graft is delivered into the sinus with simultaneous implant placement.

infection, prescription of antibiotics such as clindamycin with a loading dose of 600 mg followed by 300 mg four times daily is recommended. Metronidazole can be added for anaerobic coverage at 500 mg three times daily. Most of the time, a localized infection will respond to the treatment. However, in case of persistent symptomatology it is imperative to pursue aggressive treatment, which includes incision and drainage over the original incision line. In addition,

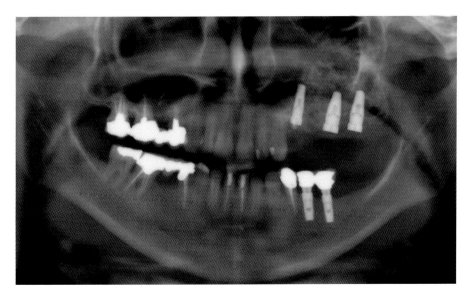

Figure 11.12 Four months later prior to uncovering.

aerobic and anaerobic cultures could be used as a supportive adjunct to determine future treatment. Sometimes local debridement is appropriate and sufficient. If the graft needs to be completely removed, a long-lasting collagen membrane should be used to cover the window. After a healing period of three to four months, the site can be re-entered for an additional grafting procedure. In response to an infection, oroantral fistulae can form which are treatable with antibiotics and oral chlorhexidine rinses. Nevertheless, large and persistent fistulae require surgical intervention. In case of a premature exposure of the membrane, it has been shown that oral bacteria can penetrate the membrane surface within four weeks (Simion et al. 1994). Thus, it is advised to continue the use of chlorhexidine mouth rinses until the final implant surgery. In any case, the patient should be closely followed in order to intervene if an infection develops and the membrane needs to be removed.

Taken together, infection should be treated in a comprehensive way to minimize the risk of spreading and maximize the success of the grafting procedure.

REFERENCES

Arnold, U., Lindenhayn, K., and Perka, C. (2002). In vitro-cultivation of human periosteum derived cells in bioresorbable polymer-TCP-composites. *Biomaterials* 23: 2303–2310.

Berengo, M., Sivolella, S., Majzoub, Z., and Cordioli, G. (2004). Endoscopic evaluation of the bone-added osteotome sinus floor elevation procedure. *Int. J. Oral Maxillofac. Surg.* 33 (2): 189–194.

Block, M.S. and Kent, J.N. (1997). Sinus augmentation for dental implants: the use of autogenous bone. *J. Oral Maxillofac. Surg.* 55 (11): 1281–1286.

Boyne, P.J. and James, R.A. (1980). Grafting of the maxillary sinus floor with autogenous marrow and bone. *J. Oral Surg.* 38 (8): 613–616.

Breitbach, A.S., Grande, D.A., Kessler, R. et al. (1998). Tissue engineered bone repair of calvarial defects using culture periosteal cells. *Plast. Reconstr. Surg.* 101: 567–574.

Cammack, G.V. 2nd, Nevins, M., Clem, D.S. 3rd et al. (2005). Histologic evaluation of mineralized and demineralized freeze-dried bone allograft for ridge and sinus augmentations. *Int. J. Periodontics Restorative Dent.* 25 (3): 231–237.

Charkawi, E., Hussein, G., Askary, E. et al. (2005). Endoscopic removal of an implant from the maxillary sinus: a case report. *Implant Den.* 14 (1): 30–35.

Davarpanah, M., Martinez, H., Tecucianu, J.F. et al. (2001). The modified osteotome technique. *Int. J. Periodontics Restorative Dent.* 21 (6): 599–607.

Doud Galli, S.K., Lebowitz, R.A., Giacchi, R.J. et al. (2001). Chronic sinusitis complicating sinus lift surgery. *Am. J. Rhinol. Allergy* 15 (3): 181–186.

Duttenhoefer, F., Hieber, S.F., Stricker, A. et al. (2014 Apr 1). Follow-up of implant survival comparing ficoll and bone marrow aspirate concentrate methods for hard tissue regeneration with mesenchymal stem cells in humans. *Biores Open Access* 3 (2): 75–76.

Froum, S.J., Tarnow, D.P., Wallace, S.S. et al. (1998). Sinus floor elevation using anorganic bovine bone matrix (OsteoGraf/N) with and without autogenous bone: a clinical, histologic, radiographic, and histomorphometric analysis--part 2 of an ongoing prospective study. *Int. J. Periodontics Restorative Dent.* 18 (6): 528–543.

Fugazzotto, P.A. and De Paoli, S. (2002). Sinus floor augmentation at the time of maxillary molar extraction: success and failure rates of 137 implants in function for up to 3 years. *J. Periodont.* 73 (1): 39–44.

Garg, A.K. (1999). Augmentation grafting of the maxillary sinus for placement of dental implants: anatomy, physiology, and procedures. *Implant Dent.* 8 (1): 36–46.

Hutmacher, D.W. and Sittinger, M. (2003). Periosteal cells in bone tissue engineering. *Tissue Engineering* 9 (Suppl 1): S45–S64.

Jensen, O.T., Shulman, L.B., Block, M.S., and Iacono, V.J. (1998). Report of the sinus consensus conference of 1996. *Int. J. Oral Maxillofac. Implants* 13 (Suppl): 11–45.

Lazzara, R.J. (1996). The sinus elevation procedure in endosseous implant therapy. *Curr. Opin. Periodont.* 3: 178–183.

Perka, C., Schultz, O., Spitzer, R.S. et al. (2000). Segmental bone repair by tissue-engineered periosteal cell transplants with bioresorbable fleece and fibrin scaffolds in rabbits. *Biomaterials* 21 (11): 1145–1153.

Pikos, M.A. (1996). Chin grafts as donor sites for maxillary bone augmentation--part II. *Dent. Implant. Update* 7 (1): 1–4.

Risbud, M. (2001). Tissue engineering: implications in the treatment of organ and tissue defects. *Biogerontology* 2: 117–125.

Schimming, R. and Schmelzeisen, R. (2004). Tissue-engineered bone for maxillary sinus augmentation. *J. Oral Maxillofac. Surg.* 62 (6): 724–729.

Schmelzeisen, R., Schimming, R., and Sittinger, M. (2003). Making bone: implant insertion into tissue-engineered bone for maxillary sinus floor augmentation-a preliminary report. *J. CranioMaxillofac. Surg.* 31: 34–39.

Simion, M., Trisi, P., Maglione, M., and Piattelli, A. (1994). A preliminary report on a method for studying the permeability of expanded polytetrafluoroethylene membrane to bacteria in vitro: a scanning electron microscopic and histological study. *J. Periodont.* 65 (8): 755–761.

Sittinger, M., Hutmacher, D.W., and Risbud, M.V. (2004). Current strategies for cell delivery in cartilage and bone regeneration. *Curr. Opin. Biotech.* 15 (5): 411–418.

Summers, R.B. (1994). A new concept in maxillary implant surgery: the osteotome technique. *Compendium* 15 (2): 152, 154-6, 158 passim; quiz 162.

Vercellotti, T., De Paoli, S., and Nevins, M. (2001). The piezoelectric bony window osteotomy and sinus membrane elevation: introduction of a new technique for simplification of the sinus augmentation procedure. *Int. J. Periodontics Restorative Dent.* 21 (6): 561–567.

Wheeler, S.L. (1997). Sinus augmentation for dental implants: the use of alloplastic materials. *J. Oral Maxillofac. Surg.* 55 (11): 1287–1293.

Zimbler, M.S., Lebowitz, R.A., Glickman, R. et al. (1998). Antral augmentation, osseointegration, and sinusitis: the otolaryngologist's perspective. *Am. J. Rhinol. Allergy* 12 (5): 311–316.

Zitzmann, N.U. and Scharer, P. (1998). Sinus elevation procedures in the resorbed posterior maxilla. Comparison of the crestal and lateral approaches. *Oral Surg. Oral Med. Oral Pathol. Oral Radiol. Endod.* 85 (1): 8–17.

Chapter 12   Extraction Site Management in the Esthetic Zone: Hard and Soft Tissue Reconstruction

Sherif Said

INTRODUCTION

When considering implant therapy in the esthetic zone, replicating the natural soft tissue frame may present challenges for the treating clinician. A harmonious gingival form and architecture are not only fundamental for adequate peri-implant pink esthetics but also for simulating a natural emergence for the future restoration. When dealing with clinical situations in which adequate tissue architecture and volume are present, preserving or further enhancement of the available support may provide an improved esthetic outcome with less associated morbidity and treatment duration. Nevertheless, reconstruction of atrophic sites due to lost hard and soft tissue volume is often inevitable in the anterior zone, which may necessitate more complex grafting procedures with varying degrees of predictability in achieving ideal peri-implant soft tissues. This chapter will highlight clinical scenarios and evidence-based treatment of cases in which the lack of hard and soft tissue volume poses difficulty in achieving optimal peri-implant esthetics. Contemporary clinical strategies and minimally invasive techniques will also be discussed in order to provide clinicians with different options to better manage hard and soft tissue deficiencies when dealing with implant therapy in the esthetic zone.

THE INFLUENCE OF TISSUE VOLUME ON THE PERI-IMPLANT "PINK" ESTHETICS

Solely relying on objective criteria for osseointegration and functional aspects of dental implants may not be sufficient in modern day implant dentistry. Esthetics and patient-centered outcomes have evolved to become integral components of our daily practice, especially in the esthetic zone. The clinician must consider that esthetics are also highly subjective and should be suited towards providing treatment that is tailored to each individual patient depending on their particular situation (Figure 12.1).

Implant esthetics can be further segmented into pink and white esthetics. The "pink" refers to the soft tissue form, contour, color, and texture surrounding the implant while the white focuses on the implant supported crown. Objective assessment criteria have been introduced in the literature (PES/WES) in an attempt to standardize how clinicians and researchers evaluate the esthetics of implant supported restorations. For anterior implant therapy, evaluation of both the pink and white esthetics is imperative, and consequently surgical therapy should be geared toward optimizing functional and biological outcomes without neglecting the esthetic component. This chapter will focus on management and correction of deficient sites through combined hard and soft tissue volume augmentation procedures to offer improved peri-implant pink esthetics and functional long-term outcomes (Figure 12.2).

TISSUE VOLUME AVAILABILITY AND REQUIREMENTS

Preservation of the existing architecture of the soft tissues prior to tooth extraction offers clinicians a simple method of obtaining a more "natural" appearance of the final implant restoration The soft tissue "curtain" that surrounds implant supported crowns requires sufficient, three-dimensional hard and soft tissue volume to attain a long-term stable result. Unfortunately, the tissue volume requirements for dental implants is often more than what is needed for maintenance of the natural dentition. Consequently, preservation of the tissue architecture alone following tooth extraction may not always be adequate to maintain tissue stability around the future implant and thus additional soft and hard tissue augmentation is often required. Spray and colleagues (2000) demonstrated the importance of sufficient buccal bone in implant dentistry. It was found that when the bone buccal to an implant fixture was less than 1.8 mm, bone remodeling and possible implant dehiscence was observed at the time of second stage uncovering. Other authors have corroborated these findings with recommendations of a minimum of 2 mm of bone buccal to the implant with a range of 2–4 mm (Grunder 2000, 2011) for maintenance of

Practical Advanced Periodontal Surgery, Second Edition. Edited by Serge Dibart.
© 2020 John Wiley & Sons, Inc. Published 2020 by John Wiley & Sons, Inc.
Companion website: www.wiley.com/go/dibart/advanced

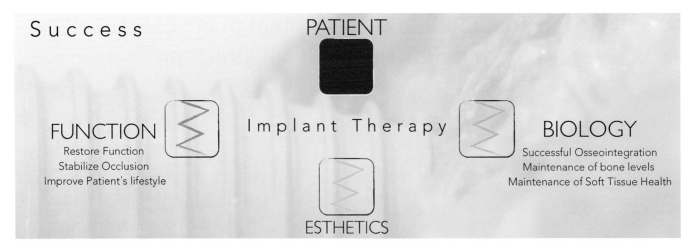

Figure 12.1 Triad of contemporary implant dentistry (Buser et al. 2017; Linkevicius et al. 2009).

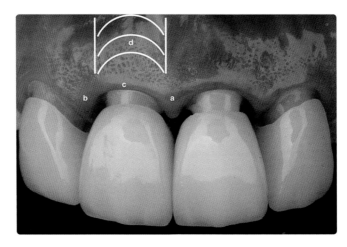

Figure 12.2 : Pink and white esthetic score. (a) Mesial Papilla. (b) Distal Papilla. (c) Soft tissue level. (d) Soft tissue color, texture, and curvature. White esthetic Score. (e) Tooth Form. (f) Tooth Outline. (g) Surface texture. (h) Color. (i) Translucency (Tettamanti et al. 2016).

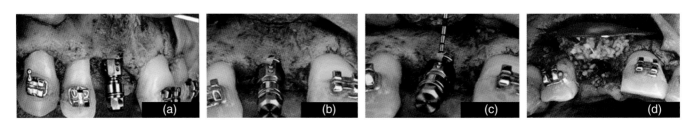

Figure 12.3 (a) Implant placement in an upper central incisor area. (b) Note the gray shadow of the implant fixture apparent through the thin buccal bone. (c) Buccal bone thickness less than 1 mm will possess minimal vascularity and is highly susceptible to further resorption following implant placement or loading. (d) Buccal veneer grafting to compensate for the remodeling of the thin buccal plate.

the peri-implant crestal bone levels and long term tissue stability (Figures 12.3 and 12.4).

With regards to the soft tissue demands, 2–3 mm of facial peri-implant soft tissue thickness has been shown to have a protective function (Figure 12.5), maintain the underlying bone integrity and avoiding visibility of the implant restorative components. Owing to its reduced vascularity and cellular content, thin peri-implant mucosa has reduced resistance to bacterial plaque and subsequently, peri-implant disease. Soft tissue recession may then result in "show through" of the underlying implant restorative components, leading to an unesthetic tissue shade or further develop to involve the implant abutment and even the implant fixture in cases where the supporting bone is compromised (Jung et al. 2009; Linkevicius et al. 2009).

Teeth with intact periodontium may require minimal augmentation (Figure 12.6). However, in cases where the integrity of the socket is compromised or in cases with severe tissue deficiencies more extensive augmentation

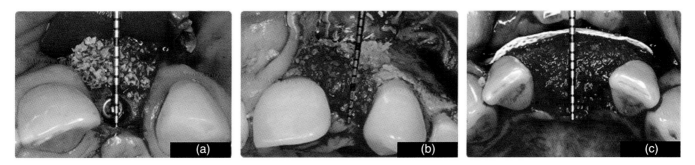

Figure 12.4 (a) Buccal veneer grafting performed at the time of implant placement with a xenograft material to further augment the buccal contour. (b) Grafting of more than 4 mm buccal to the anticipated implant position to compensate for remodeling of the bone graft material. (c) Utilizing a non-resorbable membrane to shape the bone graft to the desired ridge shape.

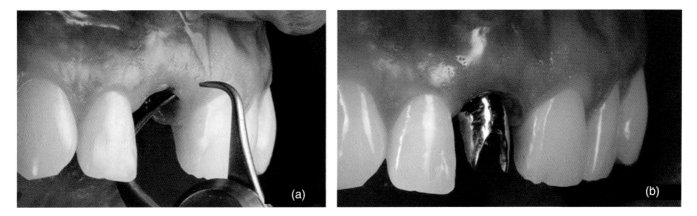

Figure 12.5 (a and b) Robust buccal volume augmentation following combined connective tissue grafting and dual zone protocols to simulate a natural emergence of the final restoration and mask any show-through of the abutment material.

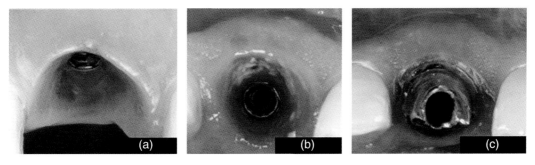

Figure 12.6 (a) Clinical situation following bone and soft tissue augmentation at the time of implant placemen (b) Note the bone graft particles encapsulated within the soft tissue. (c) Occlusal view of the final abutment in place.

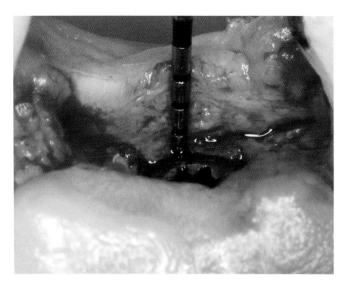

Figure 12.7 Tissue thickness augmentation following connective tissue grafting measuring 3.5 mm, providing a very stable soft tissue protective seal for the implant.

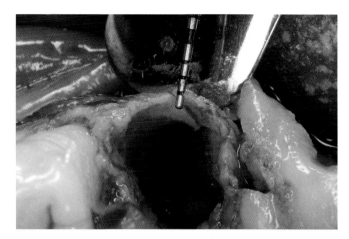

Figure 12.8 Close up view of the buccal plate of a canine socket following extraction. Flap reflection was performed revealing a green-stick fracture of the bone that was not noted at the time of tooth removal.

may be required to achieve the desired outcomes. The initial part of this chapter will focus on post-extraction tissue changes in the esthetic zone with specific focus on pre-operative tissue assessment prior to tooth extraction and implant placement (Figure 12.7).

PRE-OPERATIVE IMPLANT SITE ASSESSMENT

Due to the inherent anatomy of the alveolar topography in the anterior zone, post-extraction ridge dimension alterations are more common than in posterior sites. Tomographic studies have demonstrated that the average buccal bone thickness is less than 1 mm in 90% of anterior teeth (Braut et al. 2011).

The difficulty of management of anterior sites is compounded by the fact that the buccal plate (bundle bone) stems from the periodontal ligament of the tooth and inevitably undergoes remodeling once the tooth is removed (Figure 12.8). Araújo et al. (2006, 2008) demonstrated a 40% reduction in ridge width following tooth extractions in dogs. Buser et al. (2017) demonstrated similar findings in extraction sites that were not grafted. Such dimensional changes often require more invasive procedures to restore sufficient ridge volume to satisfy the biologic, functional, and esthetic demands. Subsequently, efforts to maximize the remaining ridge topography and tissue volume should be made at the time of tooth extraction. If residual deficiencies are still present, further augmentation may be required at the time of implant placement and/or second stage uncovering.

The clinical decision making process of the appropriate timing of implant placement and augmentation procedures will be discussed throughout the chapter. As a general

timeline, tissue augmentation may be performed at the following phases of treatment:

1. At the time of Tooth Extraction
2. At the time of Implant Placement
3. At the Time of Second Stage Uncovering or Post Implant Provisionalization

Key Factors in Diagnosis of the Surrounding Tooth Support Prior to Extraction

Accurate diagnosis of the periodontal integrity of both the tooth to be extracted and neighboring teeth must be attained in order to determine the need for prior corrective procedures and/or plan for the augmentations required prior to tooth extraction. Furthermore, analysis of the clinical situation also becomes a critical determinant in the viability of proceeding with immediate implant placement upon tooth removal.

Prior to tooth removal, the following diagnostic criteria should be considered:

- Integrity of the interproximal height of bone
- Integrity of the buccal plate of bone
- Root angulation/inclination and its relationship to the apical bone topography
- Tissue integrity or presence of mucogingival defects in the form of facial or interproximal tissue recession

Integrity of the Interproximal Height of Bone

It has been well established in the literature (Gastaldo et al. 2004) that the height of the peri-implant papilla is not dictated by the level of bone surrounding the implant

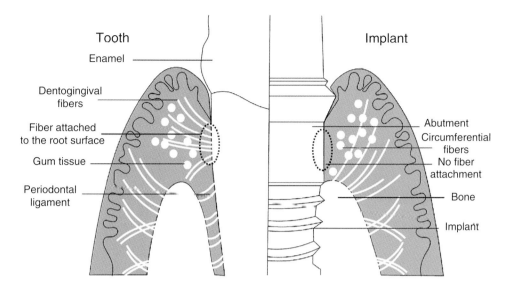

Tooth — Enamel

Dentogingival fibers

Fiber attached to the root surface

Gum tissue

Periodontal ligament

Implant — Abutment

Circumferential fibers

No fiber attachment

Bone

Implant

Figure 12.9 Schematic illustrating the differences between the peri-implant and periodontal attachment. Note the perpendicular orientation of the periodontal attachment which creates a protective barrier from physical and bacterial insults in addition to support of the supra-crestal tissue. The difference in fibers orientation histologically contributes to the difference in macroanatomy of the peri-implant papilla and gingiva.

but by the presence of the supra-crestal periodontal fibers on the adjacent teeth. It has been further shown in recent literature that the papillary height in sites of multiple adjacent missing teeth is significantly less than when the tooth is present. Therefore, the periodontal integrity and height of bone on the adjacent teeth become a key determinant in the final esthetics of the implant supported restoration. In the presence of periodontal pathology, or interproximal attachment loss on the adjacent teeth, interdisciplinary techniques such as orthodontic extrusion or changes to the tooth shape by restorative means may then be required to compensate for deficiencies in the interproximal papillary area (Figure 12.9).

Consequently, a comprehensive periodontal evaluation, radiographic analysis, and bone sounding are essential diagnostic factors prior to tooth extraction in order to anticipate the final outcome and diagnose any deficiencies that may be present. Furthermore, the clinician must be cognizant of any mesio-distal tooth mal-positioning and/or root proximity that may render the interdental bone more susceptible to resorption. The choice of flap reflection and design may also be modified in an attempt to avoid stripping of the periosteum and blood supply overlying thin (<1.5 mm) or compromised inter-radicular bone.

Integrity of the Buccal Plate of Bone

Conebeam CT scan, clinical periodontal evaluation, and bone sounding are combined to ascertain the integrity and level of the buccal plate prior to extraction (Figure 12.10). Compromise in the buccal plate integrity can ultimately yield to collapse of the tissue in the bucco-lingual aspect yielding to an unesthetic implant supported restoration

and facial tissue recession exposing the underlying restorative components. If the level of the gingival margin in relation to the adjacent teeth and in relation to the final implant supported restoration is located apically to the contralateral tooth, it may be prudent for the clinician to consider soft tissue grafting either before tooth extraction or at any time point prior to finalization of the prosthetic procedures to compensate for these discrepancies (Figure 12.11).

Root Angulation/Inclination and its Relationship to the Apical Bone Topography

Kan (Kan et al. 2011) classified sagittal tooth positions on CT scans to evaluate the viability of immediate implant placement in fresh extraction sockets based on different tooth inclination patterns (Figure 12.12). Sagittal tooth position may facilitate or hinder implant placement in the correct three-dimensional restorative driven position. Since the objective is to place the implant in a more palatal position, a buccal tooth position may offer a more favorable situation due to the increased available palatal bone for implant anchorage. If the tooth occupies most of the socket as in class IV or if there is inadequate apical bone to engage the implant, this may dictate additional hard tissue augmentation prior to implant placement. The results of Kan studies have shown that most of the anterior teeth lie in the class II and III categories, meaning that the tooth is either in the center of the socket or the root apex is angled toward the palatal aspect. These positions consequently create difficulties in placement of immediate implants in a more palatal position to facilitate a palatal screw retained access. Consequently, an angled screw channel may be utilized should a screw retained restoration be desired or the

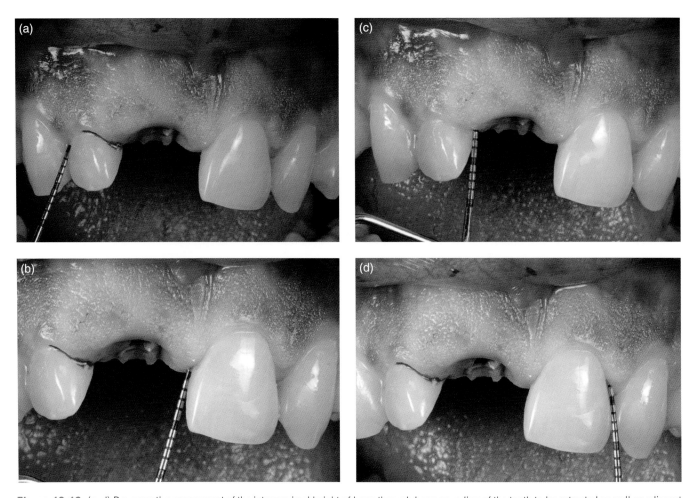

Figure 12.10 (a–d) Pre-operative assessment of the interproximal height of bone through bone sounding of the tooth to be extracted as well as adjacent dentition to determine the integrity of the periodontal attachment prior to flap reflection.

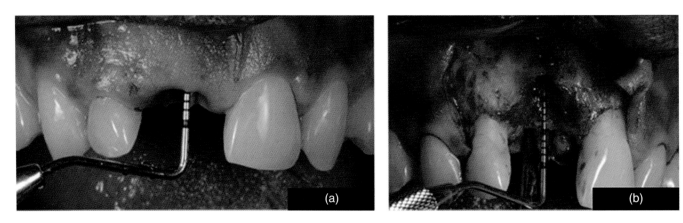

Figure 12.11 (a) Pre-operative bone sounding of the buccal plate reveals probing depths in excess of 10 mm. (b) Intra-surgical view showing complete absence of the buccal plate.

clinician may resort to a cement retained restoration with customized abutments.

It can therefore be established from the studies that the tooth position within the alveolar envelope determines the amount of apical bone to engage the implant if immediate implant therapy is considered as well as determining the need of augmentation procedures in lieu of immediate implant placement if the implant is not sufficiently encased within the alveolar envelope.

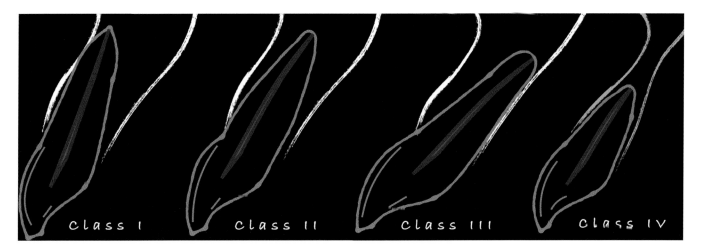

Figure 12.12 Tooth angulation in relation to the alveolar housing. Class I: the tooth is located buccal in relation to the ridge. Class II: The tooth is in the center of the ridge. Class III: The tooth is located palatal within the ridge. Class IV: The remaining ridge topography is deficient to allow adequate implant placement.

TISSUE AUGMENTATION AT THE TIME OF TOOTH EXTRACTION

Following pre-operative assessment, management of the extraction socket now becomes the focus. As a general rule, the clinician should attempt every effort to minimize invasion and morbidity to the patient. Intact sites or sites with minimal tissue deficiencies should be treated by trying to preserve as much of the available support as possible with minimal disruption of the tissue architecture, while sites with extensive deficiencies may necessitate further corrective procedures.

Salama and Salama (1993) reported on different types of extraction sites in the anterior zone with recommended extraction site management protocols. Tarnow (in Chu et al. 2012) added a modification to the type II deficiencies for the clinician to better assess the severity of the buccal dehiscence present at the time of tooth extraction. Depending on the degree of involvement of the extraction socket, the approach utilized by the clinician should allow for the best result both functionally and esthetically with the least tissue distortion.

Class I sockets have been identified as intact sockets. Those display no or minimal reduction (i.e. < 3 mm) of the buccal bone height with healthy interproximal attachment levels, and no marginal tissue recession. Class I sockets may be present in either thick or thin gingival biotype situations. Should the patient have a thin tissue biotype, soft tissue augmentation may be often mandated either at the time of tooth extraction or at second stage procedure.

In class I sockets a minimally invasive flapless approach can be utilized for both immediate implant placement and any simultaneous grafting provided that the implant is placed in the desired, restoratively driven position. Should there be anatomical deficiencies or inadequate access to achieve the desired therapeutic goal, alternative incision designs/approaches can be utilized to allow for better access and augmentation while preserving the tissue architecture (further discussed in the chapter). N.B. Implant placement in fresh extraction sockets does not prevent subsequent bone remodeling (Araujo et al. 2005), which further highlights the importance of bone augmentation at the time of implant placement (Figure 12.13). It is at the clinician's discretion and skill set to incorporate soft tissue grafting with conventional ridge preservation procedure in order to further develop the tissue volume and simplify following implant procedures.

Treatment Options for Class I Extraction Sockets

Immediate implant placement in conjunction with:

- Placement of a bone graft material in the gap between the implant and the buccal plate.
- Soft tissue graft (either free or pediculated).
- Partial Extraction Therapy (i.e. Socket Shield Technique).

All of the following options can be performed with immediate implant non-functional provisionalization, customizable healing abutments, or if inadequate implant stability is achieved a fixed tooth supported provisional with ovate pontic design may be utilized. Tissue borne provisional prostheses are not recommended during the early healing period as continuous micro-motion and pressure may have a negative impact on the underlying soft tissues and implant integration. Utilizing fixed prosthetic appliances adds a benefit of capturing the present soft tissue scallop of the interproximal papillae.

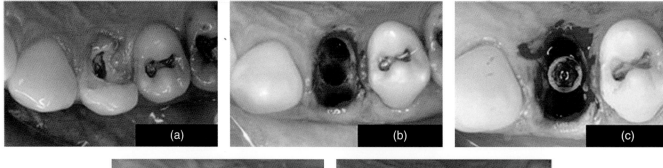

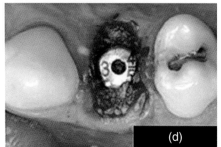

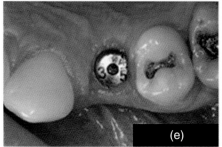

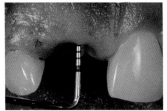

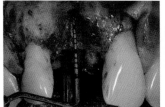

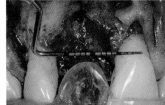

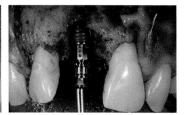

Figure 12.13 (a–e) Immediate implant placement performed following extraction of the maxillary bicuspid. Note the bucco-lingual reduction in ridge volume following tooth extraction and implant placement, despite grafting of the residual gap surrounding the implant. Further soft tissue augmentation can be utilized to enhance the bucco-lingual contour following implant integration.

Figure 12.14 Clinical example of immediate implant placement in a class II extraction socket utilizing an open approach.

Class II sockets with deficient or severely compromised buccal plates have a higher risk of bucco-lingual ridge collapse and concomitant recession defects. Therefore, flapless implant placement becomes more challenging and less predictable. These sites may be managed in either a flapless or "open" approach, depending on the clinician's experience, site topography, and ability to thoroughly access the entirety of the defect (Figures 12.14 and 12.15).

Treatment Options for Class II Extraction Sockets

Sites where the remaining bone topography allows for ideal three-dimensional implant placement within the alveolar housing. In those cases, the following management is indicated:

Immediate implant placement in conjunction with:

- Guided Bone Regeneration.

- Concomitant bone and soft tissue grafting.

- Immediate Dento-alveolar Restoration.

- Bone-ring technique.

If the site topography does not allow for implant placement, treatment options may include:

- Ridge Preservation procedures combined with either a cell occlusive membrane or growth factors.

- Ridge preservation w/ soft tissue grafting.

- Early Implant Placement.

Treatment Options for Class III Extraction Sockets

Class III sockets involve a significant compromise of the interproximal bone height or extensive circumferential alveolar bone. These defects require more elaborate surgical procedures to correct the deficiencies and involve a relatively high level of invasion and tissue alteration. Alternative options may include pre-surgical orthodontic

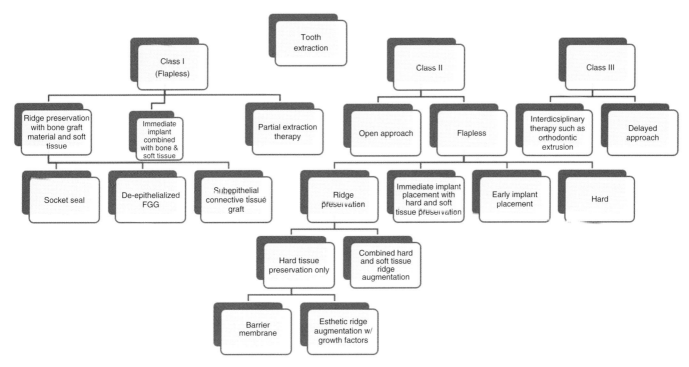

Figure 12.15 Clinical example of Class II socket. Severe compromise of the buccal plate of the socket is noted with intact interproximal bone peaks. Last picture showing immediate post-extraction implant placement within the alveolar envelope of the socket.

extrusion of the teeth to optimize the tissue architecture followed by implant placement or simply relying on restorative techniques to replicate the deficient soft tissues. Immediate implant placement in these cases is not advisable, but procedures to maximize tissue volume preservation at the time of extraction should be followed. These procedures will be discussed throughout this chapter.

MANAGEMENT OF CLASS I SOCKETS

Tissue Architecture Preservation

Flapless techniques in implant therapy have been shown to yield minimal tissue alterations. Techniques to capture the pre-operative soft tissue frame immediately following tooth removal whether through immediate implant provisional restorations, customized healing abutments, or even ovate pontics allow for better preservation of the soft tissue frame. The first step in preservation of the hard and soft tissue is atraumatic extraction utilizing appropriate instrumentation.

ARMAMENTARIUM

- Basic Surgical Kit.
- Periotomes, Extraction Forceps, and Luxating Elevators.
- Piezosurgical unit with Periotome Inserts.
- Implant Placement Kit.
- Micro-blades and Soft Tissue Tunneling Instrumentation.
- Micro tissue forceps, Castro Viejo and Scissors.

Atraumatic Tooth Extraction

Procedure:

See Figure 12.16.

1. Elevation of the tooth and luxation should be performed on all aspects except for the buccal to avoid damage to the buccal plate or greenstick fracture.

2. If the tooth is not easily luxated due to an intact periodontium or curvatures in the root, sectioning of the root may be performed utilizing a surgical length fissure carbide bur or long-shanked diamond bur. This allows the operator to reach the apex of the tooth and create room for the root fragments to be luxated within the socket. Sectioning can be performed in a mesio-distal or bucco-lingual direction, taking care not to injure the surrounding socket walls (Figure 12.17).

3. Mesio-distal and rotational movements should be directed vertically to avoid fracture of the buccal plate. N.B. Direction of elevation should never be toward the buccal aspect.

Following delivery of the tooth, thorough debridement of the socket should be performed to prevent any soft tissue encapsulation of the bone substitute material and/or implant. This can be accomplished through the use of spoon curettes or through rotary finishing diamonds or carbides with irrigation. De-epithelialization of the internal lining of the socket allows for fresh connective tissue for

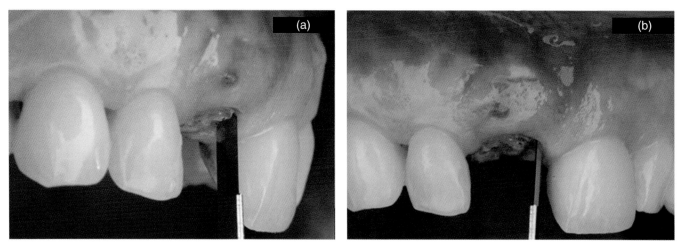

Figure 12.16 (a and b) Separation of the supra-crestal fibers with a micro-blade in order facilitate tooth luxation and instrumentation through the sulcus prior to tooth extraction.

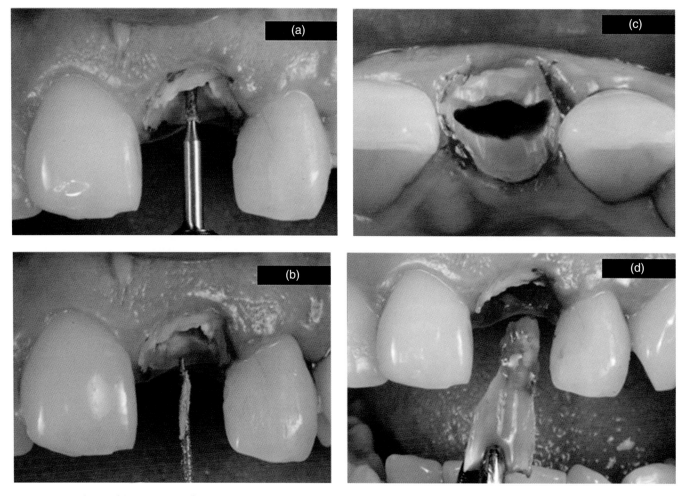

Figure 12.17 (a and b) Long shanked diamond needle bur is utilized initiate the sectioning process through utilizing the root canal as a starting point. The bur is advanced apically just beyond the tooth apex and the tooth is sectioned mesio-distally utilizing the root canal as the guide for the long axis of the sectioning process. (c) The mesial and distal walls of the tooth are thinned but not completely separated to protect the adjacent bone walls from injury. Complete separation of the root fragments may be completed delicately with the bur or manually with a small luxating elevator. (d) Removal of the palatal root fragment allows room to deliver the buccal portion of the root without risk of injuring the buccal plate.

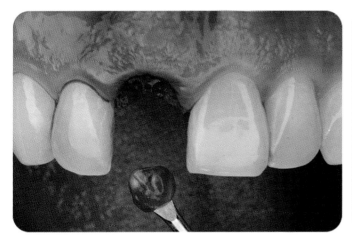
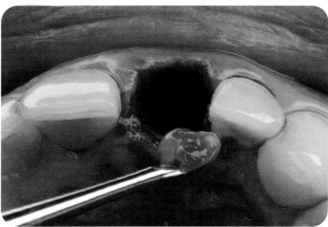

Figure 12.18 Socket degranulation may be performed by spoon currettes. N.B. The direction of socket debridement should always be toward the palatal aspect taking caution not to use the buccal plate as a fulcrum to avoid unintentional fracture of the buccal bone.

graft nourishment and union with the donor tissue (Figure 12.18).

The socket should be inspected for any fenestrations, dehiscences, and/or fracture of the buccal plate. Should there be any compromise of the socket integrity, the clinician should be ready to repair the site. If the socket walls are intact, then implant placement should be attempted and performed in the correct three-dimensional position.

THREE-DIMENSIONAL IMPLANT POSITIONING

Bucco-Palatal Position

Implant diameter and positioning are key elements in facilitating the remainder of the surgical procedure. Implant diameter should allow at least a 1.5 mm distance from the buccal plate and should not occupy the entirety of the socket as that has negative implications on the buccal plate and will not allow sufficient space for grafting the site internally. The palatal positioning of the implant fixture also offers a restorative advantage by allowing for a palatal position of the implant screw access, enabling the restorative dentist to have a final screw retained implant restoration and avoid the complications associated with sub-gingival excess cement (Figures 12.19–12.21).

Mesio-Distal Position

Sufficient implant to tooth and inter-implant distances should be preserved. Conventionally, an implant to tooth distance of 1.5 mm was required to prevent any impingement on the PDL and avoid interproximal bone loss on the adjacent tooth. Recent literature however demonstrates that when there was a proximity of 2 mm or less between an implant and adjacent tooth, the papilla failed to fully

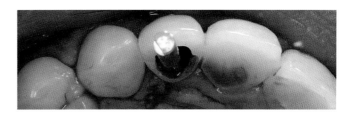

Figure 12.19 Correct implant positioning should be assessed during implant placement to emerge palatal to the incisal edge of the future restoration. An accurate surgical guide is highly valuable when it comes to esthetically sensitive implant restorations.

occupy the embrasure in all of the cases observed. It can therefore be deduced from these studies that in addition to respecting the biological limitations, one must consider the esthetic repercussions of the implant to tooth proximity. As a general guideline, a 2 mm distance between implants and adjacent teeth, and a 3 mm inter-implant should be respected to allow for adequate bone thickness to support the interproximal papilla height, knowing that there is a degree of crestal bone remodeling around the implants (Figure 12.22).

Apico-Coronal Position

With regards to implant depth, 2–4 mm from the future restorative gingival margin should be maintained. This could be referenced during surgery with an accurately constructed surgical guide simulating the final tooth form and/or the Cemento Enamel Junction (CEJ) of the contralateral tooth. The range of implant placement depth also depends on the diameter of the implant to be placed and the diameter of the tooth to be restored. Narrower implants are placed deeper to allow sufficient "running room" for developing a natural emergence profile of the final restoration (Figure 12.23).

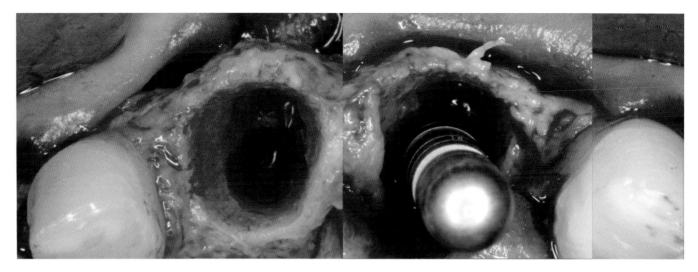

Figure 12.20 Intra-operative view of an immediate implant position in relation to an extraction socket. Note how correct anatomical implant positioning offers a confined defect for augmentation of the buccal bone. Additional contour grafting can also be performed on the buccal aspect of the socket.

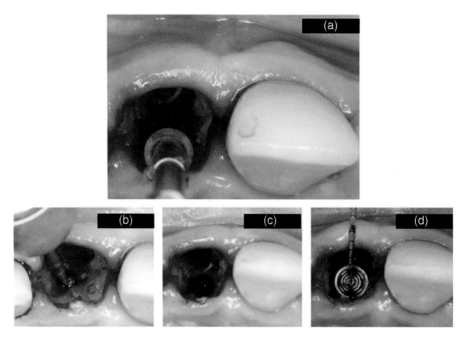

Figure 12.21 In class I (Kan) sockets, placing implants in the space occupied by the root will result in an implant that is positioned too facial. Subsequently, in order to take advantage of the available palatal bone, the osteotomy has to be initiated in a more palatal position. (a and b) This can be done by utilizing a round bur about 4 mm from the apex of the socket. The round bur is taken to a depth sufficient to have a ledge created to stabilize the pilot drill. Not having a deep enough or wide enough osteotomy for the pilot drill, will result in continuous slippage into the socket space which can result in loss of part of the bone that is critical for implant stability. (c) Picture shows the implant osteotomy (palatal) versus the buccal socket position, showing how the implant osteotomy is entirely in the palatal bone which was made possible as a result of the buccal tooth position. (d) The implant diameter utilized allows a 2–3 mm gap between the buccal plate and the implant platform to allow adequate room for graft material introduction.

SELECTION OF THE BONE GRAFT MATERIAL

Following implant insertion, the gap between the implant and the buccal plate should be evaluated for grafting with a bone graft or bone substitute material. The graft is utilized mainly to decrease the bucco-lingual remodeling of the socket, not for the purpose of osseointegration. Material properties are discussed in detail in previous editions of this book.

Mainly allogeneic and xenograft materials are utilized as the graft of choice. Utilizing allogeneic materials offers the advantage of a faster rate of turnover with more vital bone

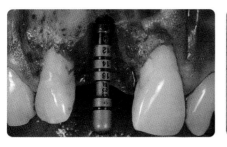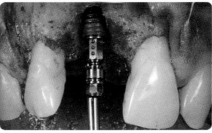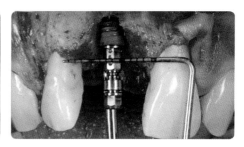

Figure 12.22 Mesio-distal positioning of implant placement in the esthetic zone, leaving 2 mm between the implant and adjacent tooth to avoid compromise of the papillary esthetics.

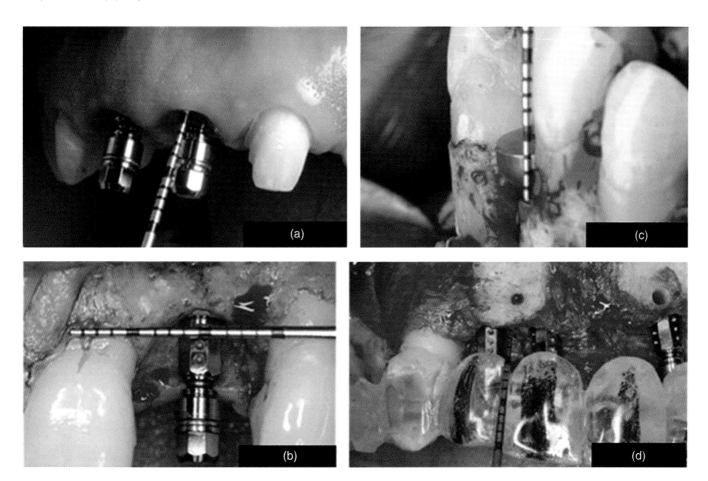

Figure 12.23 Implant depth can be measured utilizing different clinical indicators. (a) Utilizing the gingival margin of the future restoration, only possible in flapless procedures. (b and c) During flap reflection, the CEJs of the adjacent teeth can be used as a reference for implant placement depth. (d) Surgical guides that are accurately fabricated to give the clinician an accurate indicator upon implant drilling and final placement (Funato et al 2007).

compared to xenografts. However, a low turnover material may be of benefit in the esthetic zone as it offers less remodeling which provides more long term contour maintenance.

After selection of the appropriate graft material, soft tissue grafting should be considered. This may be done simultaneously with both implant placement and bone grafting or just with socket grafting as a form of hard and soft tissue volume preservation/augmentation to compensate for the expected post-extraction remodeling of the site. The tissue graft may also act as a protective barrier for the underlying bone material and/or implant.

RATIONALE

Spontaneous healing and epithelialization of the extraction site orifice usually occurs over a period of three to five weeks. However, when site preservation procedures are employed, the bone graft is left exposed to the oral cavity and is subjected to external contaminants and risk of early dislodgment. Therefore, a physical barrier may be beneficial for the purpose of protection and containment of the bone graft particles during the early phases of healing. The choice of a physical barrier may be a prosthetic one or biologic material/tissue.

Prosthetic components such as ovate pontic designed restorations have been utilized to maintain the tissue profile and architecture following tooth extractions. Regardless of the material utilized for the provisional, the surface of the material should be highly polished and clean to allow an environment conducive to healing without excessive soft tissue irritation. If an implant is placed immediately, an implant supported provisional or custom healing abutment may be utilized to allow easier tissue contouring upon implant restoration (Figures 12.24 and 12.25).

Alternatively, a barrier membrane could be utilized over the extraction site to protect the graft from epithelial downgrowth and fibrous encapsulation of the superficial layers of the graft material. The choice of membrane may be a resorbable or *nonresorbable* one. Resorbable membranes such as collagen are highly tissue compatible but undergo earlier degradation when left exposed. Nonresorbable membranes on the other hand need additional stabilization and may be associated with soft tissue retraction and dehiscences which can be unforgiving in the esthetic zone. Similar to tissue grafts, membranes can be placed only on the occlusal aspect or further stabilized underneath the buccal soft tissue by the aid of a sub-periosteal tunnel. In class I sockets, the presence of the buccal plate acts to stabilize the blood clot thereby eliminating the necessity for membranes. Should there be a buccal dehiscence defect, the use of a membrane may be required. In an attempt to

counteract early membrane resorption, closure over the fresh extraction socket can be attempted to decrease the membrane's resorption time. However, flap reflection and tissue advancement has been shown to yield inferior bone gain results in addition to having negative implications on the soft tissue architecture especially in the esthetic zone. N.B. flap reflection and periosteal reflection should be avoided in class I sockets. Flap reflection has been reported to orchestrate a series of tissue changes and bone remodeling. Therefore if a flap is reflected, osseous grafting should be performed on both the internal and external aspects of the socket to compensate for subsequent tissue changes. Subsequent to bone grafting, sealing the socket with a tissue graft may offer an advantage in the esthetic zone in terms of tissue volume augmentation and physical protection of the underlying tissue.

Options for Tissue Augmentation Procedures

- Socket Seal Approach
- De-epithelialized Free Gingival Graft
- Free Connective Tissue Graft
- Rotated Pedicle Graft

With regards to volume augmentation, a rotated pedicle graft offers the highest level of augmentation and vascularization due to maintenance of its blood supply from the palate. This procedure is usually reserved for areas with higher augmentation requirements, and not typically the first line of treatment in class I sites. More commonly, a free connective tissue graft would be sufficient to augment the buccal contours following extraction. The connective tissue graft may be harvested as

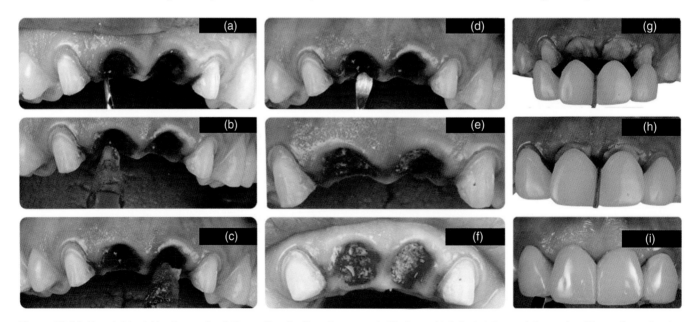

Figure 12.24 From left to right columns: (a–c) Atraumatic extraction of upper central incisors. (d–f) Socket degranulation and grafting performed up to the soft tissue margins of the socket. (g–i) Native collagen membranes were utilized over the socket orifice and sealed over with a fixed provisional restoration.

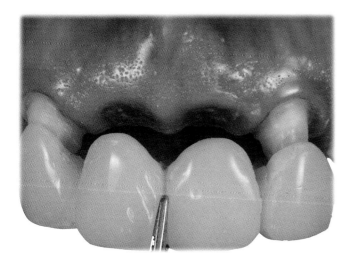

Figure 12.25 Five months follow-up of both volume and soft tissue scalloped architecture preservation by combining minimal trauma with the provisional restoration to maintain the soft tissue architecture and volume for future implant placement.

a free gingival graft and then de-epithelialized outside, or as a sub-epithelial connective tissue graft from the deeper layers of the palate. The tissue graft may be utilized to augment the buccal tissue contours as well as seal over the extraction socket. In cases where an immediate implant supported supra-structure is going to occupy the socket orifice, then the tissue graft may be placed solely on the buccal aspect. A final treatment option could be simply performing a socket seal procedure, in which the tissue graft or tissue substitute material is utilized to cover solely the extraction socket orifice. This technique provides protection of the underlying bone graft and preservation of the underlying osseous tissue volume but has the least soft tissue volume enhancement effects when compared to other techniques. Specific advantages and disadvantages of each technique will be discussed further in the following paragraphs.

SOCKET SEAL

The socket seal technique as described by Landsberg is discussed in previous editions of this book. In this edition, advanced aspects of graft adaptation and immobilization will be reviewed. As previously mentioned, this technique is mainly reserved for ridge preservation procedures when implant placement is not performed as it does not offer any significant buccal soft tissue enhancement, but merely a "seal" over the underlying graft material.

Indications

- Class I extraction sockets with Thin Tissue Biotype
- Minimal hard and soft tissue deficiencies
- Intact socket walls
- Inability to place an implant supported provisional

Contra-Indications

- Marginal tissue recession
- Compromised Periodontium
- Ability to place an implant supported restoration
- Smoking

Requirements for the Tissue/Tissue Substitute Material

- The tissue should be slightly larger than the socket orifice to allow for intimate fit between the socket walls and the graft.
- Graft should be resistant to infection and early resorption.
- The thickness of the graft should allow sufficient surface area for vascular connections to prevent early tissue necrosis. The tissue should rest passively in a stable position overlying the bone graft and in contact with the soft tissue walls of the socket.

Recipient Site Preparation

Simplicity of the recipient site is one of the advantages of the socket seal technique.

De-epithelialization of the internal socket lining is the critical step to this procedure, in order to remove the sulcular/pocket epithelium and allow access to the underlying connective tissue and vasculature. Due to the fact that the connective tissue bed is circumferential in nature and does not offer a great amount of vascularity underlying the graft it is prudent to avoid any interference of the lining epithelium with the donor tissue to maximize blood vessel anastomosis and organic union between the donor and recipient bed.

De-epithelialization can be performed with:

- A carbide finishing bur either round or flame shaped mounted on a high-speed handpiece with copious irrigation. The change between the epithelium and connective tissue will be discernible by change to the tissue appearance to a slightly more reddish color, rough texture, and appearance of bleeding points.
- A scalpel blade can also be used to internally dissect the epithelial attachment and remove it as a collar of tissue, exposing the underlying connective tissue (Figure 12.26).

Note: Care should be taken to avoid injury to the interdental papilla while performing this step.

Donor Sites

- Lateral Palate (adjacent to the premolar/molar area)
- Tuberosity Area

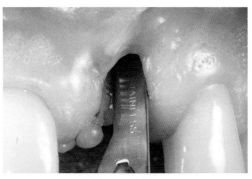
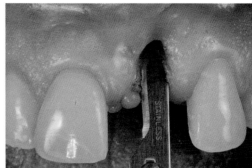
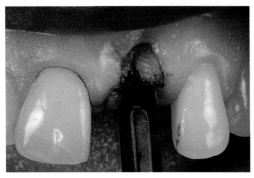
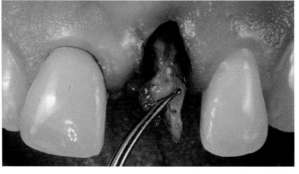
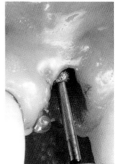

Figure 12.26 In the absence of a buccal plate or in severely compromised periodontal dentition or implants, the remaining socket walls could be lined with the pocket epithelium. In these cases, a 15 blade can be utilized for gross tissue removal and freshening of the internal socket walls. A round diamond bur can then be used to finalize the de-epithelialization of the inner lining of the socket.

- Edentulous Ridge Spans
- Collagen Based Tissue Substitute Materials

A template may be used to allow accurate dimensions in harvesting the graft. Utilizing a soft tissue punch of similar dimensions as the internal aspect of the socket offers an easier and faster harvest of the graft. The tissue is harvested in a full thickness fashion through blunt dissection using a periosteal elevator. Following which, hemostasis can be achieved with the aid of a collagen sponge or simply cyanoacrylate or a periodontal dressing over the exposed donor site.

Tuberosity tissue has the advantage of higher collagen content and dense connective tissue when compared to the lateral palate. This may be beneficial for pontic sites or for tissue augmentation around dental implants due to the absence of excessive glandular and adipose tissue.

Immediate implant placement in the extraction socket with a healing abutment that occupies most of the socket space requires a different approach other than a Free Gingival Graft (FGG) for sealing the socket as the abutment impedes the blood supply necessary for the future graft.

The soft tissue punch may be taken as a preformed tissue punch corresponding in diameter to the extracted tooth socket. However, this is not always possible as in sites of bicuspids and canines the socket orifice is not an even circle. At this point the clinician has to harvest a graft with the aid of a template to satisfy the dimensional requirements to seal the socket.

Stabilization of the Graft

The focus in stabilization of any graft is immobilization of the free tissue to allow for a stable scaffold conducive to cellular migration and union of the graft to the recipient site. Regardless of the material or technique employed the end result must always be a stable graft with minimal trauma. A clinical tip to assess graft stability is to place the graft in the position and assess both the lateral extensions of the graft as well as the vertical alignment with the adjacent soft tissue margins. The graft should rest passively in contact with the adjacent soft tissue margins laterally and at a vertical level corresponding with the surrounding gingival margins.

The most common technique to stabilize a graft uses 6–8 interrupted microsutures with 6–0 or 7–0 filaments with a microneedle. These sutures are placed in a and circumferential, opposing manner to allow for even tension over the graft and intimate, uniform contact of the graft to the donor tissue. Utilizing a microsuture filament and needle offers the added benefit of minimizing trauma of the graft while placing multiple sutures in close proximity to each other.

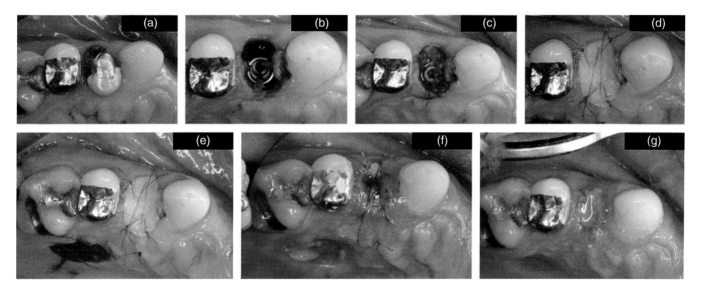

Figure 12.27 (a–d) Immediate implant placement was combined with bone grafting of the residual gap surrounding the implant. A socket seal approach was utilized to seal the extraction site. Note the adaptation of the graft to the surrounding soft tissue margins. Lower pictures show the donor and recipient sites at immediate post-op (e), one week (f) and two weeks (g) intervals.

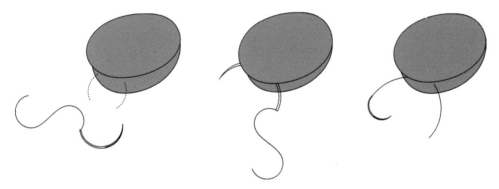

Figure 12.28 From left to right. Suture entry point: The needle is advanced within the thickness of the graft. This suture is an internal horizontal mattress suture that helps adapt the connective tissue aspects of the graft to the recipient site to enhance early revascularization.

The use of tissue adhesives may be used in lieu of multiple sutures to aid in graft stability while avoiding excessive trauma from the suture needle. N.B. tissue adhesives may not be used as the sole method of graft stabilization in this technique, but as a supplemental method to reduce the number of sutures needed to fixate the graft in place.

A compressive suture as demonstrated in Figure 12.27 offers the advantage of additional graft compression in both lateral and vertical directions. This suture is useful in cases where the graft is is too small or too thin, as stretching the graft in opposing directions may result in a dead space apical to the graft.

In addition to a compressive suture, utilizing an internal mattress suture aids in stabilization and adapting the graft to the internal socket lining (Figure 12.28).

Disadvantages of This Technique

The main disadvantage of the socket seal FGG is that there is no true augmentation of the buccal tissue volume which is critical around implants for esthetic purposes and long term stability of the underlying buccal bone. This issue may be overcome at the time of implant placement and/or second stage uncovering of the implant by either utilizing the tissue previously augmented on the occlusal aspect and introducing it onto the buccal aspect or by adding a connective tissue graft at the time of implant placement:

• The predictability of the graft taking is low

• Technique sensitive

To overcome these disadvantages a partially de-epithelialized free gingival graft or sub-epithelial connective tissue graft may be utilized (Figure 12.29). The following

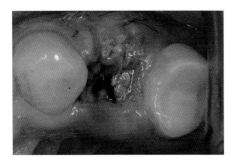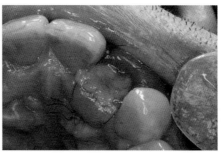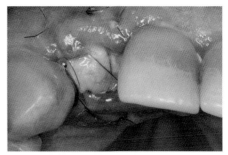

Figure 12.29 Necrosis or delayed vascularization of the exposed portion of the graft may sometimes occur at one week. Use of an antiseptic mouth wash for one more week is recommended. On the second week follow-up, any necrotic loose tissue should be removed and the site gently debrided and irrigated.

paragraphs will discuss modifications of the socket seal technique, to incorporate tissue volume augmentation of the buccal contour.

AUTOGENOUS TISSUE FOR CONCOMITANT BUCCAL VOLUME AUGMENTATION AND SOCKET SEAL PROCEDURES

Utilizing a SubEpithelial Connective Tissue Graft (SECTG) to concomitantly augment the buccal tissue volume and seal the socket offers superior buccal bone maintenance, masking materials of abutments and crowns and enhancing the peri-implant tissue contours when compared to socket seal procedures alone. The use of a connective tissue graft at the time of implant placement or ridge preservation to augment the tissue, sets up a better foundation for a more esthetic final restoration.

The lateral palate is usually the donor site of choice for procurement of sufficient tissue quantity to augment the buccal and occlusal aspects of the socket. The graft may be harvested as a subepithelial connective tissue graft or as a de-epithelialized free gingival graft. Differences in compositions of these grafts will be discussed further in this chapter. Sufficient tissue volume should be harvested to permit adequate vascularization of the graft. At least 5 mm of the tissue should be covered with the buccal tissue as well as 3–5 mm on the palatal side to allow adequate vascularization of the exposed portion of the graft overlying the socket.

The difference in these techniques is more related to the quality of tissue harvested rather than quantity. For the lateral palate, superficial layers of the connective tissue possess less adipose and glandular tissue when compared to the deeper portions. This renders de-epithelialized free gingival grafts a whitish color, with a dense, fibrous consistency when compared to a sub-epithelial connective tissue graft. The differences in consistency are due to the microarchitecture of the graft. Free grafts tend to have denser collagenous networks, with less vascular channels and loose interstitial tissue when compared to connective tissue grafts. Despite the differences in clinical handling and micro-architecture,

there has been no evidence in the literature reporting on the success rates or survival of the different graft types, or the amount of shrinkage associated with either technique.

De-Epithelialized Free Gingival Graft

The technique for graft procurement is identical to harvesting a free gingival graft as discussed in previous editions of this book. Obtaining adequate tissue dimensions have to be assessed accurately prior to proceeding with this technique so as to avoid involvement of the palatal arteries and their major branches.

N.B. Should the required tissue pose an increased risk of involvement of adjacent vital structures, then an alternative harvest technique should be utilized.

Once the graft dimensions are recorded, the graft may be harvested as a FGG and de-epithelialized outside the mouth using a fresh 15 blade. The area of de-epithelialization corresponds to the portions of the graft that will be inserted underneath the buccal or palatal gingiva. Alternatively, de-epithelialize utilizing a round diamond bur prior to graft procurement. The portion of the graft that is sealing the extraction orifice however will not be dis-epithelialized in order to maximize the thickness of the exposed part of the graft (Figure 12.30).

SUB-EPITHELIAL CONNECTIVE TISSUE GRAFT

Graft harvesting (Figure 12.31) is performed in the same way that has been described in previous editions of this book. The advantage offered by this technique is mainly related to achieving primary closure of the donor site.

Requirements

Graft dimensions are determined by:

- Augmentation volume on the buccal aspect of the socket: Not less than 5 mm

- Bucco-palatal dimension of the extraction socket orifice.

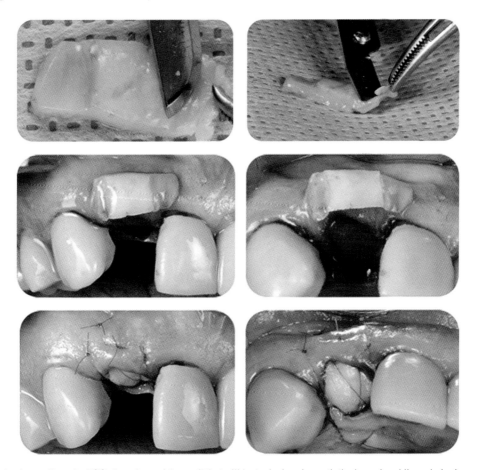

Figure 12.30 Following harvesting of a FGG, the edges of the graft that will be tucked underneath the buccal and lingual gingiva are de-epithelialized using a 15 blade. The graft is inserted with the epithelial portion over the exposed socket orifice and the connective tissue "tails" or dis-epithelialized portions are inserted underneath the gingiva to enhance the blood supply to the graft. A combination of internal mattress sutures and criss-cross compressive suture is utilized to enhance the graft stability and revascularization.

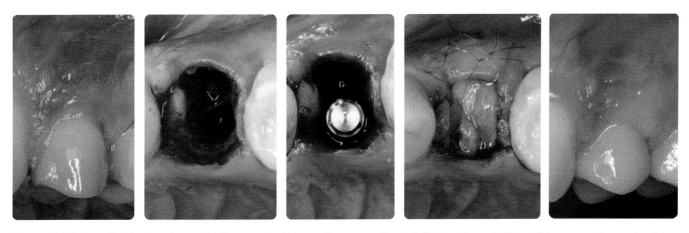

Figure 12.31 Immediate implant placement with connective tissue grafting augmenting both the buccal aspect of the soft tissue as well as sealing the socket. Post-op two years follow-up showing gingival marginal stability around the implant restoration.

- At least 3–5 mm of the graft should be covered by the palatal tissue.
- Width is determined by the mesio-distal width of the extraction orifice.

If buccal plate dehiscences are present, the dimensions of the graft may be modified to allow the graft borders to rest on sound bone margins whenever possible (Figure 12.32).

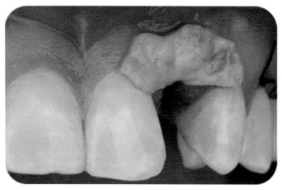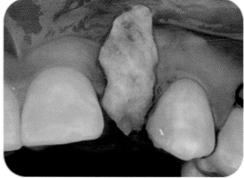

Figure 12.32 Graft orientation may be horizontal or vertical depending on the augmentation needs of the case.

Recipient Site Preparation

It is important to note that the buccal plate of anterior dentition is less than 1 mm in thickness in the majority of maxillary anterior sites and is consequently devoid of any cancellous or marrow components. This translates into minimal vascularity to the buccal cortical bone which is further compromised by severing the periodontal ligament attachment upon tooth removal and micro-fractures that can occur during tooth luxation. Therefore, in cases with intact or minimally involved sockets, it may prudent to avoid flap reflection as excessive tissue manipulation can result in tissue distortion, scarring, and recession that is less forgiving in the esthetic zone. Subsequently tunneling procedures have been introduced and further developed to offer a less invasive approach for tissue reconstruction in more sensitive and esthetic sites. The tunnel preparation can be initiated either from a crestal (sulcular) or vestibular approach, depending on the ease of access and desired area to be regenerated. The vestibular approach was introduced as a submarginal incision. Modifications have been proposed for vestibular access for horizontal ridge augmentation in the esthetic zone without affecting the soft tissue architecture and avoiding visible scarring in patients with a high smile line (Dibart et al. 2009; Nevins et al. 2009a; Zadeh 2011). The same approach may be utilized for both hard and soft tissue augmentation.

Tunnel Preparation

The plane of dissection may be performed in either a supra- or sub-periosteal fashion. If the purpose of the procedure is hard tissue augmentation, then it is necessary to perform a sub-periosteal tunnel to avoid soft tissue ingrowth into the graft material. For soft tissue augmentation procedures, supra-periosteal dissection is advocated but should be avoided in thin biotype cases to prevent excessive thinning of the outer flap and compromising the blood supply to the grafted tissue. This requires specialized, sharp tunneling instruments and micro-blades that allow maneuvering over the convexity of the buccal plate. The tip of the instrument should be aimed toward the bone and not the

tissue in order not to overly thin the buccal tissue or perforate it which could result in decreased vascularity to the soft tissue graft and subsequent tissue necrosis (Figure 12.33).

Requirements of Tunnel Preparation

- The tunnel should be performed in a single plane of dissection to allow for passive introduction of the graft.
- Usually the extension of the tunnel should be larger than the tissue to be harvested by 2 mm circumferentially.
- Ensure adequate tunnel extension to avoid ischemia of the buccal tissue and subsequent flap necrosis.

N.B. over-extension of the tunnel can compromise the stability of the grafted tissue, leading to inadequate vascularization and integration of the graft. This can be overcome with additional stabilizing sutures to immobilize the graft.

If the tissue allows, the graft may be introduced with the aid of the tunneling instruments or serrated tissue packers; however, this may not be always possible as it depends on the consistency and thickness of the graft. If the graft is too thick, or is high in adipose contents, it can be often hard to manipulate. In such cases the use of anchoring sutures can aid the clinician in guiding, positioning, and adapting the tissue graft within the tunnel.

Suturing Techniques

- Apical guiding "marionette" suture
- Horizontal adaptive mattress suture
- Positioning mattress sutures

The purpose of these techniques is to aid in navigating the tissue graft to its desired position within the prepared tunnel. Appropriate selection of the suture needle and material are critical, as this suture will be pulling the graft through an entry point that could be narrower than some aspects of the graft.

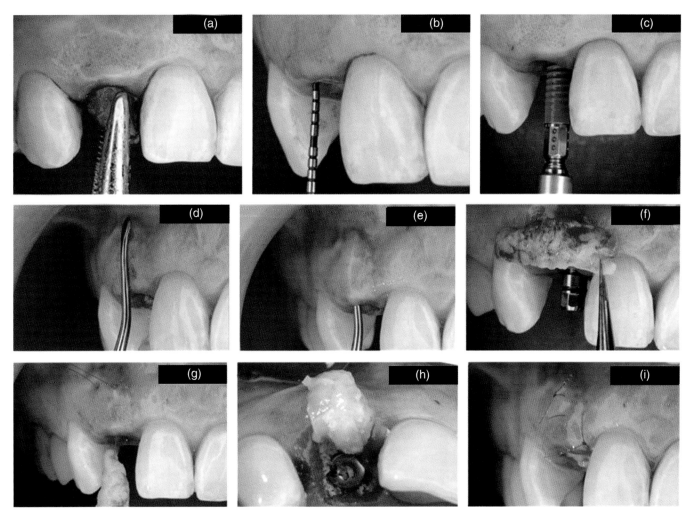

Figure 12.33 (a) Atraumatic extraction of the lateral incisor. (b) The buccal plate integrity is inspected. (c) Immediate implant placement is performed in a flapless approach. (d) Note the contra-angles in the tunneling instrument that facilitates by-pass of the buccal plate, while still having the tip of the instrument toward the bone to decrease the incidence of perforation of the buccal soft tissue. (e) The same tunneling instrument is inserted into the tunnel to provide the space necessary for graft introduction. (f and g) Connective tissue graft insertion into the tunnel with the aid of a guiding suture (h) The palatal portion of the connective tissue graft is left unsecured until the bone grafting procedure is complete. (i) Final suturing from apical to coronal: Guiding suture, horizontal mattress suture, and final criss-cross suture.

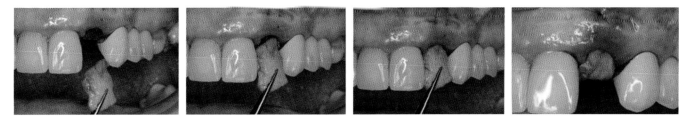

Figure 12.34 Apical guiding suture for introduction of the connective tissue graft into the prepared soft tissue tunnel. An instrument is utilized to keep the suture taut and guide the graft in place from the other aspect.

Apical Guiding "Marionette" Suture

This suture is beneficial in guiding the soft tissue graft into the prepared tunnel, ensuring that the graft is not displaced or creased during its introduction into the tunnel. The technique is used to correlate the apical border of the graft to the corresponding apical end of the area to be augmented and may be used with either free or pediculated grafts (Figure 12.34).

Suture Requirement

- A 3/8 16–19 mm suture needle is advocated in this technique in order to facilitate by-pass of the buccal bone
- Suture material with adequate tensile strength
- Monofilament material is preferred to avoid excessive drag and friction through the tissue upon pulling.

Steps

- Following inspection of the tunnel extension, the graft is placed on the buccal aspect of the socket to aid the clinician in visualizing the size and position of the graft in relation to the prepared area.
- Depending on the predetermined desired position of the graft, the first suture bite is initiated from the buccal aspect of the oral mucosa at the site corresponding to the most apical corner of the final graft position.
- The needle is exited from the buccal sulcus of the socket. This can be facilitated by introducing a micro-periosteal elevator to help slide the needle along the smooth instrument surface.
- Two purchase points are then performed to anchor the graft at its most apical portion. The purchase points are done in a horizontal fashion from within a distance of 2–3 mm between the suture bites.
- The needle is then entered once again through the buccal sulcus to exit in the same horizontal point as the initial entry point in the buccal oral mucosa to avoid uneven pull on the graft. It is preferred to have the two purchase

points of the buccal mucosa slightly wider than those performed in the graft to stretch the graft and avoid creasing at the apical ends.

- A needle holder is then used to hold both ends of the suture thread coming out of the buccal to pull the graft apically into the sulcus and desired position. Simultaneously from the coronal aspect, a tunneling instrument or tissue packer can assist in graft introduction and adaptation process during insertion (Figure 12.35).

Horizontal Adaptive Mattress Suture

This technique is utilized to allow an intimate adaptation between the graft and the overlying buccal tissue, to aid in graft stabilization as well as guiding the graft through the tunnel. The suture is performed in the same steps as the apical anchoring suture with two modifications:

- The position where the suture is initiated is in a more coronal aspect, and engages a more centralized portion of the graft to offer better graft stability.
- Purchase points in the graft and corresponding buccal gingiva are larger (3–4 mm) and equidistant to engage a larger portion of the graft and add conformity to the suture pulling vectors.

Positioning Mattress Suture

This technique is essentially a combination of the previous two methods. For longer grafts it is often difficult to stabilize the entirety of the tissue with one suture. This technique offers the flexibility of positioning the sutures

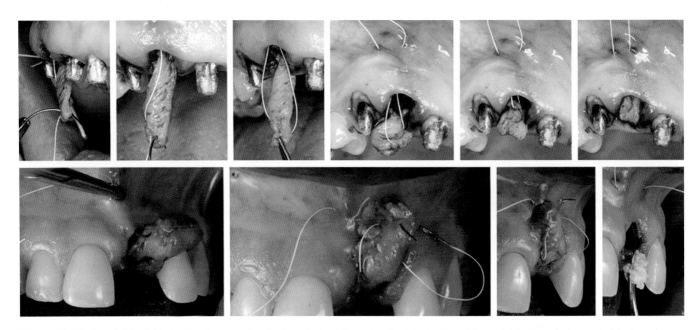

Figure 12.35 From left to right, step by step procedure for the apical guiding suture for introduction of the graft into the apical aspect of the tunnel. Depending on the desired area of graft insertion, the buccal purchase points are initiated at that level.

where they are needed depending on the site and extension of the graft. It involves utilizing smaller (2mm) internal mattress sutures which can be either vertical or oblique in orientation to help position the graft at two or more remote points (Figure 12.36).

Technique

- Following inspection of the tunnel extension, the graft is placed on the buccal aspect of the socket or tunnel preparation to aid the clinician in visualizing the size and position of the graft in relation to the prepared area.
- The first purchase point is performed from the buccal aspect on the most mesial aspect of the tunneled tissue.
- Apico-coronally, the purchase point is approximately 6mm from the gingival margin.
- The suture needle is passed to engage the graft at its most mesial portion from the lingual to the buccal aspect.
- The needle is then returned in the opposite direction 2mm coronal to that point and back through the buccal gingiva at a point 2mm coronal to the initial entry point.
- Utilizing a needle holder, the two ends of the suture thread are pulled taut. With the aid of a micro-tunneling instrument, the graft is introduced into the tunneled buccal tissue and the knot is secured following adequate positioning of the graft.

- The same procedure is then repeated on the distal aspect in the same fashion to ensure stretching of the graft and avoid any dead space that may form due to inadequate graft adaptation underneath the tunnel.
- Additional sutures may be performed in the same fashion should there be the need for additional graft stability.

Bone Graft Procedure

Following soft tissue stabilization, the bone graft of choice is packed either in the socket or between the buccal and the implant to bridge the gap. According to Tarnow (Chu et al. 2012) the bone is packed in two zones. The first zone is up to the level of the buccal plate followed by overfilling of the bone particles up to the level of the soft tissue margins. The dual zone technique can be used in lieu of the tissue graft as the particles placed in the tissue zone are encapsulated and allow for thickening of the supra-crestal implant mucosa providing augmentation of the tissue without the need of additional soft tissue grafting. This technique of overfilling may also be selected in cases where a soft tissue graft is utilized (Figure 12.37).

Closure of the Extraction Socket

To continue with sealing the socket with the tissue graft, another anchoring suture may be utilized to engage the

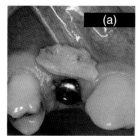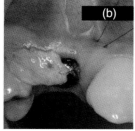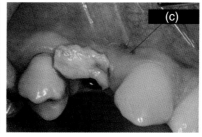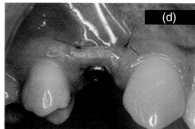

Figure 12.36 Two positioning mattress sutures are utilized to precisely position the graft at the mesial and distal aspects of the implant. The sutures offer an anti-rotational factor to the soft tissue graft and it is beneficial when utilized with longer grafts to be able to better position the tissue in the desired location at different sites.

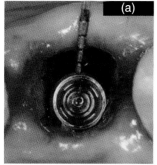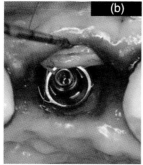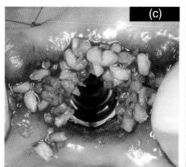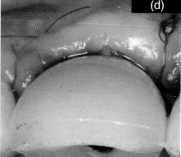

Figure 12.37 (a) Palatal placement. (b) Connective tissue graft placement and internal mattress positioning sutures. (c) Bone grafting was performed up to the level of the soft tissue margin. (d) A provisional restorarion was utilized to prosthetically seal the socket.

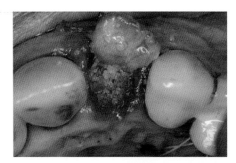
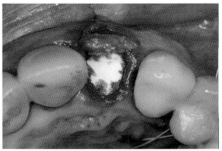
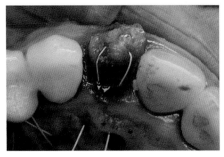
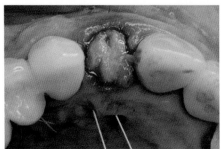
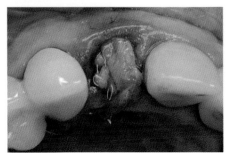

Figure 12.38 Flapless Ridge preservation.

free end of the graft and adapt it underneath the palatal tissue. Reflection of the palatal tissue is often necessary to allow adequate room for the graft (Figure 12.38).

COMPROMISED SOCKETS

As previously mentioned, adequate pre-operative diagnosis of the bone topography and root morphology/angulation is critical prior to tooth extraction. Teeth with peri-radicular endodontic lesions that are chronic in nature are not a contra-indication to bone grafting or immediate implant placement (Waasdorp et al. 2010). However, active infections should be resolved prior to proceeding with any regenerative protocols. Inspection of the socket is critical following tooth removal. Should any deficiencies be detected additional osseous regenerative procedures should be employed to allow for adequate site preservation for future implant placement.

This section will focus on management of extraction sockets with compromised buccal plate integrity, whether in the form of a dehiscence or fenestration defects. For labial dehiscence up to 5 mm, a simple bone graft combined with a collagen barrier can be combined with implant placement in a flapless approach. If additional access is needed, a minimally invasive, site specific incisional technique may be employed to maximize the soft tissue architecture and integrity. The following sections will focus on cases with complete loss of the buccal plate commencing with flapless ridge volume preservation and moving to more complex cases where open procedures are utilized

for implant placement in conjunction with hard and soft tissue augmentation.

FLAPLESS RIDGE PRESERVATION

Absence of the buccal plate poses a challenge for the clinician as additional support is required to maintain the bone within the alveolar envelope and isolate it from the soft tissues. Such defects are common in sites of fractured teeth and/or teeth with significant infections. Absence of the buccal plate support to the overlying soft tissue may have significant repercussions on the final esthetics of the implant. The same considerations in implant placement should be taken into account in compromised sites but that implant placement may pose a risk if performed sub-optimally (Figure 12.39) or if careful pre-operative case selection is not made.

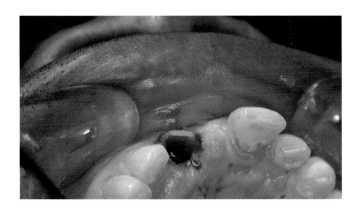

Figure 12.39 Flapless ridge preservation membrane insertion.

However, hard and soft tissue volume preservation remains essential in sites with pre-existing deficiencies as the post-extraction remodeling results in more severe defects.

Key Points

Thorough debridement of the lesion is mandatory. If there are areas that are hard to access from the socket opening, a vestibular incision (explained later) may aid in accessibility. Following thorough degranulation of the site a membrane should be placed either buccal to the socket walls or internally within the socket as an "ice-cream cone" technique (previously described).

Techniques

- Ridge Preservation with a resorbable or nonresorbable barrier.
- Esthetic ridge preservation utilizing growth factor enhanced bone matrix.
- Concomitant hard and soft tissue augmentation through free or pediculated soft tissue grafts.

Armamentarium

- Basic Surgical Kit.
- Implant Placement Kit.
- Micro-blades and Soft Tissue Tunneling Instrumentation
- Micro tissue forceps, Castro Viejo and Scissors.

RIDGE PRESERVATION UTILIZING BARRIER MEMBRANES

Deficiencies in the socket buccal plate may be reconstituted through the use of barrier membranes to aid in bone graft containment and isolate the graft particles from soft tissue encapsulation. The ice-cream cone technique proposed by Tarnow (in Chu et al. 2012) involves placing a collagen membrane that is trimmed to mimic the missing portion of the buccal plate and is placed within the socket palatal to the borders of the buccal bone peaks. This technique offers a simple approach and may be modified to address apical deficiencies in the same manner through the extraction socket opening. However, mere reconstitution of the previously lost socket topography may not be sufficient for future implant placement. Subsequently a modification of this technique can be performed by placement of the membrane on the outer aspect of the buccal socket walls.

Surgical Procedure

- Extraction is performed in the same steps as previously mentioned.

- Following adequate debridement of the internal aspect of the buccal tissue, preparation of the buccal aspect of the socket is then commenced.
- Utilizing a microtunneling instrument, the buccal gingiva overlying the socket is reflected in a full thickness fashion.
- Reflection is initiated from the apical aspect. The reason for starting with the apical portion offers several advantages:
  - Simplicity of access from the extraction site orifice in a straight downward direction
  - The bone topography apical to the extraction socket is usually depressed or concave and subsequently allows an easier and safer access corresponding to the periosteal elevator's curvature.
  - Once the buccal tissue is reflected, in the apical direction, it allows some "give" to the buccal flap, facilitating instrumentation to the adjacent areas.
- Following adequate reflection of the apical portion to allow for adequate membrane placement, the proximal areas are reflected.
- Different contra-angles of tunneling instruments offers versatility in the areas to be reached and therefore allows for easier reflection of the interproximal attached gingiva underlying the papilla.
- The dissection is continued from an apical to coronal direction reaching the base of the interproximal papilla.
- There is no need to elevate the interproximal papilla in order to avoid excessive remodeling of the underlying bone which may lead to loss of the papillary height.
- If the coronal portion of the buccal plate is completely absent, then it may be necessary to involve the interproximal papilla. N.B. care should be taken when lifting the papillary complex to avoid separation of the buccal and lingual aspects of the interdental tissue.
- Once the tunnel is prepared circumferentially on the buccal aspect, a micro-back-action chisel or piezo ultrasonic back-action tip is used to ensure complete removal of any soft tissue remnants that may be left behind during tunnel elevation.
- The tunnel is then measured, and a collagen membrane is trimmed to cover 2–3 mm of the peripheral boundaries of the socket (Figure 12.40).
- N.B. it is not advisable to utilize a native cross-linked membrane in these techniques for two reasons:
  - Non-cross-linked membranes are softer and have no structural memory, consequently these membranes do not offer sufficient resistance to allow its introduction into tight spaces without wrinkling and folding.
  - Cross-linked membranes offer more structural durability and resistance to resorption when left exposed.

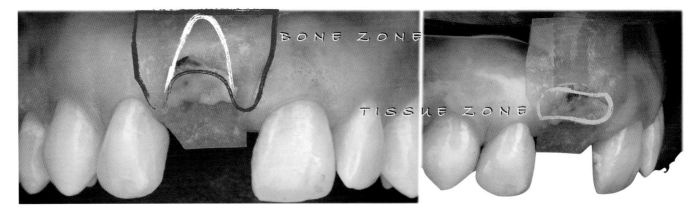

Figure 12.40 Outline of the membrane placement underneath the prepared tunnel. The membrane is trimmed to circumferentially cover the peri-implant defect 2–3 mm circumferentially. Above the crestal bone, the soft tissue graft is placed to boost the soft tissue profile without impediment of the underlying bone.

- Since the objective of this technique is to perform an in-situ bone augmentation beyond the confines of the previous socket housing, it may be prudent to trim the membrane slightly larger (1 mm circumferentially) than what is needed to compensate for the additional bone volume that will stretch the membrane and soft tissue toward the buccal direction.

- Once the membrane is secured and stabilized, a tissue plier is utilized to hold the visible occlusal portion of the membrane taut to avoid displacement or folding of the membrane during the bone grafting procedure.

- Typically, an allograft material would be the one of choice for this technique.

- The bone graft particles are packed in increments both in an apical direction and toward the buccal aspect to counteract the compression resulting from the buccal soft tissue falling into the empty socket.

- A third blunt instrument can also be utilized from the outer aspect of the tunnel at the apical position to prevent displacement of the bone graft apically.

- Finger molding of the outer surface of the site can help spread and adapt the bone in a more uniform fashion.

- The bone graft is condensed up to a coronal level at the bone crest level if a soft tissue graft is utilized. If no soft tissue graft is combined at the time of bone augmentation, the graft may be packed up to the level of the soft tissue margins to support the supra-crestal soft tissue volume.

- Following which the free occlusal tail of the membrane can be simply tucked underneath the palatal tissue with the aid of an instrument or anchoring suture as described for the soft tissue graft procedures.

- An additional criss-cross securing suture can be performed entering 3 mm from the midline of the socket and 3 mm from the gingival margin on the mesio-buccal aspect of the socket. The suture needle is then passed over the membrane and exited on the disto-palatal aspect with the same distance from the gingival margin and mid-line of the socket. The returning suture points are done from the mesio-palatal to the disto-buccal with the knot placed on the buccal. This technique offers additional security and compression of the membrane coronally without compression of the suture thread over the free gingival margin of the socket which may end up with depression and clefting of the socket margins (Figure 12.41).

- Peri-acryl can be used to seal over the socket or an ovate pontic provisional can also be utilized provided that the pontic does not extend on to the buccal aspect of the socket or form excessive compression onto the bone graft material (See Figure 12.42).

ESTHETIC RIDGE AUGMENTATION

Utilizing a membrane has been reported to be effective in Guided Bone Regeneration (GBR) techniques with proven long-term results (Figure 12.43). However, basic GBR principles demand passive primary closure for an environment that is conducive to bone regeneration. In addition to the complexity in handling, stabilizing, and shaping membranes, in the anterior zone, primary closure over extraction sockets often results in an unnatural soft tissue architecture by distorting the position of the muco-gingival junction. Subsequently, the pursuit for development and improvement of minimally invasive technologies has been widely researched over the past decades. Among those advancements is utilizing recombinant growth factor technology to enhance regenerative outcomes and minimize the use of additional barrier membranes for guided tissue regeneration (Nevins and Said 2018).

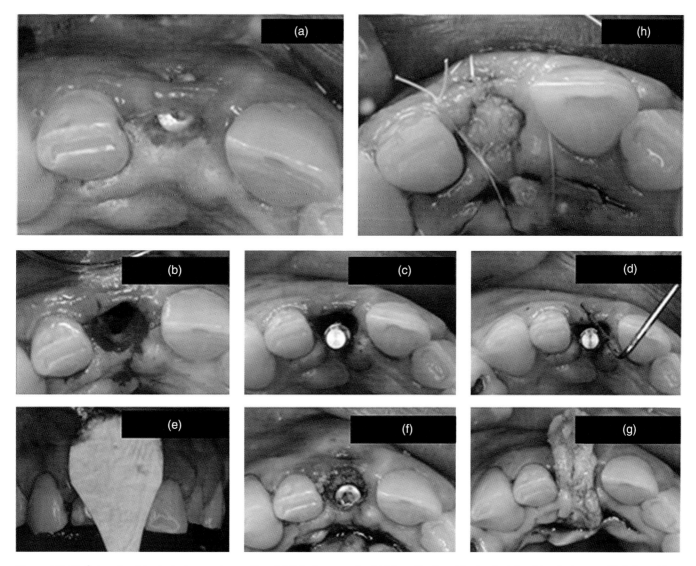

Figure 12.41 Sub-optimal implant placement correction. (a) Note the excessive labial positioning of the implant. (b–d) Implant removal is followed by replacement with a new implant in a more palatal position. (e–f) A resorbable collagen membrane is trimmed according to the defect shape combined with an allograft material and a rotated pedicle soft tissue graft to augment the labial contour of the site as well as seal over the socket (g).

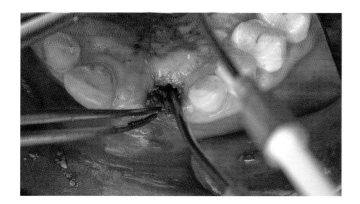

Figure 12.42 Flapless ridge preservation and implant replacement.

Rationale

Recombinant technology allows for the availability of synthetically engineered pure human growth factors. Recombinant human bone morphogenic protein-2 (rhBMP-2) has been extensively studied for extraction socket preservation and sinus elevation in multi-center randomized controlled trials (RCTs). (Fiorellini et al. 2005; Triplett et al. 2009). Recombinant human platelet-derived growth factor-BB (rhPDGF-BB) has been approved for periodontal regenerative procedures to enhance the periodontal attachment apparatus (Nevins et al. 2003a, 2005, 2013). Human histologic studies support the ability of rhPDGF-BB to induce periodontal regeneration (Nevins et al. 2003a, b). In addition, rhPDGF-BB has demonstrated

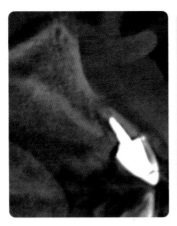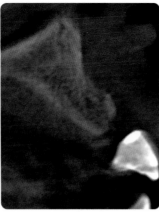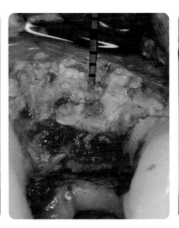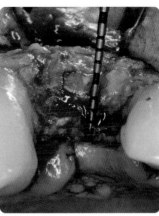

Figure 12.43 Esthetic Ridge Augmentation with growth factor induced bone matrix (Nevins and Said 2018).

positive results in pre-clinical models and human case reports for management of extraction socket preservation, sinus elevation, and vertical ridge augmentation procedures (Cooke et al. 2006; Kaigler et al. 2011; McAllister et al. 2010; Nevins et al. 2009b, 2013; Simion et al. 2007). The direct mechanism of action of platelet-derived growth factor is on the osteoblast population of cells by recruiting them to the wound and stimulating their proliferation and production of matrix. Indirectly, rhPDGF-BB stimulates the elevation of vascular endothelial-cell growth factor which upregulates neovascularization into the wound (Cooke et al. 2006).

Advantages

- Eliminate need for barrier membranes
- Reconstruction of large alveolar defects with less invasion
- Simpler and less time consuming compared to the use of a membrane
- Earlier soft tissue healing
- Linear bone growth

Disadvantages

- Additional expenses
- Long term data is still not documented for the use of this technique
- Off-label FDA use

Procedure

- Prior to beginning the surgical procedure, 1.0 g freeze-dried bone allograft (FDBA) (Regeneross Particulate Allograft, Zimmer Biomet, Palm Beach Gardens, FL) was combined with 0.5 ml of rhPDGF-BB (Gem21S, Osteohealth, Shirley, PA) and sterile water to hydrate the graft and allowed to soak for at least 10 minutes.

- Tooth Removal and Degranulation are performed in the same manner
- The growth-factor enhanced bone matrix is incrementally condensed into the extraction socket defect.
- The graft is over-filled to the level of the gingival margin.
- A collagen membrane (Bio-Gide, Geistlich Pharma North America Inc., Princeton, NJ) was trimmed to fit within the outline of the gingival margin.
- Membrane was stabilized with 6-0 chromic gut suture or medical grade cyanoacrylate (GluStitch Inc. BC, Canada). The provisional appliance was delivered and adjusted to relieve any contact pressure at the surgical site.

If the peri-radicular pathology is inaccessible from the socket orifice, a vestibular approach is utilized.

Decision Making in Soft Tissue Augmentation Following Bone Graft Procedure

Although the importance of soft tissue augmentation has been highlighted throughout the chapter, combining adequate site selection with the appropriate technique is essential. Due to their inherent limited access and space for augmentation, flapless approaches could offer limitations when combined hard and soft tissue grafts are attempted simultaneously. In sites where the buccal bone is intact, the buccal plate acts as a rigid space maintainer for the graft material. If the integrity of the buccal plate is compromised, the soft tissue flap will tend to compress the bucco-occlusal aspect of the graft material and subsequently lead to a depression in the soft tissue profile and underlying regenerated bone. It is therefore advised that flapless ridge preservation procedures are to be performed with this concept in the back of the clinician's mind. In moderately compromised sites, a barrier membrane may be utilized to augment the missing portion of the buccal plate and the bone grafting should be done actively against the buccal soft tissue to counteract for the future remodeling of that site. If a tissue

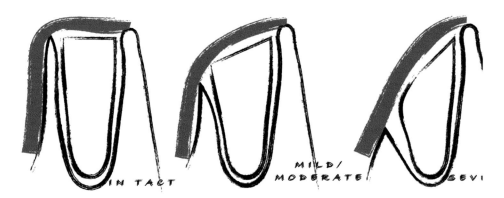

Figure 12.44 Simultaneous soft tissue grafting with ridge augmentation in severely compromised sites may actually hinder the amount of bone augmentation possible when utilizing flapless approaches.

graft is placed at the time of augmentation, the volume of the graft may compromise the hard tissue augmentation, yielding insufficient reconstitution of the alveolar defect for implant placement (Figure 12.44). It therefore may be beneficial to stage such procedures and focus on hard tissue augmentation and perform soft tissue enhancement procedures at the time of implant placement or second stage uncovering.

OPEN FLAP APPROACH FOR EXTRACTION SITE MANAGEMENT

Conservative approaches in the esthetic zone are recommended; often times however, limitations in access for adequate debridement and augmentation are encountered. It is up to the operator to determine the need for additional access to the site if required. At that point, incision design becomes critical not only to allow sufficient access to the site, but must also consider the esthetic endpoint of the case. Consequently, certain requirements for incision design in the esthetic zone must be taken into consideration.

Incision Design Requirements

- Flaps should be planned to allow for adequate access to the site to be addressed, this is pre-determined through adequate pre-operative diagnosis of the defect topography and the augmentation needs.

- Papilla reflection should be only performed on periodontally healthy dentition to avoid the compromise of the interproximal papilla. If extension of the flap to the adjacent teeth is required, papilla sparing incisions should be considered in periodontally compromised patients.

- Vertical releasing incisions are not contra-indicated in the esthetic zone, but it is preferable to avoid vertical incisions in the inter-canine area, to avoid tissue scarring or clefting in a highly visible area.

- Vertical releasing incisions should be performed in remote sites, at least one tooth away from the

augmentation site. Alternatively, if the operator opts to avoid vertical incisions, the intra-sulcular incisions then have to be extended two teeth away from the site to be augmented.

- Avoid vertical incisions directly over root prominences.

- Minimal access flaps with singular or multiple vestibular sub-marginal incisions should only be performed following accurate assessment of the entire defect extension, and still maintain a remote location to avoid having the incision line rest over the augmented site.

Incision Designs Diagram

SITE ANALYSIS AND CLASSIFICATION

Determining the type and extent of augmentation is performed mainly based on the pre-operative assessments. The operator should determine:

- Orientation of the defect:
  - Horizontal
  - Vertical
  - Combined
- Augmentation needs for the site:
  - Simple
  - Moderate
  - Complex
- Intra-bony and extra-bony
- Type of tissue to be augmented
  - Hard Tissue
  - Soft Tissue
  - Combination

The following information is most accurately determined based on the pre-operative diagnostic wax-up. The wax-up aids the clinician in visualizing the final restoration in relation to the present tissue clinically. The mock-up has to replicate the final restoration contours with respect to the tooth position and more importantly, the proposed CEJ position. This step is essential in obtaining an accurate guide for both the regenerative procedure and implant position. The mock-up is then transferred into a radiographic guide to allow for correlation of the tooth position to the underlying bone topography. If the pre-operative wax-up indicates the necessity for soft tissue augmentation, this should be also replicated in the radiographic guide utilizing a material of lower radio-density. The difference in radio-densities between the tooth and soft tissue replica aids the clinician in determining the augmentation needs and treatment sequence. Finally the pre-existing radiographic guide can be transferred into a surgical guide conventionally, or scanned and milled or printed with the aid of digital techniques. As provisional restorations act as a blue-print for the final prosthetic restorations, accurate diagnostic wax-ups offer the clinician an accurate guide for treatment planning and execution of surgical procedures (Figures 12.45, 12.46, and 12.47).

SURGICAL PHASE

Time of Tooth Removal

Management of immediate post-extraction sites poses two main challenges to the clinician

- The lack of primary closure resultant from the tooth being present.

- Obtaining primary closure will result in displacement of the muco-gingival junction position.

One of the possible methods of addressing these problems is incorporating a soft tissue graft with the regenerative bone procedure whether free or pediculated. A combined approach provides both additional volume augmentation as well as protection over the exposed regenerative site. However, this technique is only recommended with resorbable membranes, as lack of primary closure over nonresorbable membranes may cause post-operative infections and site contamination, leading to significant soft tissue esthetic defects. The section will focus on simultaneous hard and soft tissue augmentation of sites with deficient buccal plates at the time of tooth extraction.

Utilizing a combination therapy requires a more advanced skill set, and is not intended for beginner operators.

Surgical Procedure

- Extraction of the tooth can either be performed prior or following flap elevation. It may be useful to remove severely decayed or fractured teeth following flap elevation and reflection.

- Reflection should be extended to allow access of the entirety of the defect and surrounding area. Full thickness

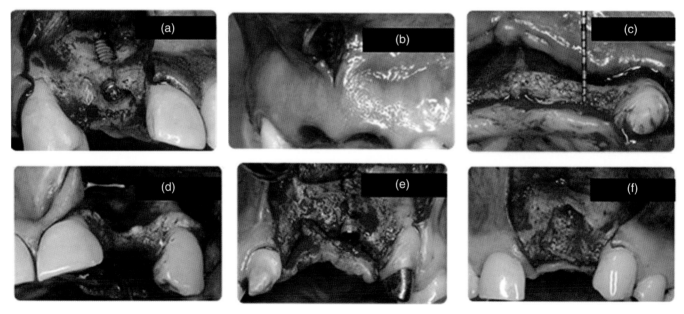

Figure 12.45 Left column top: Dehisence defects with different severity levels. (a) shows a significant implant dehiscence defect which requires more extensive flap reflection and management. (b) shows how minor dehiscence defects can be managed in a less invasive approach. Middle column shows two horizontal type defects. (c) shows a non-contained horizontal deficiency in which augmentation is required outside of the alveolar envelope. (d) shows a horizontal deficiency that is more confined and provides a higher regenerative potential and a less demanding augmentation. The last column shows the difference between two vertical defects with different regenerative potentials due to the amount of bone walls surrounding the defect. (e) Extra-bony. (f) Intra-bony.

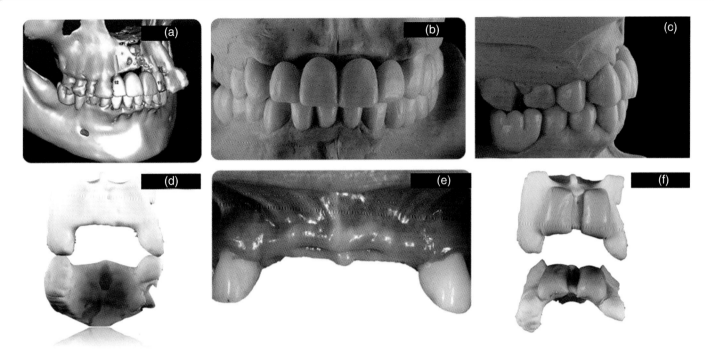

Figure 12.46 (a) CT scan with digital wax-up and virtual implant placement exhibiting inadequate bone to stabilize the proposed implants. (b) shows the vertical tissue deficiency in relation to the proposed future restoration. (c) The horizontal ridge deficiency can also be evaluated and augmentation preplanned utilizing 3d printed models (d) to plan the case surgically. These models can also be sterilized to allow pre-shaping membranes and block grafts prior to surgical exposure of the site (e and f).

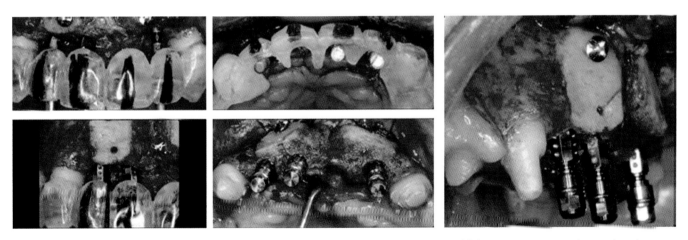

Figure 12.47 The diagnostic wax-up is then converted into a surgical guide to aid the clinician to establish the correct augmentation needs and adequately place the implants conforming to the desired restorative position.

reflection is carried out until sufficient access is achieved to expose the defect in addition to about 4 mm circumferentially around the defect.

- Tooth extraction and site debridement is performed as previously described.

- Implant placement may also be attempted if correct implant positioning can be achieved.

- The surgical guide is utilized to give the operator the ideal CEJ/gingival margin position for adequate implant placement.

- The guide is also utilized to aid the clinician with the amount and location of the site to be augmented in relation to the future implant supported restoration.

- If the defect is only horizontal in nature, a collagen membrane has been proven to be sufficient in obtaining adequate horizontal augmentation for either a veneer graft buccal to the implant or reconstitution of sufficient alveolar dimensions for future implant placement.

- The key to obtaining a predictable regenerative outcome is adequate extension of the membrane and stability of the blood clot.

Membrane Placement and Stabilization

Depending on the operator preference, the membrane may be stabilized by different techniques. Stability of the membrane is critical regardless of the membrane choice. Stabilization through use of fixation tacks and pins allows immobilization of the membrane and also permits packing the bone graft against the membrane. Depending on the preference of the operator anchoring the membrane may be done on the buccal or palatal aspects first followed by bone packing. Care has to be taken when packing the bone as there is usually a tendency to pack the bone apical to the ridge crest if the membrane is stabilized palatally. This may result in the bone graft particles being displaced vertically which makes closure more difficult, as well as displacing the graft. A high degree of cross-linking of collagen membranes produces stiffer membrane. Therefore, appropriate selection of the material becomes critical when performing these procedures. If mini-screws are utilized for fixation, the rotation may cause the membrane to become "curled" around the screw. Therefore, it is advisable to utilize an additional instrument to fixate and stretch the membrane while the screw is inserted.

Regardless of the type of membrane or amount of augmentation stability is a mandatory requirement for a successful bone graft. This is a function not only of membrane stabilization but also is the result of packing the bone and securing it under the membrane. The membrane must be stretched to fully encompass the bone graft particles and keep it in place to avoid excessive micro-motion during the initial healing phase. Failure to immobilize the graft may lead to excessive graft resorption or infection.

Techniques for Membrane Stabilization

1. Periosteal Suture
2. Fixation pins and/or screws

The membrane is trimmed to cover 2–3 mm circumferentially around the area to be augmented.

The shape of the membrane can be customized with the use of one membrane to extend on the buccal as well as occlusal aspects.

Alternatively, the membrane can be trimmed in two separate pieces to have part of the membrane dedicated for the buccal augmentation while the second piece is trimmed into an hourglass shape to extend from the palatal to the buccal aspect covering the occlusal portion of the socket. This technique offers the advantage of having a double layer of membranes over the bucco-occlusal aspect of the augmentation which increases the resorption time of the membrane in that area. Resorbable collagen membranes are trimmed to fit snug around the teeth conforming to classical GTR principles. Should the clinician decide to utilize a nonresorbable membrane, a 1.5 mm distance should be left away from the adjacent tooth roots (Figure 12.48).

Important note: Membrane trimming should be performed knowing that the bone graft material will tent the membrane overlying it, causing it to shift away from the adjacent margins. Native collagen membranes (bioguide) may be trimmed to be relatively snug over the graft material as they are more elastic and stretchable than cross-linked or nonresorbable membranes. Cross-linked membranes do not allow "give" and should be trimmed slightly larger (about 15%) prior to the augmentation.

Technical tip: Oversizing the membrane by about 15% and fixating it on one side first utilizing a tack. The bone graft material is then packed to replicate the desired ridge contours and is then pulled with tension over the graft to the opposite aspect and fixated with another tack. This ensures stability of the graft and sufficient coverage of the bone graft material.

Once the membrane is trimmed, the choice of stabilization technique would dictate the sequence of procedures. In cases where internal stabilizing sutures are to be utilized, periosteal releasing incisions should be performed prior to membrane fixation (Figure 12.49).

Requirements and Evolution of the Periosteal Releasing Incisions

- The periosteal release is composed of a continuous horizontal incision to separate the tightly bound periosteal lining of a full thickness flap.

- The incision should extend through the entire width of the flap. Partial separation of the periosteum prevents passive release of the flap leading to uneven tension and difficulty in coronal flap mobilization.

- The incision has to be performed apical to the muco-gingival junction to allow access to the elastic fibers of the oral mucosa.

- The depth of extension of the incision has evolved with the introduction of different techniques. The incision depth should extend only past the periosteal layer on average (0.8 mm). If thicker muscular structures or scar tissue exists within the internal aspect of the flap, sharp dissection may be continued slightly deeper until the submucosal area is accessed. Following which, utilizing a hemostat or periosteal elevator with blunt dissection, a coronal brushing motion is performed to allow stretching of the flap and spreading apart the periosteal incision margins to allow coronal advancement. This technique offers two advantages:

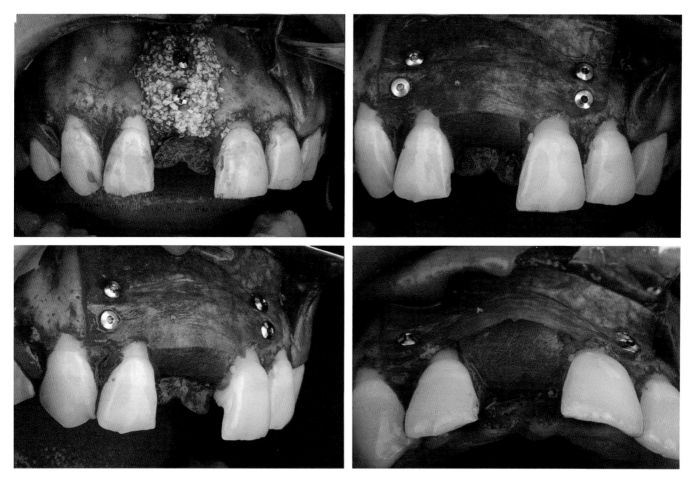

Figure 12.48 Example of membrane fixation with tacks placed to stabilize one horizontal membrane with a second membrane placed on the occlusal aspect to completely seal off the regenerative site.

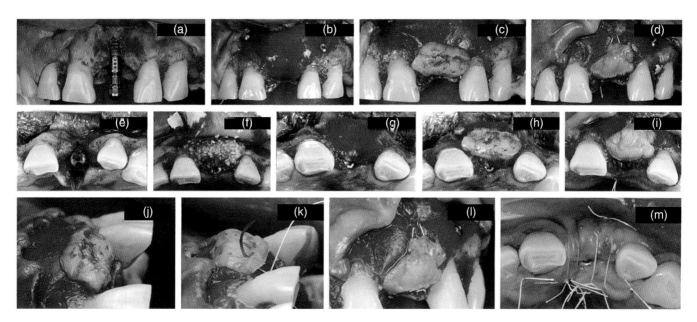

Figure 12.49 (a–d) (a) Frontal view implant placement, guided bone regeneration was performed on the buccal aspect, with fixation tacks for added membrane stability. A connective tissue graft was performed to further augment the tissue volume. The membrane and tissue graft were secured with a stabilizing periosteal suture. (e–h) occlusal view of the procedure. (j–m) Showing the graft being engaged prior to periosteal anchoring as well as the periosteal anchorage done with the same suture to stabilize the graft in place. Closure is done above the healing abutment.

- Deep sharp dissection into the submucosa causes excessive trauma, post-operative swelling, and pain as dissection into the deeper muscle layers involves more nerves and larger vessels.

- Blunt dissection offers a safer alternative when in close proximity to main nerves and vessels as this technique can be used to release the buccal flaps in other areas of the mouth.

- This form of dissection will result in the flap being split into two portions:

  - Apical to the periosteal incision line: This portion remains bound to the underlying bone.

  - Coronal to the periosteal incision line: Passive portion of the flap.

- Once the flap is checked for sufficient mobility, the corresponding palatal portion of the membrane is tucked under the palatal flap and the bone graft material is packed on the buccal aspect. The periosteal stabilizing suture is commenced.

Steps for Periosteal Stabilizing Suture

- The suture is entered from the palatal tissue about 5 mm apical to the palatal gingival margin and off set to either mesial or distal about 3 mm from an imaginary line running through the center of the site.

- The suture needle is passed to the buccal to engage the connective tissue/periosteum attached to the bone, which allows a stable anchorage to the suture.

- The suture is passed to the opposite edge of the grafted site to anchor the periosteum.

- It is then returned to the palatal flap to exit at a point symmetrical to the entry point.

- This suture exerts pressure on the edges of the membrane, adapting it to the underlying bone whilst avoiding compression of the graft material.

- If the suture bites are taken too close to each other, the suture thread creates pressure on the regenerating bone and may end with a depression of the buccal contour (Figure 12.50).

- Regardless of the membrane fixation technique, this same suture may be utilized to stabilize the soft tissue graft, whether the graft is engaged in the suture or allowing the suture thread to compress it apically.

Tacks and Pin Fixation

For a more rigid form of membrane stabilization, fixation tacks and pins may be utilized. Membrane fixation screws may also be utilized, but usually reserved for non-resorbable membranes or areas with a thick cortical plate (example: posterior mandible). When utilized with resorbable collagen membranes, the membrane tends to rotate and wrinkle owing to the rotational motion of the screw insertion. Therefore, in the anterior maxilla, fixation tacks are both simple and predictable in their use but not without drawbacks:

Advantages

- Immobilization of the membrane and underlying graft

- Precise placement with narrow diameter, can be used in between roots of the teeth

- No creasing or wrinkling of the membrane

- Have different lengths, with the same diameter which can help in cases with softer bone

Disadvantages

- Need a mallet for insertion, which is uncomfortable for the patient and may even cause paroxysmal vertigo

- Need for retrieval

- May cause minor tissue dehiscence

- Longer lengths 5 mm tend to bend easier

- Access for palatal placement may not always be possible

Procedure for Tack Insertion

- Following membrane trimming, the membrane fixation is commenced either on the buccal or lingual aspect.

- The membrane is positioned in the desired orientation.

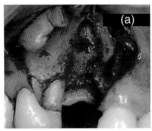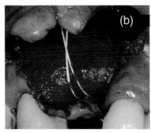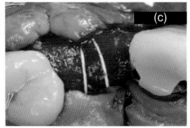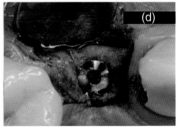

Figure 12.50 (a–c) Incorrect choice of suture material and placement compressing the graft right in the mid-buccal portion of the grafted site. (d) note the point of depression of the buccal bone related to the previously performed suture.

- An instrument is utilized to fixate the membrane in place, and the pin applicator is utilized to position the tack pin onto the membrane to prevent its movement.

- The holding instrument is then left to the assistant and the free hand is utilized to operate the mallet.
  - Note the long axes of the tack, applicator, and mallet have to be parallel. If the mallet and applicator are offset to where the tack is directed, the forces will be directed to the peripheries of the pin and will either cause it to bend or dislodge from the applicator.

- The mallet is gently tapped while maintaining the proper angulation until complete seating of the tack is observed.

- At which point an instrument such as the back edge (non-cutting side of the blade) is inserted in between the grooves of the applicator head, with pressure over the tack.

- The applicator is then bent in the opposite direction of the instrument insertion. N.B. attempting to pull the applicator in a direction opposite to the tack insertion will often result in dislodgment of the fixation pin.

- Once the membrane is fixated on one side the bone is then packed into the defect site.

- A common mistake is incorrectly *packing the bone*.

- The membrane is pulled taut over the packed bone. Tip: An instrument such as a periosteal elevator can be utilized to maintain the bone in the desired shape to maintain the space underneath the membrane.
  - Common errors: If the membrane is tacked on the palatal initially, the bone particles will have a tendency to fall apically during the buccal fixation.
  - If fixation is performed from buccal to the palatal, the bone will tend to rise crestal and result in an inadvertent vertical augmentation which makes closure much more difficult.

- If the implant was placed the implant cover screw/healing abutment can act as the palatal anchorage and a small slit performed with a 15 blade can allow for securing the membrane around the implant platform.

- The membrane is pulled taut over the bone particles and fixation is continued in the same fashion at the apical corners of the augmentation site.

- Multiple tacks can be placed along the membrane periphery to minimize any voids between the bone and membrane, ultimately leading to complete clinical immobilization of the membrane/graft complex.

- The same can be applied when the membrane is trimmed in two segments. The membrane is fixated in a horizontal orientation initially followed by insertion of the second portion of the membrane from the palatal to occlusal aspect.

- Should additional stabilization of the second portion of the membrane be needed, a stabilizing suture can be used but usually is not necessary (Figure 12.51).

Soft Tissue Stabilization

Once the bone graft is performed, the connective tissue graft is introduced to the site.

The connective tissue graft can be situated horizontally or vertically. In cases where there is an extraction socket orifice it may be advantageous to place a portion of the graft to protect the underlying bone graft during the initial healing as well as prevent excessive distortion of the MGJ. However, the graft must have no more than 20% of its surface exposed, in order to attain sufficient blood supply and avoid necrosis. If primary closure is planned then the graft can be oriented horizontally, i.e. mesio-distally to allow for augmentation of the interproximal papillae in a horizontal dimension in addition to the buccal contours.

SUTURING OF THE GRAFT

The tissue graft may be sutured utilizing different areas for its anchorage.

The Buccal or Palatal Flap

Anchoring Periosteal Suture

Depending on the homogeneity of the graft thickness the graft can be sutured to either the buccal or palatal flaps. If sutured to the buccal flap a horizontal mattress suture is used to ensure that the graft is stabilized in the desired position in relation to the ridge and the flap. Following graft stabilization, the site must be inspected for any lack of conformity, excessive folding, or lack of adaptation of the graft prior to flap closure.

Steps (Figure 12.52):

1. Suturing is started from the vestibular aspect of the flap, by holding the graft and flap with tissue forceps (Figure 12.52).

2. The suture needle is passed to engage the buccal flap and connective tissue about 2mm from the center of the graft.

3. The needle is then passed back through the connective tissue graft and inner aspect of the flap to emerge about 3mm away from the initial entry point on the same horizontal plane.

4. Securing the suture should be done in a manner that is not too tight, as excessive pulling will cause the graft and flap to curl toward the center of the suture. The same might occur if the suture bites are too far apart horizontally. Visual assessment is needed during this step.

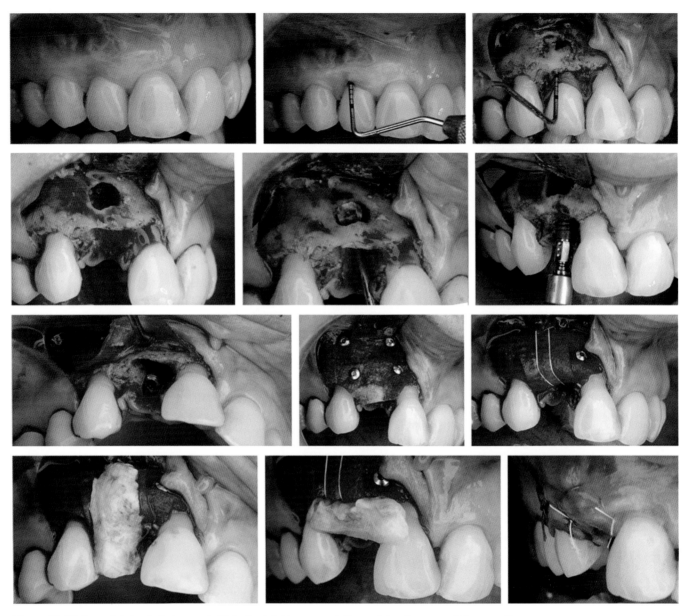

Figure 12.51 Immediate implant placement with horizontal ridge augmentation and simultaneous soft tissue grafting.

The purchase points should be 3mm apart, sufficient to adapt the graft well to the flap. If the bite sizes are too wide apart or the suture too tight, the graft will have a tendency to curl toward the center. Sutures bites that are too close will not encompass sufficient surface area of the graft to prevent its rotation and adequately stabilize it.

The graft could also be stabilized to the palatal flap though the same approach. However, reflection of the palatal flap is required to successfully accomplish closure of the flap as the space occupied by the tissue graft elevates the buccal flap (positions it more coronal), preventing adequate approximation of the buccal and lingual tissues. By elevating the palatal flap adequate closure with connective tissue contact between the two flaps allows earlier union and better healing.

Suturing of the Graft and Simultaneous Flap Closure

In single tooth sites, where soft tissue grafting is performed, graft fixation can be combined with initial flap approximation. This approach is essentially composed of two vertical mattress sutures performed at the mesial and distal interproximal papillae.

Surgical Steps

In contrast to horizontal mattress sutures, vertical mattress sutures allow coronal positioning and eversion of edges of the flap if needed.

The suture entry point is from the palatal aspect below the base of the palatal interproximal papilla.

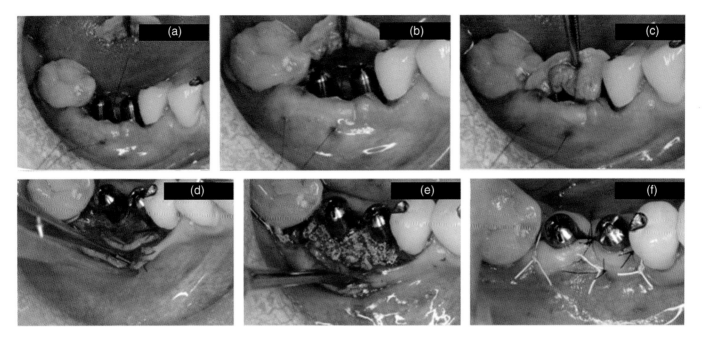

Figure 12.52 (a–c) A mattress suture is used to anchor the graft to the flap. (d) showing the graft sutured to the flap. (e) Buccal bone grafting was performed. (f) Closure of the site.

The needle is passed through the palatal tissue, through the graft and in through the buccal flap at about 5 mm from the tip of the buccal surgical papilla.

The needle is then returned through the buccal flap approximately 2 mm coronal to the initial exit point and then passed straight to the corresponding site on the palatal aspect without engaging the graft.

The end result of this suture is coronal repositioning of the flap and stabilization of the graft.

N.B. if the graft is engaged on the return passes of the suture, both the graft and flap will become coronally positioned which will result in interference of the connective tissue graft with the flap edges and subsequently lack of adequate adaptation of the tissue.

STABILIZATION OF THE GRAFT

An alternative approach stabilizes the graft prior to flap closure which offers the advantage of having more control of the buccal flap and less mobility of the tissue during the suturing process. The most stable tissue is usually the attached periosteum and overlying connective tissue below the level of the periosteal releasing incision. The tissue is anchored into the periosteum by either a horizontal mattress or vertical mattress type of suture.

Suturing is started from the palatal aspect and is offset to either the mesial or distal side and at least 3 mm from the crestal incision in a vertical plane. The graft is engaged, and the needle is then passed into the connective tissue perpendicular to the buccal bone to ensure at least 2–3 mm of tissue for anchorage. For single tooth sites one suture is usually sufficient. One or more of these sutures may be used for larger spans and bigger tissue grafts depending on the clinician's judgment of the graft stability. A third alternative is engaging the periosteum in two different points along the same horizontal plane consequently obtaining a larger surface area to stabilize the graft. N.B. depending on the accessibility, the suture may be criss-crossed. The needle is then passed through the graft from a buccal to palatal aspect and finally exits through the palatal tissue at the same horizontal plane as the entry point (Figure 12.53).

The vertical approach is the same concept except in a vertical orientation, meaning that at least two sutures are necessary to stabilize the graft, one on either side of the graft at the mesial and distal edges.

CLOSURE

Closure of the flap should re-approximate the tissue to its original position while utilizing the tissue to offer a protective barrier to the underlying augmentation complex. Should a prosthetic component be placed such as a stock or customized healing abutment, additional fine interrupted sutures should be utilized to achieve good adaptation around the abutment.

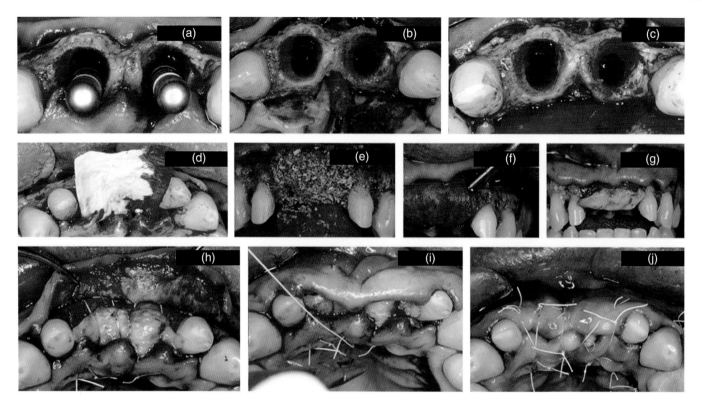

Figure 12.53 (a–c) Extraction and implant preparation osteotomies. (d) Membrane fixation is performed on the palatal aspect. (e and f) Contour bone grafting was performed combined with a collagen membrane. (g) Positioning of a free connective tissue graft on the buccal aspect prior to suturing. (h) Horizontal mattress sutures overlapping the grafts and engaging the periosteum on the buccal flap. (i) Note how tightening of the mattress sutures allows for coronal advancement of the flap while exerting downward pressure on the soft tissue to ensure adequate stability of the free graft. (j) Closure of the flap, showing minor areas of the underlying connective tissue used to cover the extraction site openings.

MANAGING IMPLANT TISSUE DEFICIENCIES

Regardless of efforts employed to preserve and augment the tissue volume, certain deficiencies resulting from surgical complications, inadequate tissue management/augmentation, or simply severe anatomical deficiencies may compromise implant placement and long-term implant function.

As previously discussed, correct three-dimensional implant placement may not always be possible at the time of tooth extraction. Efforts to reconstitute the deficient tissue volume should then be maximized at the time of tooth extraction, often requiring significantly larger procedures. However, certain patient related factors such as esthetics, patient refusal of more invasive procedures, and healing potential can often hinder clinicians in achieving the optimal results in one surgery. Therefore, alternative less invasive techniques may be performed in stages to specifically address deficient sites or complications.

Case Study: Apical Topography (Vestibular Approach)

1. A 37 year old medically healthy patient presented with severely decayed maxillary central incisors and failed root canal therapy.

2. CBCT evaluation revealed Class IV type sockets with inadequate socket or apical topography for immediate implant placement (Figure 12.54).

3. Teeth extraction was performed atraumatically with FDBA allograft placed to the level of the soft tissue.

4. Prosthetic sealing of the socket was performed with a fixed tooth supported provisional bridge.

5. Four months post extraction, note the preservation of the gingival architecture and support of the interproximal the soft tissue profile (Figure 12.55).

6. Five months CBCT scan revealed adequate bone fill, but residual apical concavity preventing adequate implant placement (Figure 12.55).

7. Implant placement was planned through a digitally guided approach to avoid flap reflection and disruption of the tissue architecture

8. Based on the pre-operative planning, the site of implant fenestration was accounted for prior to the surgical procedure.

9. Tissue punch and flapless implant placement was performed. Note the bone graft encapsulation within the soft tissue. (Figure 12.56).

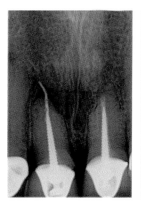
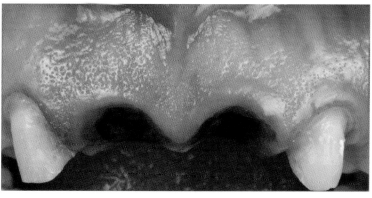
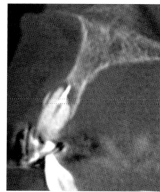

Figure 12.54 Class IV type sockets with Inadequate socket or apical topography for immediate implant placement.

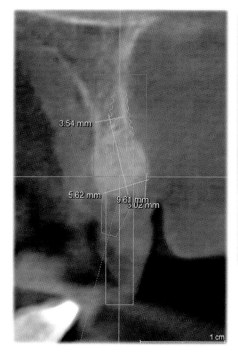
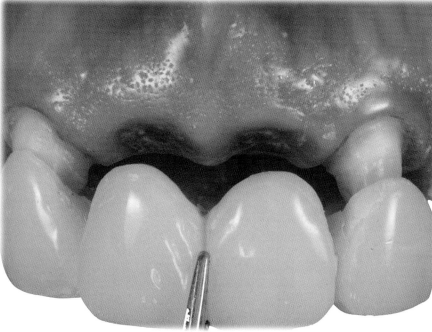

Figure 12.55 Note the bone preservation of the ridge with maintanence of the soft tissue architecture.

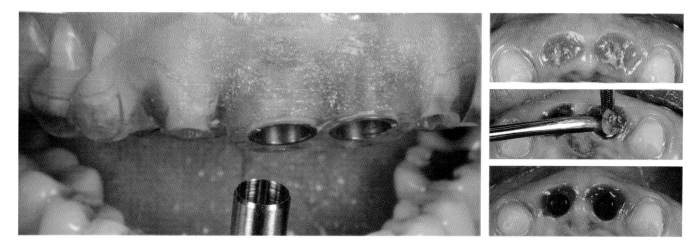

Figure 12.56 Soft tissue punch performed for flapless implant placement. Note the bone graft particle encapsulation within the soft tissues which act to preserve the tissue volume in the area.

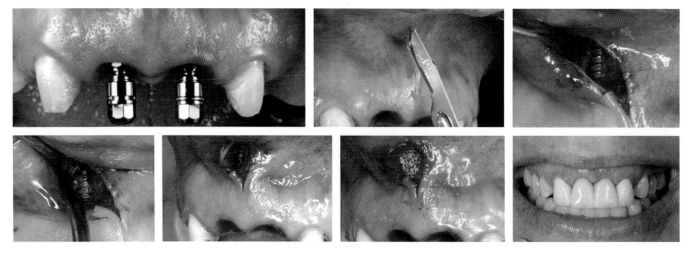

Figure 12.57 Implant placement and guided bone regeneration performed through a vestibular tunnel procedure.

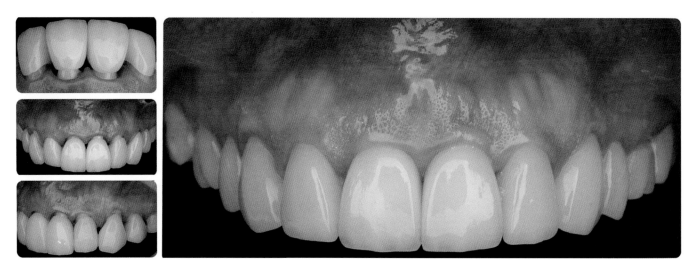

Figure 12.58 Final implant restoration and veneers to mask the congenitally missing laterals.

10. A small vestibular incision was utilized to address the site without the need for reflection of a full thickness flap that may have compromised the esthetics of the case.

11. Full thickness reflection was performed to expose the defect entirety with sufficient space to accommodate for membrane placement and bone graft material.

12. Site closure with microsutures (Figure 12.57).

13. Final case following finalization of the restoration.

14. Post-operative CT scan revealed adequate buccal bone both in the coronal and apical portions.

Lessons learned: Staging procedures with less invasive augmentation techniques may provide an alternative to larger reconstructive procedures with more esthetically acceptable results (Figure 12.58).

• Dual zone bone grafting protocols combined with prosthetic socket sealing may provide better maintenance of the soft tissue architecture and volume, offering a less invasive approach to soft tissue grafting procedures.

• The same philosophy can be performed with simultaneous implant sites and in more compromised sites, provided that:

1. The implant is not placed outside of the alveolar envelope as the avascular implant surface will hinder cellular migration and subsequent bone formation buccal to the implant.

2. Excessive buccal inclination or poorly positioned implants should be removed and replaced with a more palatally positioned implant either immediately or in staged fashion. A more palatal relocation of the implant will also allow more space for the buccal hard and soft tissue augmentation.

3. The operator is able to operate with the correct instrumentation within the confines of the performed access tunnel whether from a crestal or vestibular approach.

Same-Site, Minimally Invasive Surgery

In cases where soft tissue augmentation was performed at the time of extraction and adequate reconstitution of the hard and soft tissue contours has been achieved, a flapless approach may be utilized for implant placement procedure provided there is sufficient keratinized tissue. In these cases, the soft tissue augmented socket orifice can be an excellent donor site for additional buccal soft tissue augmentation.

Procedure

Whether the area is being performed utilizing guided surgery or conventional techniques, the outline of the soft tissue punch should be slightly greater than the diameter of the final implant to be used. If a customized healing abutment or provisional crown are planned, the soft tissue punch may be performed to replicate the root/restoration cross-section. The benefit of applying these technical tips is to maximize the amount of tissue to be utilized for the soft tissue augmentation.

1. The outline of the soft tissue punch is performed in a partial thickness outline with the use of a scalpel blade or a pre-standardized tissue punch of the corresponding diameter.

2. A large round diamond bur is utilized to de-epithelialize within the outline of the punch.

3. The incisions are then continued full thickness and the soft tissue is removed with the aid of a periosteal elevator.

4. Depending on the shape and thickness of the soft tissue harvested, the tissue can be trimmed to the desired shape and size.

5. Following implant placement, a tunnel preparation is made to allow introduction of the graft. The tunnel in these cases will be coronal to the crest of bone as the purpose of this procedure is to enhance the coronal soft tissue thickness and quality (tissue zone). Should any additional bone grafting be needed, this can be performed on the buccal aspect up to the implant platform (bone zone) (Figure 12.49f–i).

6. The soft tissue is secured in place utilizing one of the pre-mentioned securing sutures or even the healing abutment and/or provisional restoration to secure the graft in place (Figure 12.49j).

Combining this technique with a vestibular incision on the buccal aspect can provide the clinician with an alternative for management of hard of soft tissue defects of a more

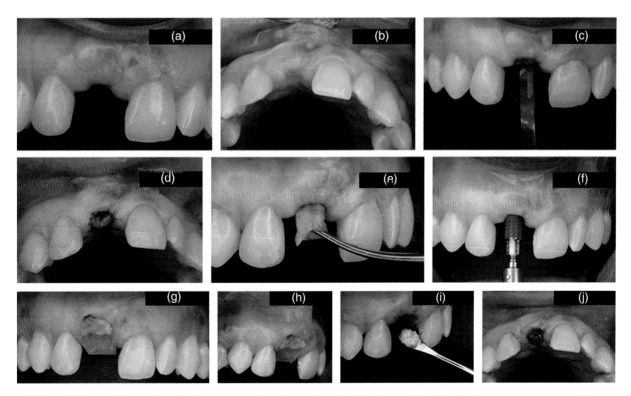

Figure 12.59 (a–j) Sequential procedures for the treatment of a failed implant site with a "same-site minimally invasive surgical approach."

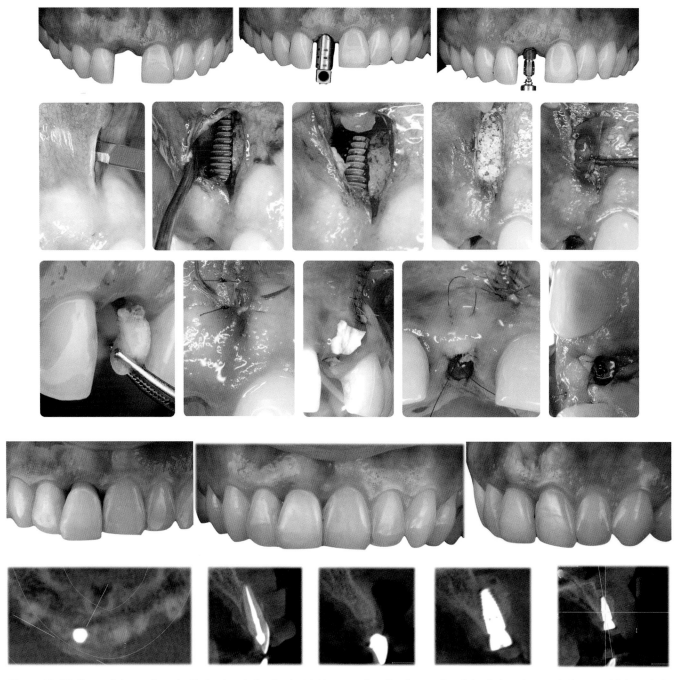

Figure 12.60 Sequential procedures for the treatment of an implant dehiscence site with a "same-site minimally invasive surgical approach" through the aid of a vestibular incision.

severe nature in the esthetic zone with a single incision. This is especially useful in esthetically sensitive areas with complex peri-implant deficiencies (Figures 12.59 and 12.60).

CONCLUSION

The purpose of this chapter was to illustrate the different components of establishing optimum peri-implant esthetics through correct implant positioning, reconstitution of tissue volume, as well as minimizing soft tissue architecture distortion through less invasive approaches. As clinical practice becomes more demanding our techniques have evolved to involve less invasion while simultaneously enhancing the overall results. Therefore, as clinicians, our approaches to more complex sites should be tailored to minimize the invasiveness to the patient without compromising the end result (Figure 12.61).

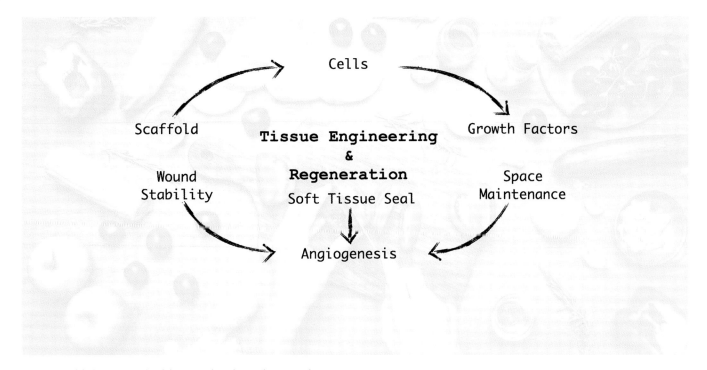

Figure 12.61 Fundamentals of tissue engineering and regeneration.

REFERENCES

Araujo, M., Linder, E., Wennström, J., and Lindhe, J. (2008). The influence of Bio-Oss Collagen on healing of an extraction socket: an experimental study in the dog. *Int. J. Periodontics Restorative Dent.* (2): 28.

Araujo, M.G., Sukekava, F., Wennstrom, J.L., and Lindhe, J. (2005). Ridge alterations following implant placement in fresh extraction sockets: an experimental study in the dog. *J. Clin. Periodont.* 32 (6): 645–652. https://doi.org/10.1111/j.1600-051X.2005.00726.x.

Araújo, M.G., Sukekava, F., Wennstrom, J.L., and Lindhe, J. (2006). Tissue modeling following implant placement in fresh extraction sockets. *Clin. Oral Implant Res.* 17 (6): 615–624. https://doi.org/10.1111/j.1600-0501.2006.01317.x.

Braut, V., Bornstein, M.M., Belser, U., and Buser, D. (2011). Thickness of the anterior maxillary facial bone wall-a retrospective radiographic study using cone beam computed tomography. *Int. J. Periodontics Restorative Dent.* 31 (2): 125–131.

Buser, D., Chappuis, V., Belser, U.C., and Chen, S. (2017). Implant placement post extraction in esthetic single tooth sites: when immediate, when early, when late? *Periodontology 2000* 73 (1): 84–102.

Chu, S.J., Salama, M.A., Salama, H. et al. (2012). The dual-zone therapeutic concept of managing immediate implant placement and provisional restoration in anterior extraction sockets. *Compend. Contin. Educ. Dent.* 33 (7): 524–532. 534.

Cooke, J.W., Sarment, D.P., Whitesman, L.A. et al. (2006). Effect of rhPDGF-BB delivery on mediators of periodontal wound repair. *Tissue Engineering* 12 (6): 1441–1450. https://doi.org/10.1089/ten.2006.12.1441.

Dibart, S., Sebaoun, J.D., Surmenian, J. (2009). Piezocision: A minimally invasive, periodontally accelerated orthodontic tooth movement procedure. *Compend. Con-tin. Educ. Dent.* 30: 342–350.

Fiorellini, J.P., Howell, T.H., Cochran, D. et al. (2005). Randomized study evaluating recombinant human bone morphogenetic protein-2 for extraction socket augmentation. *Journal of Periodontology* 76 (4): 605–613.

Funato, A., Salama, M.A., Ishikawa, T. et al. (2007). Timing, positioning, and sequential staging in esthetic implant therapy: a four-dimensional perspective. *Int. J. Periodontics Restorative Dent.* 27 (4): 313–323.

Gastaldo, J.F., Cury, P.R., and Sendyk, W.R. (2004). Effect of the vertical and horizontal distances between adjacent implants and between a tooth and an implant on the incidence of interproximal papilla. *J. Periodont.* 75 (9): 1242–1246. https://doi.org/10.1902/jop.2004.75.9.1242.

Grunder, U. (2000). Stability of the mucosal topography around single-tooth implants and adjacent teeth: 1-year results. *Int. J. Periodontics Restorative Dent.* (1): 20.

Grunder, U. (2011). Crestal ridge width changes when placing implants at the time of tooth extraction with and without soft tissue augmentation after a healing period of 6 months: report of 24 consecutive cases. *Int. J. Periodontics Restorative Dent.* 31 (1): 9.

Jung, R.E., Windisch, S.I., Eggenschwiler, A.M. et al. (2009). A randomized-controlled clinical trial evaluating clinical and radiological outcomes after 3 and 5 years of dental implants placed in bone regenerated by means of GBR techniques with or without the addition of BMP-2. *Clin. Oral Implant Res.* 20 (7): 660–666.

Kaigler, D., Avila, G., Wisner-Lynch, L. et al. (2011). Platelet-derived growth factor applications in periodontal and peri-implant bone regeneration. *Expert Opin. Biol. Ther.* 11 (3): 375–385. https://doi.org/10.1517/14712598.2011.554814.

Kan, J.Y., Roe, P., Rungcharassaeng, K. et al. (2011). Classification of sagittal root position in relation to the anterior maxillary osseous housing for immediate implant placement: a cone beam computed tomography study. *Int. J. Oral Maxillofac. Implants* 26 (4): 873–876.

Linkevicius, T., Apse, P., Grybauskas, S., and Puisys, A. (2009). The influence of soft tissue thickness on crestal bone changes around implants: a 1-year prospective controlled clinical trial. *Int. J. Oral Maxillofac. Implants* (4): 24.

McAllister, B.S., Haghighat, K., Prasad, H.S., and Rohrer, M.D. (2010). Histologic evaluation of recombinant human platelet-derived growth factor-BB after use in extraction socket defects: a case series. *Int. J. Periodontics Restorative Dent.* (4): 30.

Nevins, M., Camelo, M., Nevins, M.L. et al. (2003a). Periodontal regeneration in humans using recombinant human platelet-derived growth factor-BB (rhPDGF-BB) and allogenic bone. *J. Periodont.* 74 (9): 1282–1292. https://doi.org/10.1902/jop.2003.74.9.1282.

Nevins, M.L., Camelo, M., Nevins, M., et al. (2009a). Minimally invasive alveolar ridge augmentation procedure (tunneling technique) using rhPDGF-BB in combination with three matrices: A case series. *Int. J. Periodontics Restorative Dent.* 29: 371–383.

Nevins, M., Garber, D., Hanratty, J.J. et al. (2009b). Human histologic evaluation of anorganic bovine bone mineral combined with recombinant human platelet-derived growth factor BB in maxillary sinus augmentation: case series study. *Int. J. Periodontics Restorative Dent.* 29 (6): 583–591.

Nevins, M., Giannobile, W.V., McGuire, M.K. et al. (2005). Platelet-derived growth factor stimulates bone fill and rate of attachment level gain: results of a large multicenter randomized controlled trial. *J. Periodont.* 76 (12): 2205–2215. https://doi.org/10.1902/jop.2005.76.12.2205.

Nevins, M., Kao, R.T., McGuire, M.K. et al. (2013). Platelet-derived growth factor promotes periodontal regeneration in localized osseous defects: 36-month extension results from a randomized, controlled, double-masked clinical trial. *J. Periodont.* 84 (4): 456–464. https://doi.org/10.1902/jop.2012.120141.

Nevins, M.L., Camelo, M., Lynch, S.E. et al. (2003b). Evaluation of periodontal regeneration following grafting intrabony defects with bio-oss collagen: a human histologic report. *Int. J. Periodontics Restorative Dent.* 23 (1): 9–17.

Nevins, M.L. and Said, S. (2018). Minimally invasive esthetic ridge preservation with growth-factor enhanced bone matrix. *J. Esthet. Restor. Dent.* 30 (3): 180–186. https://doi.org/10.1111/jerd.12357.

Salama, H. and Salama, M. (1993). The role of orthodontic extrusive remodeling in the enhancement of soft and hard tissue profiles prior to implant placement: a systematic approach to the management of extraction site defects. *Int. J. Periodontics Restorative Dent.* 13 (4): 312–333.

Simion, M., Rocchietta, I., and Dellavia, C. (2007). Three-dimensional ridge augmentation with xenograft and recombinant human platelet-derived growth factor-BB in humans: report of two cases. *Int. J. Periodontics Restorative Dent.* 27 (2): 109–115.

Spray, J.R., Black, C.G., Morris, H.F., and Ochi, S. (2000). The influence of bone thickness on facial marginal bone response: stage 1 placement through stage 2 uncovering. *Ann. Periodont.* 5 (1): 119–128. https://doi.org/10.1902/annals.2000.5.1.119.

Tettamanti, S., Millen, C., Gavric, J. et al. (2016). Esthetic evaluation of implant crowns and peri-implant soft tissue in the anterior maxilla: comparison and reproducibility of three different indices. *Clin. Implant Dent. Rel. Res.* 18 (3): 517–526. https://doi.org/10.1111/cid.12306.

Triplett, R.G., Nevins, M., Marx, R.E. et al. (2009). Pivotal, randomized, parallel evaluation of recombinant human bone morphogenetic protein-2/absorbable collagen sponge and autogenous bone graft for maxillary sinus floor augmentation. *Int. J. Oral Maxillofac. Implants* 67 (9): 1947–1960.

Waasdorp, J.A., Evian, C.I., Mandracchia, M. (2010). Immediate placement of implants into infected sites: a systematic review of the literature. *J. Periodontol.* 81 (6): 801–808.

Zadeh, H.H. (2011). Minimally invasive treatment of maxillary anterior gingival recession defects by vestibular incision subperiosteal tunnel access and platelet-derived growth factor BB. *Int. J. Periodontics Restorative Dent.* 31: 653–660.

Chapter 13 Digital Technologies in Clinical Restorative Dentistry

Vygandas Rutkūnas, Rokas Borusevičius, Agnė Gečiauskaitė, and Justinas Pletkus

FROM CONVENTIONAL TO DIGITAL TECHNOLOGIES

Dental technologies are undergoing constant development influencing current treatment modalities and founding a basis for the new diagnostic, treatment, and follow-up concepts. In the past dentistry underwent considerable changes with invention and application of anesthesia, X-ray units, turbine handpieces, new restorative materials and many other devices. These changes were associated with economic, social, and technological improvements, which were altered by several industrial revolutions. Introduction of the biological fusion of bone to a foreign material, or osseointegration, a concept first described by Bothe et al. in 1940 and later developed by Prof. P. I. Branemark, reinvigorated the realm of implant dentistry.

The above mentioned developments have relied on analog techniques involving physical means, mechanical and electrical tools (negative and positive molding, hand modeling, lost wax casting technique, etc.), with no digital component and are called conventional or analog techniques. Many of them have been improved to the level of high precision and even today serve as a gold standard.

However, with the third industrial revolution, came the rise in electronics, computers, telecommunications, and other fields, which opened the doors to the digitalization of healthcare. The first dental CAD/CAM was invented in 1973 by French professor François Duret, who first described the principles of optical dental impressions. The Nobel Prize in Physiology or Medicine 1979 was awarded jointly to Allan M. Cormack and Godfrey N. Hounsfield "for the development of computer assisted tomography." Digital dentistry consistently evolved, continuously integrating with the conventional workflow and forming an array of dental devices:

- Intraoral scanners (IOS) including photogrammetry-based intraoral scanning;
- Laboratory and chair-side CAD/CAM systems;
- Face scanners;
- Caries diagnosis devices;
- Computer-aided implant dentistry and oral surgery (designing and production of implant placement guides, cutting guides, etc.);
- Surgical and restorative navigation systems with augmented reality (AR);
- Digital radiography, cone beam computed tomography (CBCT), magnetic resonance imaging (MRI);
- Piezoelectric handpieces;
- Occlusion and TMJ analysis and diagnosis tools;
- Extraoral and intraoral photo and video cameras;
- Spectrophotometers and colorimeters for shade matching;
- Dental lasers;
- Computerized dental anesthesia;
- Practice and patient record management – including digital patient education;
- Haptic devices;
- Additive manufacturing (AM) devices;
- Robotics;
- Others.

Practical Advanced Periodontal Surgery, Second Edition. Edited by Serge Dibart.
© 2020 John Wiley & Sons, Inc. Published 2020 by John Wiley & Sons, Inc.
Companion website: www.wiley.com/go/dibart/advanced

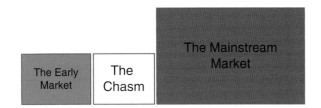

Figure 13.1 Adapted from technology adoption life cycle. Source: http://www.insightsquared.com/2016/01/the-saas-startup-guide-to-crossing-the-chasm.

These technologies in general follow the technology adoption life cycle which vary in duration and intensity (Figure 13.1). It is not clear if some of the currently developed technologies will cross the so-called "chasm" and will be used by the majority of practitioners.

Nowadays, IOS, CBCT, CAD/CAM, and other systems are used extensively in daily practice. Merging of the images from various sources (IOS, lab scanner, CBCT, face scanner, digital camera) make the foundation for the "digital patient" concept. Fully-digital workflow now is a reality, especially for less extensive cases. While more extensive cases (e.g. full-arch restorations) still involve hybrid digital–conventional procedures.

Digital technologies have empowered the conventional techniques giving the opportunity for less invasive, more controlled, faster, cheaper, and longer-lasting treatment modalities, such as full-arch four implant-supported restorations (Ayub et al. 2017).

Currently available digital technologies are changing the face of dentistry, forming new diagnostic (combining the CBCT and ultrasonography data) (Chan et al. 2017), treatment (accelerated orthodontic treatment) (Piezocision™ 2016), lab production (3D printing of dental ceramics) (Dehurtevent et al. 2017), follow-up (superimposition of IOS data) (Hartkamp et al. 2017), and educational (AR) (Kwon et al. 2018) tools. It is a huge challenge for practitioners to adapt to these changes and to decide which technology is worth the investment and can provide reasonable return on investment (ROI). Switching from analog to digital workflow comes with the need to update professional terms. The American College of Prosthodontics (ACP) has issued the Glossary of Digital Dental Terms (Grant et al. 2016). Dental practices are facing demands to collect and store large amounts of 2D and 3D images. Due to increased sharing of sensitive data, adhering to guidelines, such as the Health Insurance Portability and Accountability Act (HIPPA) Privacy Rule and Security Rule becomes more crucial.

DIGITAL SOLUTIONS FOR PLANNING AND MANUFACTURING OF TEETH-SUPPORTED RESTORATIONS

Digital Tools for Analysis and Treatment Planning

The first papers discussing utilization of photography for smile analysis were published in the 1990s (Wichmann 1990). Over the years it has evolved to advanced techniques for design of restorations in the esthetic zone using Powerpoint, Keynote, or Photoshop software packages (Arias et al. 2015; Sundar and Chelliah 2018). In this way the 2D design was planned based on the facial and dental landmarks, such as:

- facial midline;
- inter-pupillary, commissural line;
- upper teeth exposure during rest, speech, and smiling, which in turn depends on: (i) mobility of the lips; (ii) vertical length of upper lip; (iii) clinical crown length; (iv) skeletal relationships (Ritter et al. 2006);
- buccal corridor;
- smile line;
- lower lip line during smiling;
- exposure of the incisal edge;
- dental midline;
- proportions of the width and length of the teeth;
- progressive axial inclinations of the anterior teeth;
- papilla and teeth height ratio;
- some others, including anterior teeth contact areas, incisal frames, etc.

Subsequently, terms such as digital smile, virtual smile, digital smile design, etc. and protocols have been reported by different authors (Ackerman and Ackerman 2002; Coachman and Paravina 2016; McLaren et al. 2013). Sets of standardized facial and dental photographs are taken and imported to the above mentioned programs or special software, dedicated to digital smile design (e.g. DSD App, Smile Designer Pro, Romexis smile design, 3Shape smile design, etc.). Based on the facial midline, inter-pupillary, commissural, and additional lines the rotational calibration of the image is done (Figure 13.2.1). Preferred reference points are selected in order to calibrate the photos of retracted and non-retracted smile (Figure 13.2.2). In order to do the measurements at the design stage, the calibrated ruler should be used indicating real intraoral measurements (e.g. length of the central incisor, width of the central incisors, etc.) (Figure 13.2.3). Based on the preferred esthetic landmarks and biological aspects the esthetic framework of the anterior teeth is defined and outline of the restorations is selected in frontal, occlusal and 12 o'clock projections (Figure 13.2.4). To facilitate the process, different libraries of the teeth shape can be used and adjusted based on the patient or dentist preferences. The simulation of the final result can also be done in order to better communicate the planned result to the patient (Figure 13.2.5). The concept of visagism is also used and allows clinicians to design the shape of the teeth that blends the patient's physical appearance, personality, and desires (Visagism: The Art of Dental Composition 2018). Patients can evaluate the planning and 2D dental after final adjustments, which can then be transferred to the lab for further procedures: wax-up (digital or analog), model or mock-up, or restoration fabrication (Figure 13.2.6).

However, it should be understood that such 2D planning should be taken as guidance, rather than a precise and final treatment plan. The shortcomings of such 2D planning are related to the fact that only static images are taken, under certain lighting conditions and projection. It has been shown that lighting conditions can affect the buccal corridor appearance on smile photography (Ritter et al. 2006). Another disadvantage is that planning is done based mainly on esthetic criteria and fails to address biological and functional circumstances. Despite these aspects, 2D digital design is a very informative tool enhancing communication between dentist, patient, and dental technician.

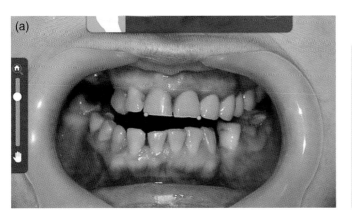

Figure 13.2.1 Rotational calibration of the face photo based on the facial horizontal and vertical lines.

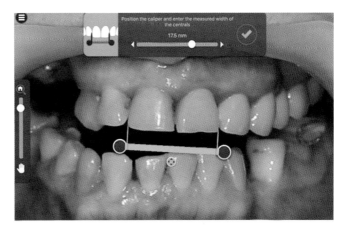

Figure 13.2.3 Calibration of the dimensions is done with the ruler, in order to indicate measurements on the final smile design version.

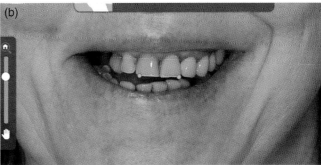

Figure 13.2.2 Photos of retracted and non-retracted smile are calibrated by selecting reference points.

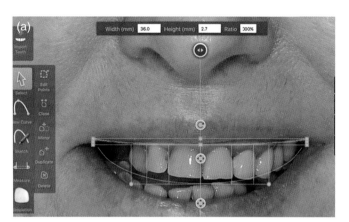
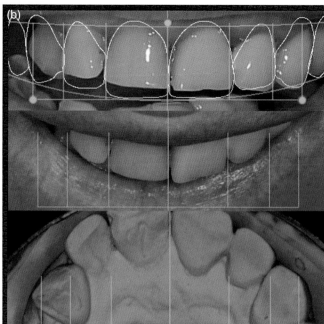

Figure 13.2.4 Esthetic framework has been determined from the frontal, 12 o'clock, and occlusal aspects considering esthetic and biologic aspects.

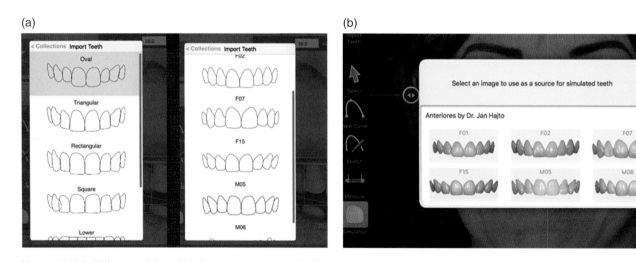

Figure 13.2.5 Different teeth form libraries can be employed to facilitate the smile design process and to create realistic simulation of the planned result.

After completion of the 2D design, it is transferred to the 3D design step, which can be done either on a conventional model or a digital model. There are different ways to align a 2D model to a 3D model, however these techniques inevitably involve a certain level of inaccuracy. For this reason, it would be more beneficial to proceed straight to 3D design, avoiding limitations of 2D treatment planning.

Merging of several 3D images obtained from face scanner, CBCT, IOS, combining it with virtual articulator and 2D intraoral and extraoral photographs, currently provides the maximum diagnostic potential for complex treatment planning (Figure 13.2.7). Based on this, not only esthetic,

but also biological and functional aspects can be addressed in a more detailed way.

Based on 3D planning, mock-ups, or temporary restorations can be fabricated paying much attention to the smile design. Mock-up is a very powerful tool helping to evaluate esthetics, phonetics, and occlusal relationships and gives a perfect opportunity for the patient to evaluate planned final results (Simon and Magne 2008). Moreover, it is very useful for guiding preparations of the teeth and ensuring minimal invasiveness during this and subsequent steps (Figure 13.2.8). The application of the mock-up can be limited in cases where extensive crown lengthening and reduction of the tooth structure is anticipated.

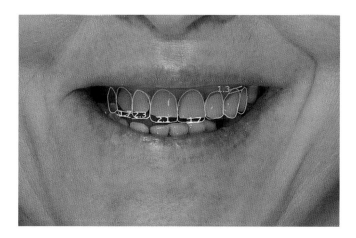

Figure 13.2.6 Planned smile design of upper anterior teeth with calibrated measurements of anticipated modifications.

Surgical crown lengthening can be planned in a similar way by using patients' CBCT, IOS data, and digital photographs. Fusion of these images can provide valuable information about the needed extent of the gingivectomy and bone reduction. Based on 2D design, digital wax-up can be accomplished and a 3D printed model produced. Silicon index can be prepared on the 3D printed model and mock-up or directly made temporary restorations applied at the same visit (Figure 13.2.9).

Clinical Applications of Digital Techniques in Tooth-Supported Restorations

Currently, the digital workflow can cover production of all types of indirect restorations from partial crowns to removable dentures. However, extended and complex cases

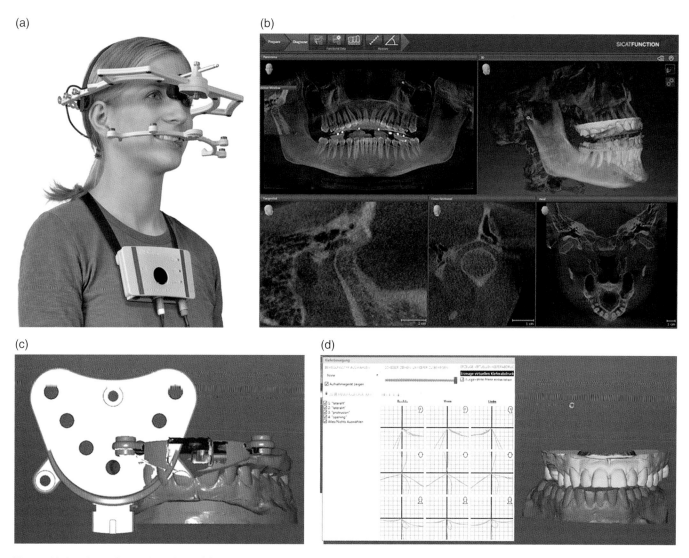

Figure 13.2.7 Lower jaw tracking device (a) can be used with CBCT data, allowing capability of functional CBCT, where individual patient movements can be simulated on the mandible (b). With the aid of a special fork (c), the position of the maxilla as well as mandibular movement data file can be imported to the CAD system, enabling reproduction of individual mandibular movements on virtual articulator and manufacturing dental prostheses with functional occlusion design (d).

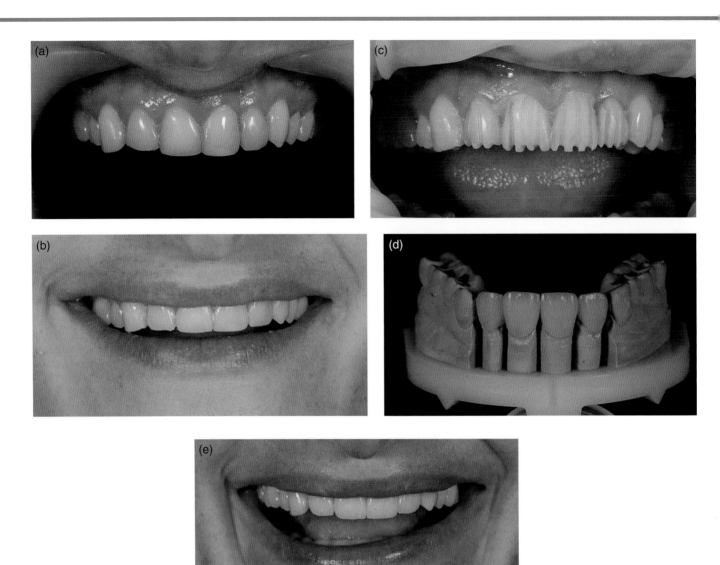

Figure 13.2.8 Restorative treatment for upper incisors (a) was planned using smile design and mock-up (b). Tooth reduction through mock-up (c) enabled controlling reduction of the teeth and thickness of the restorations (d). Final result (e) was achieved in a controlled way based on the initial plan.

can still be challenging. Therefore, hybrid workflow including both analog and digital techniques can be employed.

Three-dimensional accuracy of digital impression with IOS is of crucial importance. In addition, the ability of different IOS algorithms to interpret finish lines is also essential. It has been reported that color output from IOS may enhance the identification of the finish line due to contrasting colors, but is still dependent on the underlying technology (Nedelcu et al. 2018). Many studies have been published reporting similar accuracy level at the margin of digitally and conventionally produced single crowns (Boeddinghaus et al. 2015). However, some of them have reached conclusions, that conventional impression and pressed restorations produced more accurate 2D and 3D margin fits (Anadioti et al. 2014).

The procedure for the single crowns is straightforward – digital impression with IOS is taken after preparation. CAD design can be done chairside or in the lab using the pre-preparation method, mirroring the opposite tooth form and designed individually using automated processes (Arslan et al. 2015). Many features, including occlusal surface anatomy, cut-back technique, cement gap, distance to margin and others, can be controlled during the CAD design phase (Figure 13.2.10a). A virtual articulator can be used to simulate mandibular movements and automatically adjust the shape of the prosthesis (Figure 13.2.10b). Master cast is an obligatory step in conventional restoration fabrication workflow. While in digital workflow full-contour restorations can be made, avoiding this step. A 3D printed or milled model is needed in order to proceed with layered restorations and/or adapt the margins (Figure 13.2.10c). However, 3D printed models still need to be validated considering 3D accuracy in general, finish line accuracy, die repositioning, resulting inter-arch relationship of the models, occlusal contacts, etc. Some studies have indicated, that the conventional method of die fabrication was more reliable than that of investigated 3D printers (Park and Shin 2018).

Due to the increased optical features (natural shade, translucency, multi-layered blank, etc.) of ceramic CAD/CAM materials, full contour restorations became more esthetically appealing and a standard procedure for the posterior teeth.

More complex restorations involving multiple teeth, reorganization of occlusion, and layered restorations currently are more reliably implemented through the mixing of

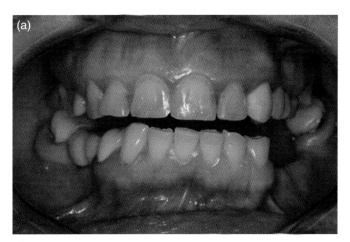

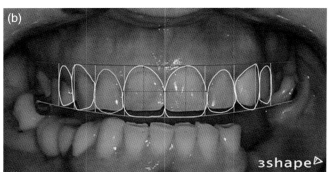

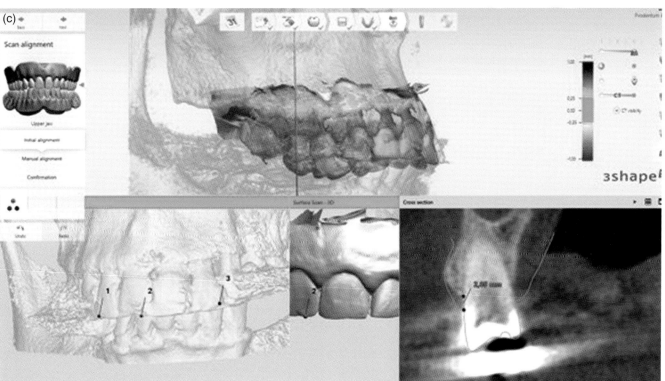

Figure 13.2.9 Patient with worn dentition had esthetic demands (a), therefore 2D digital planning of the smile was done (b). Based on CBCT and IOS data, prospective margin of the restoration was planned and need for the bone reduction estimated (c). 3D printed surgical guide for crown-lengthening was produced (d). Digital wax-up was done, taking 2D planning as guidance (e and f) and models produced with a 3D printer. Silicon indexes were produced on 3D printed models (g and h) and used for mock-up, in order to evaluate esthetics, phonetics, and occlusion (i). Later, surgical guide was used as the reference in order to perform crown lengthening.

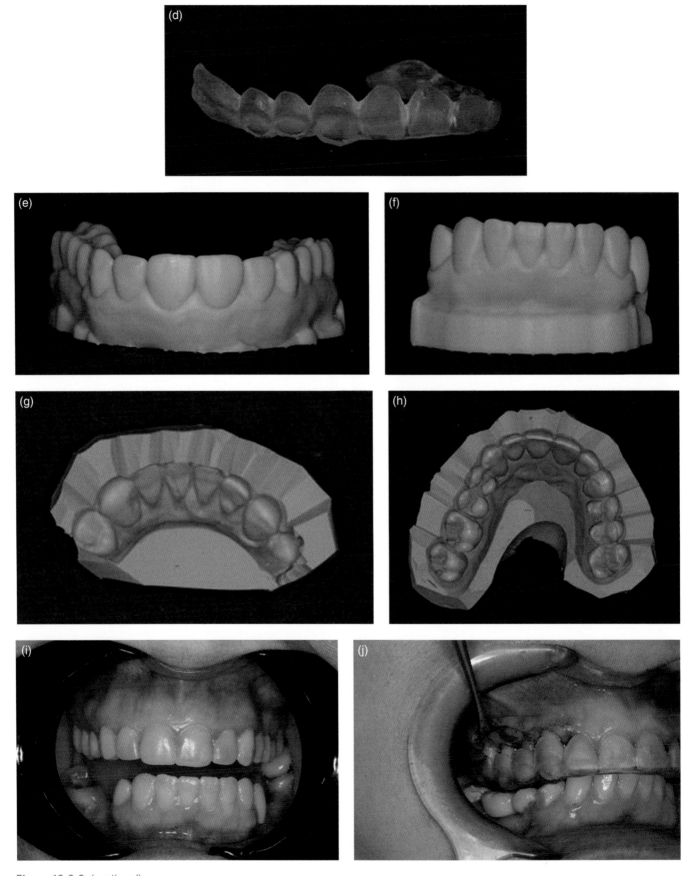

Figure 13.2.9 *(continued)*

(a)

(b)

(c)

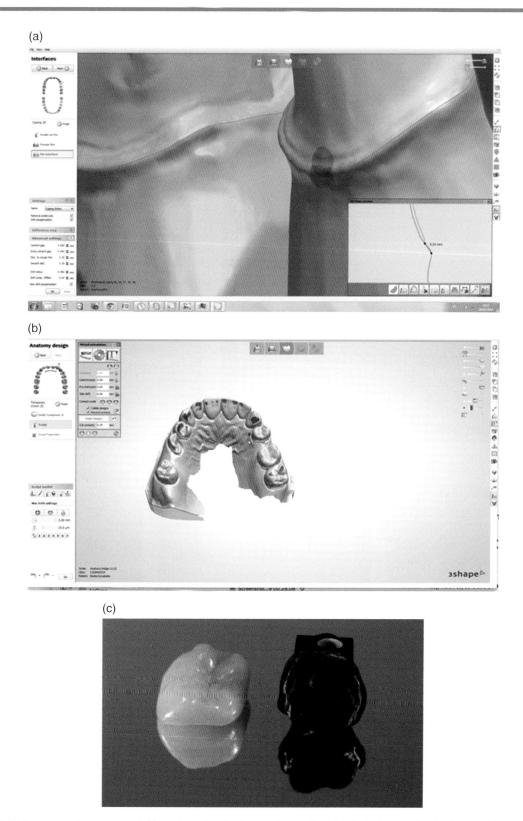

Figure 13.2.10 CAD software offers many useful tools to control the design of restorations (a), including the virtual articulator (b). A monolithic full-contour crown from translucent multi-layered zirconia blank was milled, infiltrated, stained, and glazed after taking digital impression and using CAD design. Die was printed using a 3D printer in order to adjust the margins of the restoration (c).

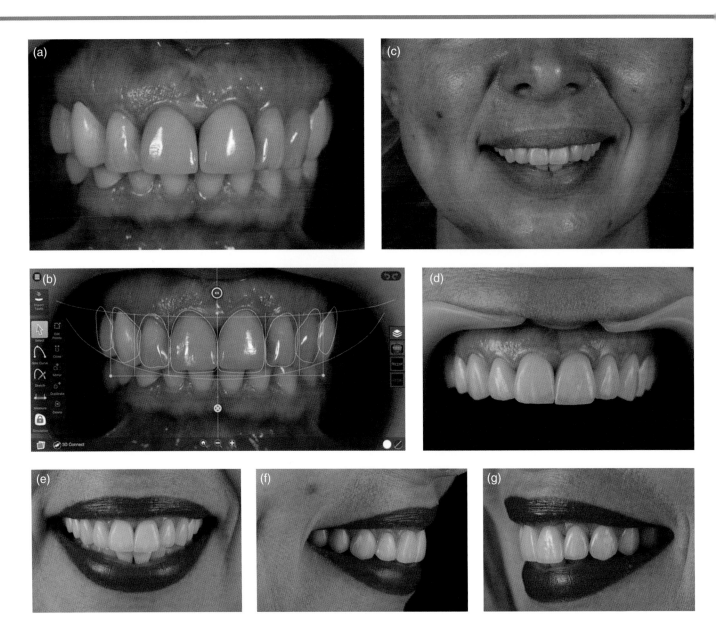

Figure 13.2.11 Hybrid conventional-digital method was utilized to restore upper and lower dentition. After initial situation evaluation (a), digital design and mock-up (b and c) was made. Conventional impressions were used to fabricate master models, and CAD design was applied based on data from digital design, mock-up, or temporary restoration phase. Restorations were finalized (d–g) according to the initial treatment plan.

conventional and digital techniques. Digital smile design in 2D can be done during initial examination and used for the digital wax-up, which through the 3D printed model can be used to fabricate mock-up and evaluate esthetic and functional aspects (Figure 13.2.11). Mock-up can be modified and scanned with IOS. This data can be used for the fabrication of temporary CAD/CAM restorations maintaining the 3D shape of the tested mock-up. After endodontic and periodontal treatment, conventional impressions and bite registrations are done and a plaster cast is scanned with a laboratory scanner. Shade determination is done using digital photography and spectrophotometry. During the CAD process, 3D data of mock-up and temporary restorations can be superimposed and used as the

reference. To control the contour of the restorations during the layering of ceramics, silicon indices should be used.

Digital technologies are increasingly applied to aid fabrication of the removable prostheses. The classic approach is to use CAD software to design the framework of the removable partial denture (RPD), to print it from the wax and cast the metal alloy framework. A combination of digital and analog techniques is more common due to many reasons. Firstly, muco-static or muco-compressive impression taking techniques and border molding could be employed only with conventional impression techniques. Secondly, in cases where fixed and removable prostheses are combined, the digital workflow is not well established, especially when extracoronal attachments are planned to be used. Thirdly, not all clinical situations allow the use of artificial teeth that are available in digital libraries. However, with the advances in new CAD/CAM and materials, attachment components and major connectors as well as denture bases can be milled and 3D printed (Figure 13.2.12).

Advantages and Limitations

Digital workflow offers many new opportunities in diagnostic, treatment, and follow-up stages. Merging of data from various devices (CBCT, face scanner, digital camera, IOS) provides an ultimate possibility for comprehensive diagnosis and treatment planning. From the perspective of the dentist, the preparation for the impression taking remains the same: proper preparation design and retraction techniques are still prerequisite for an excellent impression. However, verification of the quality of the impression can be performed during the procedure and digital impression can be corrected at ease by re-scanning specific areas of the teeth and soft tissues. Clearance at the occlusal and axial surfaces can also be verified instantly. Some IOS have an integrated shade measurement tool, allowing selection of the shade of the restoration at the same step of impression taking. Also, there is no risk of 3D distortion when data is kept digitally. Moreover, digital data is easy to share, which save the costs of transportation. With advances in ceramic materials, monolithic restorations are becoming more and more popular. Avoiding the layering step enables better fulfillment of the planned shape of the restorations and takes dentist–technician–patient communication to the next level. In this way the CAD design phase can be also facilitated as standard and custom teeth shape libraries can be employed. Fabrication of full-contour restorations from the digital impressions allows dental technicians to avoid master-cast fabrications, hence the laboratory step takes less time and productivity is increased. Patients can benefit from the digital workflow as their situation is better visualized, and their final treatment plan is better communicated and controlled. They can also benefit from more comfortable impression taking procedures and reduced treatment time. Digital workflow does not eliminate the human factor completely; however, it enables an increase in the level of standardization of restorative procedures, as well as reliability. Digital tools can be very efficient for follow-up procedures, e.g. visualizing the wear of the teeth.

However, the high price of digital technologies prevents some practitioners from using them. Due to rapid improvements, time span for the ROI could be too short. The learning curve for some of the devices could be steep and the workflow sometimes cannot be integrated between different devices and software packages. Current levels of digital impression techniques, do not allow to completely get rid of elastomeric impression materials, as they are still needed for more complex fixed and removable situations. In case of deep subgingival margins, elastomeric materials, in contrast to optical impressions, are able to displace the soft tissues and record it. A recent study stated that the curvature (sharpness) of the margin recorded by a commercial IOS is significantly affected by clinical factors obscuring visibility (close interproximal contacts, etc.) (Arslan et al. 2015). Using CAD/CAM systems, it could be complicated to mill thin margins of the ceramic restorations. If the master cast is needed (e.g. layered restoration), the model should be 3D printed, which inflicts additional cost and potential problems of accuracy. Strict regulations should be followed to ensure secure sharing and storing of digital records.

DIGITAL SOLUTIONS FOR PLANNING AND MANUFACTURING OF IMPLANT-SUPPORTED RESTORATIONS

Implant and Implant-Supported Restoration Planning with Digital Tools

Planning, Analysis (CBCT, Radiological Guides, Dual-Scan, Surgical Guides, Dynamic Guidance)

Treatment planning is of foremost importance for the prosthetically driven dental implant placement. Technologies, including CBCT, IOS, enabled clinicians to evaluate soft and hard tissues with an accurate precision prior to any surgical intervention. This data in combination with improving computer software allows to plan implant position regarding these tissues and future prosthesis. Finally, surgical guidance systems are used to transfer the planned implant position to the patient's mouth.

CBCT with specially made radiological guides or existing prostheses converted to radiological guides, is of great diagnostic value, helping to decide more favorable implant location, which is also suitable from the prosthetic point of view.

CBCT and IOS data can be merged and virtual tooth set-up accomplished, followed by production of the surgical guide for dental implant placement. The surgical guide can be used only for the pilot drill during implantation, as well as for fully-guided implant insertion. Many studies have evaluated the accuracy of fully-guided implant insertion. A recent systematic review reported a mean implant deviation at the entry point of 1.25 mm, 1.57 mm at the apex, and 4.1° in angle with fully-guided implantation protocol. A totally guided system using fixation screws with a flapless protocol demonstrated the greatest accuracy (Zhou et al. 2018). This level of accuracy in general is not adequate for the fabrication of final restorations based on planned implant positions. Nonetheless, this principle can be applied to a limited extent with less

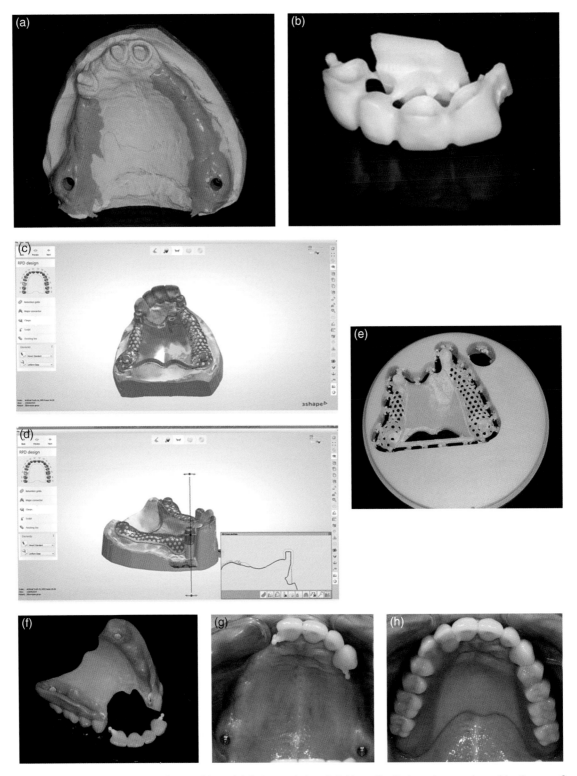

Figure 13.2.12 Tooth- and implant-supported removable partial denture and zirconia bridge with attachments were planned for the case. Conventional impressions were taken and master cast fabricated (a). CAD software was used to design zirconia fixed partial denture with extracoronal attachments, according to the selected path of insertion, which was done using digital parallelometer (b). Traditional pick-up impression was taken with seated FPD and overdenture attachments on implants. Master cast was scanned and CAD design or RPD was made (c). Using digital tools, isolation in the area of minor connectors, finish lines, and thickness of the RPD framework can be easily controlled (d). High performance polymer PEEK blank was used to mill RPD framework (e). Denture teeth were set and acrylics heat processed in a traditional way. Corresponding parts of the RPD attachments were glued to the RPD and prosthesis finalized (f). Prosthesis was delivered to the patient and currently in service for four years (g and h).

extensive rehabilitations. Besides static dental implant placement, dynamic navigation surgery is also a possibility (Block and Emery 2016).

Digital implant impressions (DII) with IOS can be taken at the implant and multi-unit abutment level using specific scan bodies. DII can also be taken from the custom prosthetic abutment. 3D scan body position recorded by DII is very important, as dental implants lack periodontal ligament and cannot compensate even minor misfit due to the absence of mobility. The level of misfit that could be acceptable clinically is fiercely debated in the literature. Marginal gaps and static strains due to screw tightening were not found to have negative effects on initial osseointegration or peri-implant bone stability over time (Katsoulis et al. 2017). A few clinical studies reported that the risk for technical screw-related complications was slightly higher. Clinical tools are lacking in order to evaluate objectively the fit of implant-supported restorations. Therefore, it is useful to combine several techniques to assess the accuracy of fit (Abduo et al. 2010).

Clinical Applications of Digital Techniques in Implant-Supported Restorations

Similar principles as with tooth-supported restorations can be employed in the diagnostic and treatment planning phase of implant-supported restorations.

Digital techniques are very useful in producing temporary restorations on implants, as teeth form before the extraction can be used as a reference, peri-implant tissue thickness and possibility to shape it can be evaluated well during the 3D design (Figure 13.3.1). Later, the shape of temporary restorations can be duplicated into the final restoration. Spectrophotometers can be used in order to accurately reproduce the shade of the neighboring teeth, as well as to evaluate the color change of the peri-implant tissues with different types of abutment materials.

One abutment–one time concept may be offered in order to avoid the irritation of the peri-implant tissues during re-insertion of the healing abutment. For this purpose, split file of the custom abutment and temporary restoration can be designed and fabricated using CAD/CAM (Figure 13.3.2). This approach can be used in different stages of the treatment: during implant planning, shortly after implant placement, and during the second stage surgery. Custom abutment can be made from different materials: metal alloy, zirconia, or polymer.

One abutment–one time can be used in combination with fully-guided implant placement, when final abutments and temporary restorations on them are produced before surgical procedures (Figure 13.3.3). Deviation of implant positions from the planned one will prevent prosthetic components from being placed. Therefore, this technique is limited to cases of one or two missing teeth. Best practice should be used in order to increase accuracy of fully-guided implant surgery.

As accuracy of fully-guided surgery is still not satisfactory and does not enable producing screw-retained implant-supported restorations before the surgery, selected cases with adequate primary implant stability can be treated using one crown–one time concept (Figure 13.3.4). This technique became available due to improved accuracy of DII and CAM techniques, allowing usage of pre-milled blocks of ceramic materials.

Integration of digitally planed implant positions and CAD/CAM temporary and final restorations can be accomplished in full-arch cases as well. However, DII, bite registration, and 3D printing accuracy is not well documented for full-arch implant-supported cases. Therefore, parts of the workflow still have to rely on conventional techniques (Figure 13.3.5).

Advantages and Limitations

Based on CBCT data, challenging anatomical situations can be addressed and a proper treatment plan selected. Radiological and surgical guides allow placing implants in a prosthetically oriented manner. With increased accuracy of implant placement and improvements in digital prosthesis fabrication techniques, treatment time can be shortened, risks minimized, and more predictable results achieved.

However, CBCT images can be distorted by metallic artifacts, patient movement, etc. complicating alignment with the images obtained from IOS. Due to multiple factors (IOS, 3D printing accuracy, movement of the teeth, mobility of mucosa, sleeve related factors, etc.) fully-guided implant placement is still lacking the accuracy level needed in order to integrate it better with prosthodontic procedures.

Despite IOS continuously being improved, there are still limitations to their use. IOS accuracy could be compromised by many aspects: movements of the object, saliva, fogging of the optics, occlusion registration challenges, and other patient-, operator-, and device-related limiting factors (Rutkūnas et al. 2017). Scanning location can be important, as distant regions could be difficult to reach in a real clinical situation. Length of the edentulous ridge, lack of attached gingiva, tongue, and cheek mobility could also negatively affect the ability to stitch images. Scanning strategy and mode have also been demonstrated to be important aspects (Müller et al. 2016). Repositioning accuracy of scan bodies and other prosthetic components could be another source of limitations.

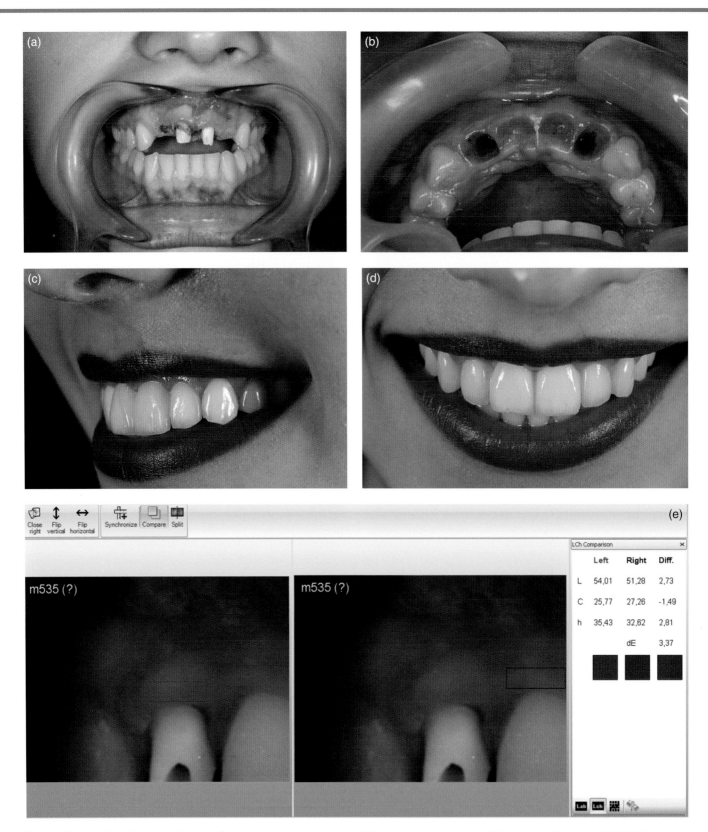

Figure 13.3.1 Initial clinical situation resulting from previous dental trauma (a). Implant placement and soft tissue formation using CAD/CAM temporary restorationas (b). Final restoration was produced taking temporary restorations as a reference (images from the frontal and side aspect – c and d). Abutment material effect on the color of the peri-implant tissues can be selected by using spectrophotometry readings (e).

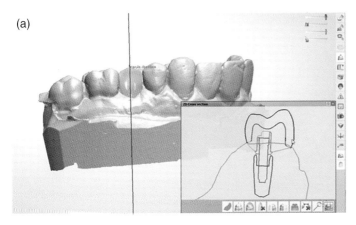

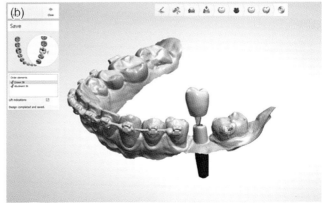

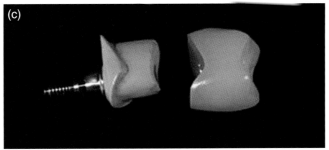

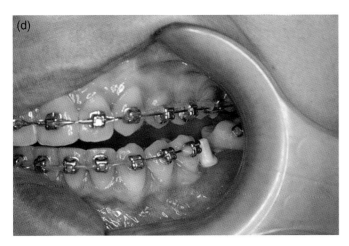

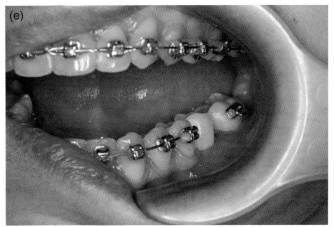

Figure 13.3.2 Custom abutment and temporary cement-retained crown is designed in the CAD (a and b). Abutment can be milled from zirconia and cemented on the titanium base (c). Temporary crown on the abutment can be cemented extraorally. Custom abutment is placed in the mouth and attached permanently using the final torque indicated by the manufacturer (d). Temporary crown is placed on custom abutment (e). After soft tissue healing, margin on the custom abutment can be modified and abutment level impression taken for the final restoration.

Complex cases would need 3D printed models, which still lack the required level of accuracy. Conventional techniques today still have the edge with certain procedures: edentulous cases, VDO increase, implant-supported overdentures, etc.

FUTURE PERSPECTIVES

The currently developing fourth industrial revolution (4IR) is about to affect and disrupt all kinds of industry. Fusion of digital, physical, and biological realms is characteristic for 4IR. Developments in fields of robotics, nanotechnology, biotechnology, 3D printing, artificial intelligence (AI), virtual, and AR are very common, including the fact that available knowledge nowadays is shared between billions of people.

Fusion of 3D and 2D data from various sources made the foundation for the concept of "the virtual patient" and has further improved. This enables diagnostic, treatment, and follow-up capabilities at much better level. Due to this, requirements to store, share, and protect huge amounts of data continue to increase. Large amounts of medical information create a challenge of correct interpretation of the

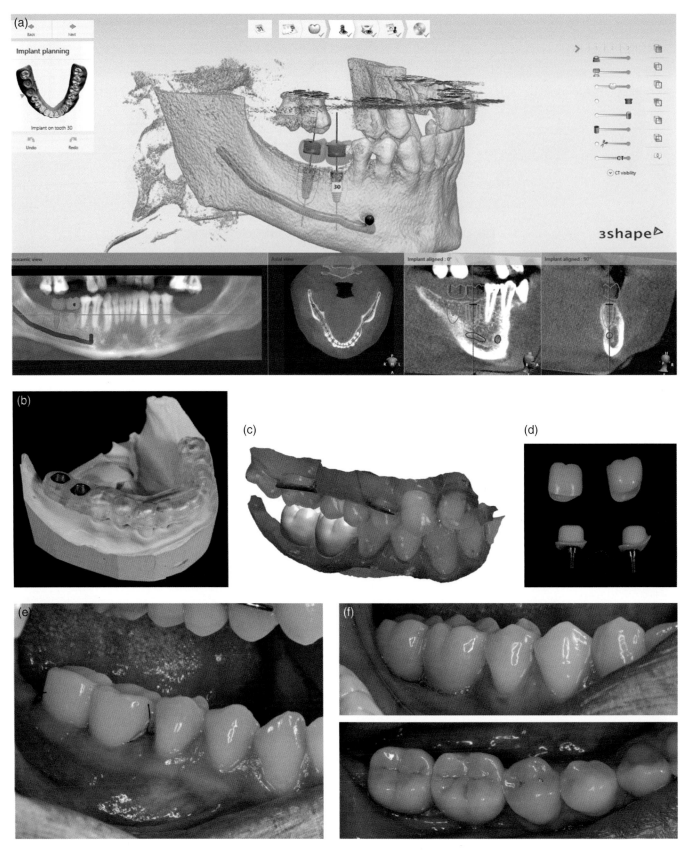

Figure 13.3.3 A two implant placement was planned as a fully-guided procedure (a and b). Using the planned implant positions, final zirconia abutments and temporary crowns were planned using split file (c and d). After fully-guided implant placement, custom zirconia abutments were tightened and temporary crowns placed and evaluated for the need for adjustment (e). Final full-contour zirconia crowns were made two months after implant placement (f).

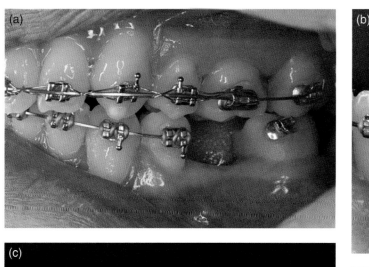

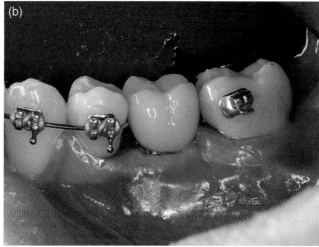

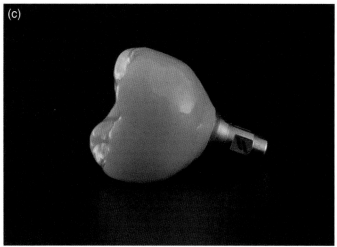

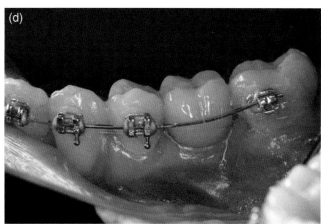

Figure 13.3.4 Implant was planned in the site of missing molar tooth (a). Right after the implant placement DII was taken to record implant position and the occlusion relationship. During the next few hours full-contour ceramic crown was produced and cemented to the titanium base (b). Screw-retained crown was delivered on the same day under functional loading conditions (c). Restoration is now followed for a period of one year (d).

data. Moreover, static images are more and more supplemented with dynamic 3D data, e.g. dynamic face scanner, filming of mandibular movements with IOS, integrating data from jaw tracking devices with CAD and CBCT software. New to dentistry, future imaging technologies like OCT (optical coherent tomography), MSCT (multi-slice computerized tomography), traditional, and dynamic MRI and others are making their way in to clinical applications.

AR is used to show the planned esthetic outcome to the patient in real time (Figure 13.4). There is huge potential for integrating AR into surgical and restorative procedures.

IOS usage for taking impressions revolutionized prosthodontics. However, clinical procedures before taking digital impressions from the teeth remain virtually the same, including proper gingival retraction techniques and fluid control. Ability to supplement optical impression with OCT, ultrasound, or other technology enabling avoidance of gingival retraction could substantially change this clinical step. Accuracy of IOS for full-arch scanning and bite

registration techniques should be further improved as currently complex cases belong more to the conventional side. Digital workflow should further be supplemented with more accurate and faster 3D printing technology.

Many advantages of digital workflow come from the array of dental materials that can be conveniently used only with CAM equipment. CAM techniques enable high precision and standardization of the work, minimizing the human factor. Multi-layered restorations are becoming more and more popular as this allows for dental restorations with a more natural appearance, with zones of different translucency and color. This potential could be further increased with additive technologies (e.g. 3D printing of ceramic materials) enabling production of different mechanical, physical, and optical features at different volumes of the restoration. AMF and other similar production file formats will be used for this instead of STL. Subtractive and additive technologies are expected to be able to produce ultrathin restorations of good mechanical properties in order to reduce invasiveness of restorative procedures.

Digital Technologies in Clinical Restorative Dentistry **229**

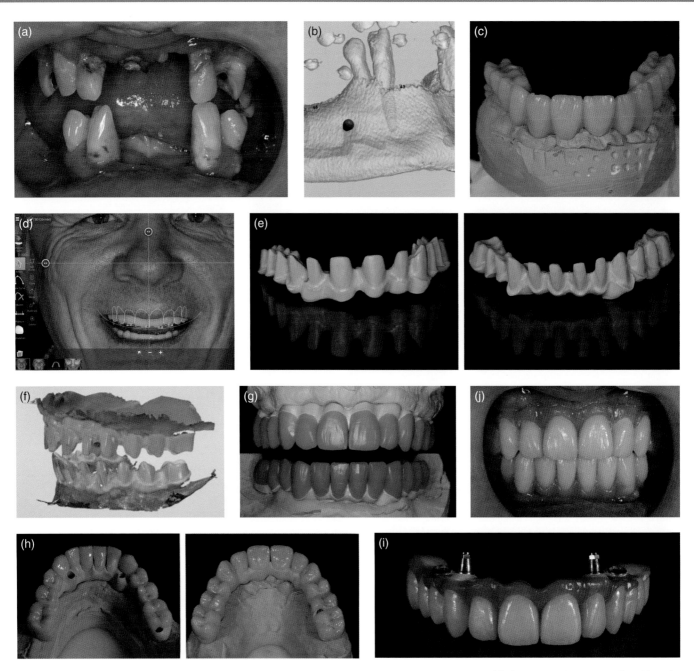

Figure 13.3.5 Full-arch implant-supported fixed prostheses were planned for a patient with failing dentition (a). Surgical guides were produced based on CBCT double scan technique with radiological guides (b). Immediately after teeth extraction and implant placement, milled temporary restorations were produced (c). Based on digital smile design (d), shape of the final restorations was designed in CAD software and substructure from high performance polymer (PEEK) was produced (e). After fitting substructure intraorally, digital bite registration with IOS was accomplished (f). Full contour individual crowns were milled from wax (g) and pressed from lithium-disilicate ceramics (h). Gingival part was modeled with composite resin (i) and prosthesis delivered to the patient (j).

Direct additive technologies allowing avoidance of laboratory steps are also under development.

Besides 3D printing of models and restorations, bio-printing of the soft and hard tissue scaffolds with and without cell cultures could offer new possibilities in cases demanding regenerative procedures which can be combined with dental implant placement and restorative procedures.

AI will increase efficiency of diagnostic and treatment algorithms and automation will be used more in the production of dental restorations. Mobile health applications will continue to improve oral public health (e.g. BruxApp application to assess awake bruxism). Telemedicine in dentistry is expanding, with some attempts to exclude local dental offices. First attempts have been demonstrated of autonomous robotic dental implant placement.

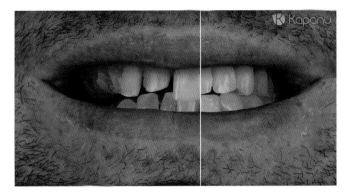

Figure 13.4 Kapanu AR application (Ivoclar Vivadent) allows visualization of planned anterior restorations in real time.

Though many advanced digital technologies are currently available in the market, high prices are limiting their wider application into clinical practice. It should be also mentioned that traditional literature is struggling to catch up with rapidly improvements in hardware and software for dental digital solutions.

ACKNOWLEDGMENTS

We thank very much dental technicians Tomas Simonaitis and Aušra Kleizienė for the laboratory work that was used in the figures, as well as for their positive and supportive attitude.

REFERENCES

Abduo, J., Bennani, V., Waddell, N. et al. (2010 Jun). Assessing the fit of implant fixed prostheses: a critical review. *Int. J. Oral Maxillofac. Implants* 25 (3): 506–515.

Ackerman, M.B. and Ackerman, J.L. (2002 Apr). Smile analysis and design in the digital era. *J. Clin. Orthod.: JCO* 36 (4): 221–236.

Anadioti, E., Aquilino, S.A., Gratton, D.G. et al. (2014 Dec). 3D and 2D marginal fit of pressed and CAD/CAM lithium disilicate crowns made from digital and conventional impressions. *J. Prosthodont. Off. J. Am. Coll. Prosthodont.* 23 (8): 610–617.

Arias, D.M., Trushkowsky, R.D., Urea, I.M. and David, S.B. (2015 Jul). Treatment of the patient with gummy smile in conjunction with digital smile approach. *Dent. Clin. N. Am.* 59 (3): 703–716.

Arslan, Y., Karakoca Nemli, S., Bankoğlu Güngör, M. et al. (2015 Dec). Evaluation of biogeneric design techniques with CEREC CAD/CAM system. *J. Adv. Prosthodont.* 7 (6): 431–436.

Ayub, K.V., Ayub, E.A., Lins do Valle, A. et al. (2017 Dec). Seven-year follow-up of full-arch prostheses supported by four implants: a prospective study. *Int. J. Oral Maxillofac. Implants* 32 (6): 1351–1358.

Block, M.S. and Emery, R.W. (2016 Feb). Static or dynamic navigation for implant placement–choosing the method of guidance. *J. Oral Maxillofac. Surg. Off. J. Am. Assoc. Oral Maxillofac. Surg.* 74 (2): 269–277.

Boeddinghaus, M., Breloer, E.S., Rehmann, P., and Wöstmann, B. (2015 Nov). Accuracy of single-tooth restorations based on intraoral digital and conventional impressions in patients. *Clin. Oral Investig.* 19 (8): 2027–2034.

Chan, H.-L., Wang, H.-L., Fowlkes, J.B. et al. (2017 Mar). Non-ionizing real-time ultrasonography in implant and oral surgery: a feasibility study. *Clin. Oral Implants Res.* 28 (3): 341–347.

Coachman, C. and Paravina, R.D. (2016 Mar). Digitally enhanced esthetic dentistry – from treatment planning to quality control. *J. Esthet. Restor. Dent. Off. Publ. Am. Acad. Esthet. Dent. Al.* 28 (Suppl 1): S3–S4.

Dehurtevent, M., Robberecht, L., Hornez, J.-C. et al. (2017). Stereolithography: a new method for processing dental ceramics by additive computer-aided manufacturing. *Dent. Mater Off. Publ. Acad. Dent. Mater* 33 (5): 477–485.

Grant, G.T., Campbell, S.D., Masri, R.M., and Andersen, M.R. (2016 Oct). American College of Prosthodontists Digital Dentistry Glossary Development Task Force. Glossary of digital dental terms: American College of Prosthodontists. *J. Prosthodont. Off. J. Am. Coll. Prosthodont.* 25 (Suppl 2): S2–S9.

Hartkamp, O., Lohbauer, U., and Reich, S. (2017). Antagonist wear by polished zirconia crowns. *Int. J. Comput. Dent.* 20 (3): 263–274.

Katsoulis, J., Takeichi, T., Sol Gaviria, A. et al. (2017). Misfit of implant prostheses and its impact on clinical outcomes. Definition, assessment and a systematic review of the literature. *Eur. J. Oral Implantol.* 10 (Suppl 1): 121–138.

Kwon, H.-B., Park, Y.-S., and Han, J.-S. (2018 Feb 21). Augmented reality in dentistry: a current perspective. *Acta Odontol. Scand.*: 1–7.

McLaren, E.A., Garber, D.A., and Figueira, J. (2013). The Photoshop smile design technique (part 1): digital dental photography. *Compend. Contin. Educ. Dent. Jamesburg NJ 1995* 34 (10): 772, 774, 776 passim.

Müller, P., Ender, A., Joda, T., and Katsoulis, J. (2016 Apr). Impact of digital intraoral scan strategies on the impression accuracy using the TRIOS Pod scanner. *Quintessence. Int. Berl. Ger. 1985* 47 (4): 343–349.

Nedelcu, R., Olsson, P., Nyström, I., and Thor, A. (2018). Finish line distinctness and accuracy in 7 intraoral scanners versus conventional impression: an in vitro descriptive comparison. *BMC Oral Health.* 18 (1): 27.

Park, M-F and Shin S-Y. (2018). Three-dimensional comparative study on the accuracy and reproducibility of dental casts fabricated by 3D printers. *J. Prosthet. Dent.* 2018 Feb 21, 2 15 0.

Piezocision™, D.S. (2016). Accelerating orthodontic tooth movement while correcting hard and soft tissue deficiencies. *Front. Oral Biol.* 18: 102–108.

Ritter, D.E., Gandini, L.G., Pinto A dos, S. et al. (2006). Analysis of the smile photograph. *World J. Orthod.* 7 (3): 279–285.

Rutkūnas, V., Gečiauskaitė, A., Jegelevičius, D., and Vaitiekūnas, M. (2017). Accuracy of digital implant impressions with intraoral scanners. A systematic review. *Eur. J. Oral Implantol.* 10 (Suppl 1): 101–120.

Simon, H. and Magne, P. (2008 May). Clinically based diagnostic wax-up for optimal esthetics: the diagnostic mock-up. *J. Calif. Dent. Assoc.* 36 (5): 355–362.

Sundar, M.K. and Chelliah, V. (2018). Ten steps to create virtual smile design templates with adobe Photoshop® CS6. *Compend. Contin. Educ. Dent. Jamesburg NJ 1995* 39 (3): e4–e8.

Visagism: The Art of Dental Composition [Internet]. [cited 2018 Mar 18]. Available from: http://connection.ebscohost.com/c/case-studies/87112467/visagism-art-dental-composition

Wichmann, M. (1990 Aug). Visibility of front and side teeth. *ZWR* 99 (8): 623–626.

Zhou, W., Liu, Z., Song, L. et al. (2018 Mar). Clinical factors affecting the accuracy of guided implant surgery: A systematic review and meta-analysis. *J. Evid-Based Dent. Pract.* 18 (1): 28–40.

Index

Note: Page numbers in *italics* refer to figures, those in **bold** refer to tables.

Practical Advanced Periodontal Surgery, Second Edition. Edited by Serge Dibart.
© 2020 John Wiley & Sons, Inc. Published 2020 by John Wiley & Sons, Inc.
Companion website: www.wiley.com/go/dibart/advanced